Sustainability, Midwifery and Birth

Environmental awareness and sustainability are vitally important concepts in the twenty-first century and, as a low environmental impact health care profession, midwifery has the potential to stand as a model of excellence.

This innovative volume promotes a sustainable approach to midwifery practice, philosophy, business administration and resource management. Drawing on an interdisciplinary body of knowledge, this international collection of experts explore the challenges, inviting readers to critically reflect on the issues and consider how they could move to effect changes within their own working environments. Divided into three parts, the book discusses:

- The politics of midwifery and sustainability
- Midwifery as a sustainable health care practice
- Supporting an ecological approach to parenting.

Sustainability, Midwifery and Birth identifies existing models of sustainable midwifery practice, such as the continuity of care model, and highlights the potential for midwifery as a role model for ecologically sound health care provision. This unique book is a vital read for all midwives and midwifery students interested in sustainable practice. Contributors include: Sally Baddock, Carol Bartle, Ruth Deery, Nadine Pilley Edwards, Ina May Gaskin, Megan Gibbons, Carolyn Hastie, Barbara Katz-Rothman, Mavis Kirkham, Nicky Leap, Ruth Martis, Zoë Meleo-Erwin, Jenny L. Meyer, Jo Murphy-Lawless, Mary Nolan, Sally Pairman and Sally Tracy.

Lorna Davies is a Midwife Lecturer at Christchurch Polytechnic Institute of Technology, New Zealand. She was formerly a Lecturer in Midwifery at Anglia Ruskin University and is Co-Director of www.withwoman.co.uk. She still carries a small midwifery caseload as a self-employed midwife.

Rea Daellenbach is a Midwife Lecturer at Christchurch Polytechnic Institute of Technology, New Zealand. She has a ministerial appointment on the Midwifery Council of New Zealand.

Mary Kensington is Co-Head of Midwifery at Christchurch Polytechnic Institute of Technology, New Zealand.

Sustainability, Midwifery and Birth

Edited by Lorna Davies,
Rea Daellenbach and Mary
Kensington

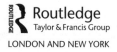 Routledge
Taylor & Francis Group

LONDON AND NEW YORK

First published 2011
by Routledge
2 Park Square, Milton Park, Abingdon, Oxon, OX14 4RN

Simultaneously published in the USA and Canada
by Routledge
270 Madison Avenue, New York, NY 10016

Routledge is an imprint of the Taylor & Francis Group, an informa business

© 2011 Lorna Davies, Rea Daellenbach and Mary Kensington.
Individual chapters; the contributors.

Typeset in Garamond by
Florence Production Ltd, Stoodleigh, Devon

Printed and bound in Great Britain by
CPI Anthony Rowe, Chippenham, Wiltshire

British Library Cataloguing in Publication Data
A catalogue record for this book is available
from the British Library

Library of Congress Cataloging-in-Publication Data
Sustainability, midwifery, and birth/edited by Lorna Davies,
Rea Daellenbach, and Mary Kensington.
       p.; cm.
    Includes bibliographical references.
    1. Midwifery.   2. Sustainability.   I. Davies, Lorna.
    II. Daellenbach, Rea.   III. Kensington, Mary.
    [DNLM: 1. Midwifery.   2. Conservation of Natural Resources.
    3. Infant Care.   4. Parturition.   5. Politics.   6. Social
    Environment. WQ 160 S964 2011]
    RG950.S87 2011
    618.2—dc22   2010015452

ISBN13: 978–0–415–56333–8 (hbk)
ISBN13: 978–0–415–56334–5 (pbk)
ISBN13: 978–0–203–84124–2 (ebk)

Contents

Notes on contributors

Sally Baddock B.Sc. Dip Tchng, Ph.D. has been involved in the SIDS (Sudden Infant Death Syndrome) research area for over 10 years. She has a B.Sc. majoring in physiology and completed her Ph.D. in 2005. She investigated the physiology and behaviour of infants while bedsharing compared to cot-sleeping. Findings from this study have been published in high-ranking international peer-reviewed journals and presented at many international and national conferences. Sally has also taught physiology at undergraduate and postgraduate level to students of midwifery and other health professions for over 20 years. She is currently Associate Head of School of Midwifery at Otago Polytechnic.

Carol Bartle RN, RM, IBCLC, PGDip. Child Advocacy, MHeal.Sc. heard E. F. Schumacher speak in England in the early 1970s, thanks to her inspiring cousin Cynthia Stein. Further exposure, to environmental issues, was also directly as a result of work by Stein who lobbied for the development of recycling systems in West Yorkshire. Later in the mid-1970s, after Carol moved to Christchurch, New Zealand, she worked as a volunteer at the Environment Centre, learning from another inspirational person, the late Rod Donald, who became the co-leader of the NZ Green Party. Carol has developed an enduring interest in optimal and safe infant feeding and women's health. Over the years she has worked as a midwife and breastfeeding advocate and is concerned about the unethical marketing of substitutes for breastmilk and the growing market push for dairy development to the detriment of the environment and health.

Pat Brodie is the Immediate Past President of the Australian College of Midwives and Adjunct Professor of Midwifery at the University of Technology, Sydney. For more than two decades, she has contributed to policy change and practice development that has enhanced continuity of care and the recognition of midwives as primary carers. Pat has had a leadership role in major reforms to midwifery education, regulation and practice throughout Australia.

Rea Daellenbach (editor), BA (Hons), Ph.D. (Sociology), was introduced to the ecology movement by her father as a small child. She became active in the Home Birth Association in the mid-1980s and, as a consumer representative, was involved in the establishment of the New Zealand College of Midwives. At the same time she completed a Ph.D. in sociology about the home birth movement in New Zealand. In 2004 she was appointed as a 'lay person' to the inaugural Midwifery Council of New Zealand. Currently, she is a Lecturer for the School of Midwifery at the Christchurch Polytechnic Institute of Technology, New Zealand.

Hannah Dahlen is an Associate Professor of Midwifery at the University of Western Sydney and is the Vice President of the Australian College of Midwives. She is well known for her commitment to the reforming of maternity care in Australia, her skills in political negotiation and her creative expertise in media liaison. Hannah has published widely about research that is focussed on improving midwifery practice and woman-centred care.

Lorna Davies (editor), RM, B.Sc. (Hons), PGCEA, MA, is a UK qualified midwife who has worked in midwifery education for the last 15 years. She has published extensively in midwifery journals and texts and has edited two midwifery titles in recent years. She has been interested in environmental issues for a considerable length of time and was an executive committee member of the Women's Environmental Network (WEN) for several years. During this time she co-edited a book on green issues and contributed to several TV documentaries. Lorna is currently a principal lecturer in midwifery at Christchurch Polytechnic Institute of Technology in New Zealand. She also carries a small caseload as a self-employed midwife and is a childbirth educator. She is presently undertaking a doctoral thesis exploring midwifery practice within a framework of sustainability.

Ruth Deery RGN, RM, ADM, B.Sc. (Hons), Ph.D., is Reader in Midwifery at the University of Huddersfield. Over a career spanning 34 years she has worked continuously as a midwife and academic. She worked for many years on a large, busy delivery suite but now works mainly in birth centres and community midwifery. As an academic her key interest at doctoral level was in applying sociological and political theory and action research methodology to the organizational culture of midwifery in the National Health Service (NHS) in England. Since then her main work has been in the maternity services and women's health in the new NHS, with particular interests in organizational change, public policy, emotions and care and critical obesity using qualitative, observational and ethnographic methods. Her work has been widely published in refereed journals

Nadine Pilley Edwards, Ph.D., has worked with the Association for Improvements in the Maternity Services (AIMS) since 1980. She has an honorary research post at Sheffield Hallam University and is one of the Directors of the Pregnancy and Parents Centre in Edinburgh, Scotland, a charity working with pregnant women and families. She lectures and writes on maternity issues in the UK and overseas. Her book, *Birthing Autonomy*, articles and chapters focus on the relationships between woman and midwives, and the political complexities of choice, home birth, safety and risk.

Ina May Gaskin, MA, CPM, Ph.D. (Hon.), is founder and Director of the internationally acclaimed Farm Midwifery Center in Tennessee where she has attended more than 1,200 births. She is a prolific writer and has authored several books including the hugely influential textbook, *Spiritual Midwifery*, and was editor of *Birth Gazette* for 22 years. She was President of the Midwives' Alliance of North America from 1996 to 2002 and has received many awards. In 2003 she was chosen as Visiting Fellow of Morse College, Yale University and more recently, in 2009, was granted honorary Ph.D. status by Thames Valley University in the UK. Now in her seventies she continues to campaign for improvements in maternity services with a current focus on maternal mortality in the US.

Megan Gibbons, M.Sc. (1st Class Hons), Dip Diet, BCApS, currently teaches nutrition, bioscience and sustainable development for the Bachelor of Midwifery at Otago Polytechnic, as well and teaching nutrition at postgraduate level and supervising Master's degree students. She is currently enrolled in a Ph.D. at Auckland University, where she is examining the role of nutrition as a risk factor for community acquired pneumonia in 0–5-year-old children. She has published a number of articles in the area of nutrition and paediatrics and during pregnancy.

Carolyn Hastie, RM, RN, Dip. Teach., IBCLC; Certificate Sexual and Reproductive Health; Grad. Dip. PHC; FACMI; M.Philosophy; Ph.D. candidate. As a result of her work with childbearing women over 35 years, Carolyn is fascinated by the role of the environment, emotions and perceptions in human behaviour, experience and relationships. In 2005, her expertise in creating the right environment for women to birth well was sought to establish a publically funded, community based midwifery service. Located in a specially designed, calm, relaxing woman-centred birth centre, the service provides women with the option to birth at home or at the centre. Carolyn is now the Senior Midwifery Lecturer at the University of Newcastle.

Barbara Katz-Rothman, Professor of Sociology at the City University of New York, serves on the faculties of Women's Studies, Disability Studies and Public Health, and is Visiting Professor at the University of Plymouth in the UK and the Charite Medical School in Berlin. Her books include *Weaving a Family: Untangling Race and Adoption*; *Genetic Maps and Human Imaginations*; *Recreating Motherhood*; *The Tentative Pregnancy*; *In Labor*; and with Wendy Simonds, *Laboring On*.

Mary Kensington (editor), RM, ADM, Dip. Tchg. Tertiary., BA, MPH, has practised as a midwife in a variety of maternity settings around the world. For the last 15 years she has worked in midwifery education at Christchurch

Polytechnic Institute of Technology and is currently a Principal Lecturer and Co-Head of Midwifery. Mary was responsible for setting up the three-year direct-entry midwifery degree in Christchurch, which commenced in 1997. Recently she led the Christchurch arm of the new innovative collaborative Bachelor of Midwifery programme with Otago Polytechnic that provides for flexible and blended delivery. Mary also carries a small caseload as a self-employed midwife and provides rural locum cover.

Mavis Kirkham is Emeritus Professor of Midwifery at Sheffield Hallam University and holds honorary professorial positions at the University of Huddersfield and the University of Technology, Sydney. She has worked continuously as a midwife researcher and a clinical midwife for nearly 40 years. She is now interested in reflecting and writing on midwifery in its wider context. Her central professional concern is with normal birth: the conditions that foster it and its enabling effects upon mothers, families and midwives. She has long been concerned with how birth stories are negotiated and adjusted and the impact of these stories on tellers and hearers.

Nicky Leap is an Adjunct Professor of Midwifery at the University of Technology, Sydney and a Visiting Senior Research Fellow at Kings College London. For over 25 years, in both England and Australia, Nicky has been involved in developing midwifery continuity of care in the public health sector. She has written extensively about the importance of community-based midwifery and woman-centred care and has led reforms in Australian midwifery education standards.

Ruth Martis, RM, RGON, ADN, Grad. Dip. Tchg., BA, MA, IBCLC, has practiced as a midwife for over 30 years in a variety of settings, including home births. She has been involved in research, particularly in South East Asia, and midwifery education for a number of years. Ruth is currently a full-time midwifery lecturer at Christchurch Polytechnic Institute of Technology (CPIT). Ruth is a fledging Cochrane Systematic Review author and interested in clinical guideline practice development. Her Master's degree thesis focused on her other passion – young pregnant women and their antenatal education needs. While active in her home birth practice she was introduced to sustainability through a home birth family. They encouraged her to critically assess what she was using in her midwifery practice.

Zoë Meleo-Erwin is a Ph.D. candidate in sociology and a MA student in disability studies at the City University of New York Graduate Center. Her research interests include the disciplinary and productive effects of discourse around the obesity epidemic; similarities and differences between disability rights, transgender and fat activist movements; and the social and bodily experiences of weight-loss surgery patients. She is the author of "Reproductive Technology: Welcome to the Brave New World" in

Redesigning Life: The Worldwide Challenge to Genetic Engineering, Brian Tokar, ed. and "Fat Activism" in *The Cultural Encyclopedia of the Body*, Victoria Pitts-Taylor, ed.

Jenny L. Meyer, RN, BA, Dip Journalism, lives on a fault line with spectacular harbour views in Wellington, New Zealand. She and her husband Mark, have three children, who were all born at home and breastfed in Auckland in the 1990s. The daughter of a blind father and partially sighted mother who are both physiotherapists, Jenny was conceived in London and born in New Zealand. Jenny has nursed for 20 years in surgical, mental health and maternity settings, and currently works two nights per week in Wellington's Neonatal Intensive Care Unit. In 2008 she trained as a journalist and now also works part time for Radio New Zealand International, researching and writing news stories from around the Pacific.

Jo Murphy-Lawless, BA, MA, Ph.D., works as a sociologist focusing primarily on the politics of birth. Much of her writing about childbirth explores the troubling levels of complexity that confront women and midwives alike. She teaches in the School of Nursing and Midwifery, Trinity College Dublin where she has been involved with the development of the four-year undergraduate direct-entry midwifery programme. She is also a member of the Birth Project Group, which comprises academics, birth activists and midwives in Dublin and Edinburgh who are seeking to build a collective approach to better support women and midwives in training.

Mary Nolan trained as a nurse in Cheltenham, England, in the 1980s and subsequently as a childbirth educator with the National Childbirth Trust, the largest European charity for birth and parenting education. She gained her Ph.D., entitled *Empowerment and Antenatal Education*, at the University of Birmingham. From the 1990s onwards she became known as a writer and speaker on choice and decision-making in maternity, education for normal birth and the role of the voluntary sector in health care, with numerous articles appearing in professional and academic journals. She has lectured across the UK, in Europe, and in New Zealand and Australia. In 2007, she became Professor of Perinatal Education at the University of Worcester.

Sally Pairman, MNZM, BA, RGON, RM, MA, D.Mid. is Head of the School of Midwifery and the Health and Community Group Manager at Otago Polytechnic, Dunedin, New Zealand; Inaugural Chair of the Midwifery Council of New Zealand; honorary member, previous President and founder member of the New Zealand College of Midwives; co-chair of International Confederation of Midwives Regulation Standing Committee and Regulation Taskforce; co-author, with Karen Guilliland, of *Midwifery Partnership: A Model for Practice*, a monograph describing a theoretical model of midwifery as a partnership between the woman and the midwife; and co-editor and author of several chapters in the midwifery textbook *Midwifery: Preparation for Practice*. In 2008 Sally was made a Member of the Order of New Zealand for her services to midwifery and women's health.

Jean Patterson, RM, RN, BA, MA, Ph.D., is a Senior Lecturer and Post-graduate Programme Co-ordinator at the School of Midwifery, Otago Polytechnic, in Dunedin. Jean came to teaching after many years in a variety of nursing and midwifery roles in rural New Zealand. The sustainability of a rural birth option for women continues to be both her passion and research interest.

Juliet Thorpe has been a midwife for 20 years and has been working as a home birth midwife in Christchurch NZ for 18 years. She completed her Master's degree in 2005, which investigated strategies for sustaining midwifery collegial relationships, and continues to be a passionate advocate for women choosing to birth at home.

Sally Tracy is Professor of Midwifery at the University of Sydney and is the research leader on two large nationally-funded three-year research projects evaluating midwifery care in the maternity system Professor Tracy is based at the Royal Hospital for Women, Sydney where she is involved in evaluating caseload midwifery care. She is a co-editor and author of several chapters in the midwifery textbook, *Midwifery: Preparation for Practice*. She is a regular presenter at conferences both nationally and internationally and is currently the Pacific representative on the ICM Taskforce on Global Standards for Midwifery Education.

Prologue

Nei rā te mihi kau atu ki kā aroaro mauka o te motu, ki a koutou hoki kā iwi e noho ana ki tēnā pito, ki tēnā pito taiāwhio i te ao tēnei te mihi a Aoraki mauka ki a koutou katoa. Nau mai, nau mai, tauti mai rā.

Greetings to all of the lofty peaks of the land, and to all peoples from around the world, from Aoraki mountain (and those that reside beneath him). Welcome, welcome, welcome.

To identify oneself as an indigenous Māori woman of Aotearoa me Te Waipounamu means to locate myself topographically, by the landmarks that simultaneously represent *who* I come from and *where* I come from. My name is not the defining landmark in the sequence of remembering but that of the mountains and rivers that physically and spiritually link me to my tupuna/ancestors. My landscape is named after particular ancestors and therefore whenever I walk the Papa/Whenua/Earth I also reconnect with those who came before me.

The earth is named Papatuanuku and is representative of the archetypal mother and also *pa-pa* (explosion), *atua* (from the ages/other dimensions) and *nuku* (shift in energy) also related to *nukunuku* (unconscious), therefore embedded through esoteric language in the naming of the mother are ideas around spirituality, motion and a powerful shift in energy or intuition. As a midwife I have also seen these states represented in the birthing woman unrestricted and connected to her own mana/prestige/power and awe, who moves through birth as a powerful state of being to welcome the next generation into this new world. For Māori there is a welcoming ceremony called the powhiri where our elder women call on the visiting peoples with a keening call we know as the kaikaranga – this creates a safe world pathway between this world and the one of each respective groups ancestors so that we might greet each other and become one for a specific time and purpose. I see the midwives' role in birth as parallel to this idea – she is the link to creating that space, the safe world pathway for this birthing journey. The overriding theme is of connection. The link between birth and the whenua/land on both a terrestrial and a celestial level are continuously reinforced in metaphoric language and stories, in the ways we walk the land and in the way we name ourselves as descendents of this birthing mama and her archetypal mama. Every time whakapapa are recited the links between the different states/times/dimensions are remembered and we are reminded of our place within this as a part of something larger and more wondrous than any one component. One where all dimensions of health must be considered as necessary for health to occur including but not limited to the physical, but also the spiritual, environmental and mental.

For me as a Māori midwife the link between the whenua/land and birthing is embodied within the symbolism and language handed down through time. For example, the word whenua denotes land and also placenta, and Māori return the whenua back to the localized place they whakapapa to as another way of recreating the link from one nurturing place to another, this allows us to claim turangawaewae, a place to stand for the rest of our time and for our future children.

Many Māori creation traditions use symbols of childbirth, the growth of trees, thought, energy and the fertile earth to convey the idea of constant, repeated creation. These symbols convey the idea of a world in a state of perpetual 'becoming'. These are statements about the nature of the world, and their repetition echoes the creation story – the world is ritually 'recreated' in them as a series of never-ending beginnings or births. This idea is a key aspect of the traditional Māori worldview. Creation stories give people a way of looking at their world. These stories tell us about individuals acting in particular ways and securing their position in the world. They stand, therefore, as a model for individual and collective behaviour and aspirations. For Māori the environment exists on several different levels at once. A mountain can be the personification of a particular atua, as well as being rock, a resource to be utilized, and having qualities such as beautiful or cold. This worldview has a number of connotations for our relationships with each other and the earth.

The creation of the Universe for Māori also mimics the movement of Birth from the darkness of all potential where the archetypal parents were locked in embrace to the movement into te ao marama, a time of light and understanding and the birth of the new world and ancestors as children. I am continually reminded of the responsibility to birthing mama as our future ancestors and in reverence to the ones before then as a continual line of their whakapapa or genealogy. In this place I too am honored and revered, I too have whakapapa and this is a reciprocal relationship.

The overriding themes for me in this book sit well therefore beside a Māori worldview because they examine how our Kaupapa/philosophies shape our interactions with each other and our papa/our world, our whenua/our mama/our earth. That the responsibility to be mindful of our connectedness as more than a rhetoric of holistic care means that we will live our lives in a way that sustains and enhances our lives and world.

I end on a whakatauaki/proverb/saying from my own tribe/Iwi of Ngai Tahu:

Mō tātou, ā, mō kā uri ā muri ake nei
– For us and our children after us

Amber Clarke
Ngai Tahu

Acknowledgements

We would like to say a big thank you to a number of people who have supported us with this project. First, to the group of contributors who have found the time and space in their busy lives to bring what we consider to be an important book into being.

To our long suffering colleagues Jacqui, Julie, Ruth and Amber who have 'midwifed' us through its gestation.

To Kelly Dorgan and Janine Puentener for their images and their 'good housekeeping' modelling by using cycles in their practice lives and to Lucy Kennett for your 'beautiful belly'. To Joanne Webber for taking on the role as official photographer. To Min and Richard at Beautiful Bellies for their wonderful placenta print image.

To our editing team at Routledge, Grace and Khanam, for having faith and encouraging us to break new ground in midwifery literature by publishing this text.

Finally, we would especially like to thank our families for their enduring patience, understanding and support. To Tom and Joe, Mark and Ruairi, and Richard and Laura.

Introduction

Rea Daellenbach, Lorna Davies and
Mary Kensington

> Our postmodern era with its values of a global consumer culture has created
> disengagement, disconnection, forgetting and discarding. Normal birth stands
> in stark opposition to these values by representing rootedness, connection and
> remembering.
>
> (Murphy-Lawless 2006: 439)

A student magazine asserts that a key action towards sustainability is 'don't
have kids' (Anon. 2008: 29). Another 'green' magazine for parents points out
that 'in the US, even having just one child creates a carbon legacy almost six
times greater than each parent's own lifetime carbon emissions' (McAleer
2009). Sustainability and birthing human children are figured as mutually
exclusive. So how do we get an edited collection of essays in a book with both
the words 'sustainability' and 'birth' in the title?

This book suggests that attention to sustainability involves more complex
thinking than is implied by the simple injunction 'do not breed'. After all,
sustainability is about attention to the future. As defined by the Brundtland
Commission, it 'meets the needs of the present without compromising the
ability of future generations to meet their own needs' (World Commission on
Environment and Development 1987: 43). Across history and cultures, people's
attention to the future has been most obvious in reproduction. Personal, family,
community and political futures have been invested in bearing children and
the creation of future generations. It is widely considered to be a biological
imperative. Thus, using the lens of sustainability to critically examine how
women give birth and nurture their babies, the shape of maternity services and
the place of midwives is vitally important.

Sustainability has been placed in the public spotlight in recent years
through the climate change debates. Documentaries such as *An Inconvenient
Truth* (2006), Yen Arthus-Betrand's *Home* (2009), fictional films such as
The Day After Tomorrow (2004) and *The Age of Stupid* (2009) and intensive media coverage of the Copenhagen Climate Change Summit in December
2009 have all contributed to growing awareness that the accumulation of
greenhouse gases in the atmosphere through human energy consumption

jeopardizes the lives of billions of people on this planet. The harmful health consequences of global warming extend beyond the loss of homes due to rising sea levels. They include increases in infectious diseases (in humans and animals), malnutrition due to food and water shortages, health risks associated with extreme weather events and the detrimental effects on mental health all these can create (Maclean and Sicchia 2004; Patz *et al.* 2005; McMichael *et al.* 2006).

The sustainability of life on this planet requires urgent attention to reducing our ecological footprint. The concept of sustainability focuses on the future of humanity and the relations between human beings and with all living things in the environment. McMichael argues that 'For human populations, sustainability means transforming our ways of living to maximize the chances that environmental and social conditions will indefinitely support human security, well-being, and health' (McMichael *et al.* 2003: 1919). Thus, attention to sustainability encompasses social, political, economic and ecological concerns.

Bioethicist James Dwyer suggests that we need to think about sustainability as an ethical framework. He states that we

> need to develop norms and institutions that will help us to share fairly the biosphere's capacity to sustain life. . . . [T]he virtues that we need are social justice, international justice, a concern for the most vulnerable, modesty of demands, and the creativity to fashion healthy and good lives with limited natural resources. The vices that we need to avoid are ignorance of our situation, the corruption of vested interests, the injustice of taking more than our share, and indifference to the plight of others.
>
> (2008: 285)

The underlying philosophy of the midwifery profession is essentially aligned with sustainability. Midwifery practice is about community-based primary health, strengthening family relationships and promoting normal birth (International Confederation of Midwives 2005). A midwifery model approach thus promotes low resource use and the minimizing of unnecessary intervention. The contribution that midwifery could make to sustainability by helping to safeguard the health and well-being of new families by modelling less exploitative health care practices is considerable. By supporting a sustainable approach to practice philosophy, resource management and personal and professional sustainability, midwifery could ultimately lead the field in health care as a truly ecological and socially responsible profession.

The book draws upon an interdisciplinary body of knowledge, including ecology, sociology, economics, political sciences and midwifery knowledge. The focus of the book is not a prescriptive recipe of 'what to do' and 'what not to do'. Instead, it invites readers to reflect critically on the issues and to consider how they could move to effect changes within their own personal and professional environment. This book features a range of internationally known authors with a longstanding interest in the politics of childbirth and midwifery. Although their names are not necessarily associated with sustainability issues, they all recognize the potential for sustainability to provide a framework in which to site midwifery philosophical and epistemological concerns. As editors, we approached these authors because we knew that their work and interests resonated with the broad principles of sustainability: the respect and commitment to protection of natural undisturbed birth (Odent 2002) and concerns with social justice for women in childbirth. We gave the authors a very open remit with regard their subject specialism.

The book begins by introducing the reader to the concept of sustainability and birth by theoretically analysing the political issues relating to midwifery and sustainability from a range of perspectives. It sets the scene for the book by exploring some of the universal ecological issues that influence birth globally in the twenty-first century. Section Two continues by exploring some of the strategies that may help to play a part in the development of midwifery as a formidable agent in sustainable health care practice. The third and final section focuses primarily on the politics and practicalities of becoming a parent in the age of neoliberalism, with its continuing drive for sustained economic growth.

The politics of midwifery and sustainability

The profession of midwifery could be viewed as an anomaly within health care practice. It provides for women who are generally in a state of health rather than disease and although the interface with clients is episodic in character, the length of contact with women is frequently of a greater duration than most health service encounters. Midwifery is based around the philosophy that pregnancy and birth are normal life events and should be situated within a social rather than a medical model (Pairman and McAra-Couper 2005). The midwife is expected to support the physical, psychosocial, cultural and spiritual well-being of the woman throughout the childbearing cycle, provide women with individualized care, education and counselling, and mitigate the involvement of technological interventions and clinical intervention (MANA Midwifery Task Force 2004). The midwife should acknowledge the woman's autonomy in her own life and respect the decisions she makes for her childbearing experience (New Zealand College of Midwives (NZCOM) 2005).

The role of the midwife is an ancient one, which predates all other health care practices (Towler and Bramall 1986). Traditionally, the midwife was a village woman who learned her trade by attending the births of her family and neighbours. Skills and knowledge were handed down through generations of women. This was the case until fairly recently from a historical perspective within Western countries, and remains to be the case in other non-Western parts of the world today. However, the medicalization of childbirth in the last century has altered the role of the midwife. It has led to an increasing tendency for women to birth their babies in hospital, an increasing reliance on technology and mounting rates of clinical intervention. Consequently the role of midwife in many countries has been reduced to that of a medical aide (van Teijlingen 2005).

The technocratic approach to childbirth has escalated the economic and resource costs of maternity services without equal gains in the safety of child-birth. This was combined with neoliberal influence of the 1980s and 1990s in the design of health services globally through the World Bank who viewed health in terms of tradable commodities and services in the marketplace rather than a public good (McCoy 2007). In this discourse, natural childbirth became viewed as an individual lifestyle choice in the maternity services market place and vested economic interests have lead to women being persuaded to pay for obstetric care even when they are experiencing a normal pregnancy (Epstein, 2008).

The issues related to the medicalization and commodification of childbirth are explored in several chapters within this section. Jo Murphy-Lawless begins setting the context by exposing the gap between the language of midwives and childbirth activists and the language of capitalism within health care practice. Ina May Gaskin is critical of the technocratic/medicalized approach to childbirth and asks where we can find alternatives that are more holistic and sustainable for the future. In Chapter 3, Sally Tracy argues that the current obstetric regime is unsustainable, economically and socially. She critiques the inequitable distribution of resources that is fostered by the neoliberal design of maternity services. Zoë Melleo-Erwin and Barbara Katz-Rothman take up this theme and examine its implication for the social meanings attached to women's bodies and fetus/babies in relation to commercial surrogacy.

Midwifery as a sustainable health care practice

In recent decades midwives, supported by the women with whom they have worked, have fought to re-establish midwifery as an autonomous profession in countries around the world (Reid 2007). This has been particularly notable in New Zealand where a renaissance of midwifery as an autonomous profession has been able to effect the establishment of a national, state-funded maternity service based on continuity of care and carer. The NZCOM 'Partnership Model' (Guilliland and Pairman 1995), which underpins the organization of maternity care in New Zealand, aims to ensure that the delivery of care is a collaborative affair, with women clearly staking their claim in the process. It is a system that enables midwives to truly work within a framework of continuity and to be with woman in a holistic sense. In Chapter 5, five authors, led by Nicky Leap, introduce and reflect upon the characteristics of some of the working models that may provide a sustainable 'habitat' for midwifery practice.

The relationship that a midwife has with a woman within the continuum of childbearing is a unique one. This is particularly so when both the woman and the midwife are privileged enough to work within a continuity of carer model, and get to know each other over a number of months, during a period where personal growth figures significantly for the woman. It is theorized that this relationship is a significant factor in achieving well being, which bestows an important role upon the midwife stretching far beyond addressing the physical needs of the woman as defined by the medical model (Thompson 2003). Mavis Kirkham refers to this concept, which she describes as 'the flow' within Chapter 7.

Midwives working within a continuity care model may be in a position to help to safeguard the health and well being of new families by modelling less-exploitative health care practices and promoting a holistic approach to care. In Chapter 11, Ruth Martis explores the 'housekeeping' practices of midwives and suggests that by promoting a sustainable approach to practice philosophy, resource management and self preservation, midwifery has the potential to provide a valuable contribution to sustainable health care.

Midwives need to find ways of working that allow them to sustain their philosophy and their practice. These include nurturing their emotional well being, supporting their fledgling practitioners and educating for sustainable practice. These areas are addressed in Chapters 6, 9 and 10 by Ruth Deery, Sally Pairman and Mary Kensington respectively.

If we consider the structural framework of ecological theory in relation to pregnancy and the immediate post-natal period, they could be said to represent a unique ecosystem. Mammals are described as developing through a series of 'habitats'. During pregnancy the habitat is the uterine environment. Within a specific habitat, the nascent organism is believed to be neurobehaviourally programmed to behave in a way that will enable it to provide for its own needs. This pre-programmed behaviour can be described as the 'niche'. Once the baby is born the habitat is embodied in skin-to-skin contact and breast-feeding represents the 'niche' or pre-programmed behaviour designed for that habitat (Bergman 2005). The midwife has a hugely important role to play in facilitating this 'econiche'. In pregnancy, the midwife can work with the woman in helping her to indentify some of the environmental and lifestyle factors that she may be advertently or inadvertently exposed to. Such identification may direct the woman to consider ways in which she could eradicate some of the risks where possible, or at least to mitigate the effects. Megan Gibbons and Jean Patterson examine some of more common hazards within Chapter 14. The actions of the midwife in protecting, promoting and preserving the significance of the mother–baby dyad in pregnancy, during labour and birth and in the early hours, days and weeks of new motherhood is of paramount importance. It has been proposed that the mother–baby relationship could be viewed as the prototype of all relationships (Odent 1999). If the baby is able to establish a reciprocal and loving relationship with its mother, it is more likely to be able to connect with others along its life's journey and to establish successful relationships (Bergman 2005). These factors are analysed by Carolyn Hastie within the context of the environment of birth in Chapter 8.

Supporting and ecological approach to parenting

Consumerism can be viewed as having an immeasurable effect on the experiences of parenting (Louv 2005). The growth in the market of 'parent related industries' could be seen to be transforming the norms of motherhood in western industrialized societies. Women appear to be faced with ever-increasing demands of juggling work/life balance in order to deal with the complexity of their lives. Many of the solutions offered seem to be based around increased use of goods and services. The dynamic relationship between consumption practices and parenthood are explored in this section of the book.

A relationship referred to in analysis around social sustainability is the relationship that we have with ourselves (Layard 2003). Various authors have suggested that our consumer-driven society has encouraged us to develop our identity around what we have and do, rather than who we are (Thomas 2007; Schwartz 2005; Travis 2000). It could be argued that this makes us dependent on others for our self esteem. It has been said that personal happiness and well being are equated with autonomy, achievement and the development of interpersonal relationships and less with the acquisition of material wealth and goods (Kahneman and Sugden 2005). Midwives, by educating, encouraging, supporting and listening to women, have the opportunity to assist women in building self esteem and personal resilience. This is explored by Lorna Davies in Chapter 12.

Childbirth and parent education sessions are another vehicle that can be used to help women to connect with others in their community. In Chapter 15, Mary Nolan suggests that this may promote relationships and encourage women to establish their own new network of friends and support. By encouraging the active involvement of the woman's partner or her family members, existing relationships may additionally be strengthened.

A simple way of promoting the 'econiche' of the mother–baby dyad is by supporting the practice of breastfeeding. This ancient practice provides an important renewable natural resource. Its production and delivery take place without the use of other resources and it creates few disposal problems. In contrast, infant formula expends a great deal in environmental costs, at every step of its life cycle. It also contributes towards the deaths of million babies every year and causes ill health in countless others (Palmer 2009). Carol Bartle describes the proliferation in the use of breastmilk substitutes as a 'global disaster' and reframes the significance of breastfeeding within an ecological context. It is believed that skin-to-skin care enhances the effects of lactogenesis and features in the establishment of attachment and co-dependence of mother and baby. Co-sleeping can be viewed as a continuation of skin-to-skin care (Newman 2008). Until relatively recently, co-sleeping constituted a prerequisite for infant survival, because it ensured that the baby had an unlimited access to breastmilk. This is still the case for many mother and baby pairings outside the western industrialized context. This significant human behaviour is therefore introduced as an ecological parenting practice by Sally Baddock in Chapter 16.

Finally, Rea Daellenbach and Nadine Pilley Edwards deconstruct contemporary challenges for contemporary childbirth activists who want to advocate for undisturbed birth. They suggest that women and midwives need to work together in order to ensure the sustainability of childbirth services not just for the individuals concerned but for the wider community as well.

The book ends with a creative piece that was originally written as a radio play that celebrates the deep connections between the woman, the baby, the placenta and the planet Earth.

References

Anonymous (2008) 'Ten ways to reduce your carbon footprint', *Capsule*, Environmental Issue: 29.

Armstrong, F. (2009) *The Age of Stupid*, Dog Woof Pictures.

Arthus-Bertrand, Y. (2009) Online. Available at: www.home-2009.com/us/index.html (accessed 21 December 2009), Good Planet Company.

Bergman, N. (2005) 'More than a cuddle: skin-to-skin contact is key', *Practising Midwife*, 8, 9: 44.

Dwyer, J. (2008) 'The century of biology: three views', *Sustainability Science*, 3, 2: 283–85.

Emmerich, R. (2004) *The Day After Tomorrow*, Twentieth Century Fox.

Epstein, A. (2008) *The Business of Being Born*, Ample Productions and Barranta Productions.

Guggenheim, D. (2006) *An Inconvenient Truth*, Paramount Classics.

Guilliland, K. and Pairman, S. (1995) *The Midwifery Partnership: A Model for Practice*, Monograph Series: 95/1. Wellington: Department of Nursing & Midwifery, Victoria University.

International Confederation of Midwives (2005) 'Definition of a midwife'. Online. Available at: www.internationalmidwives.org/Portals/5/Documentation/ICM%20 Definition%20of%20the%20Midwife%202005.pdf (accessed 21 December 2009).

Kahneman, D. and Sugden, R. (2005) 'Experienced utility as a standard of policy evaluation', *Environmental & Resource Economics*, 32: 585–87.

Layard, R. (2003) 'Happiness: has social science a clue'. Lionel Robbins Memorial Lecture. LSE. Online. Available at: http://photo.kathimerini.gr/xtra/files/Meletes/pdf/Mel011106.pdf (accessed 25 January 2010).

Louv, R. (2005) *Last Child in the Woods: Saving Our Children from Nature-Deficit Disorder*. New York: Algonquin Books.

McAleer, A. (2009) 'Maybe baby, good: New Zealand guide to sustainable living'. Online. Available at: http://good.net.nz/magazine/9/features/eco-mamas-and-papas (accessed 24 March 2010).

McCoy, D. (2007) 'The World Bank's new strategy: reason for alarm?', *Lancet*, 369, 9572: 1492–501.

Maclean, H. and Sicchia, S. (eds) (2004) 'Gender, globalization and health, excerpts from a background paper'. Ottowa: Canadian Institutes of Health, Research Institute of Gender.

McMichael, A., Butler, C. and Folke, C. (2003) 'New visions for addressing sustainability', *Science*, 302, 5652: 1919–920.

McMichael, A., Woodruff, R. and Hales, S. (2006) 'Climate change and human health: present and future risks', *Lancet*, 367, 9513: 859–69.

Midwifery Education and Accreditation Council (MANA) (2004) 'Midwifery Task Force'. Online. Available at: www.mana.org/pdfs/CPMIssueBrief.pdf (accessed 8 February 2010).

Murphy-Lawless, J. (2006) 'Birth and mothering in today's social order: the challenge of new knowledges', *MIDIRS Midwifery Digest*, 16, 4: 439–44.

New Zealand College of Midwives (2005). 'Scope of practice of the midwife'. Online. Available at: www.midwife.org.nz/index.cfm/1,178,html (accessed 7 February 2010).

Newman, J. (2008) 'The importance of skin to skin contact'. Online. Available at: www.drjacknewman.com/pdfs/Skin%20to%20skin%20contact-2008.pdf (accessed 12 January 2010).

Odent, M. (1999) *The Scientification of Love.* London: Free Association Books.

Odent, M. (2002) 'The first hour following birth: don't wake the mother', *Midwifery Today*, Spring, 61: 9–11.

Pairman, S. and McAra-Cooper, J. (2005) 'Theoretical frameworks for midwifery practice', in S. Pairman, J. Pinchcombe, C. Thorogood and S. Tracy (eds) *Midwifery: Preparation for Practice.* Marricksville: Elsevier.

Palmer, G. (2009) *The Politics of Breastfeeding: When Breasts are Bad for Business*, London: Printer & Martin.

Patz, J., Lendrum, D., Holloway, T. and Foley, J. (2005) 'The impact of regional climate change on human health', *Nature*, 438: 310–17.

Reid, L. (2007) *Midwifery: Freedom to Practice.* Edinburgh: Elsevier.

Schwartz, B. (2005) *The Paradox of Choice. Why More is Less.* New York: Harper Collins.

Teijlingen, E. van (2005) 'A critical analysis of the medical model as used in the study of pregnancy and childbirth', *Sociological Research Online*, 10, 2. Online. Available at: www.socresonline.org.uk/10/2/teijlingen.html (accessed 6 February 2010).

Thomas, S. G. (2007) *Buy, Buy Baby: How Consumer Culture Manipulates Parents and Harms Young Minds.* New York: Houghton Mifflin Harcourt.

Thompson, F. (2003) *Mothers and Midwives: The Ethical Journey.* London: Elsevier.

Towler, J. and Bramall, J. (1986) *Midwives in History and Society.* London: Routledge, Kegan & Paul.

Travis, D. (2000) *Emotional Branding: How Successful Brands Gain the Irrational Edge.* New York: Crown Business.

World Commission on Environment and Development (WCED) (1987) *Our Common Future.* Oxford: Oxford University Press, p. 43.

Section one

The politics of midwifery and sustainability

1 Globalization, midwifery and maternity services
Struggles in meaning and practice in states under pressure

Jo Murphy-Lawless

Keywords and birth policies

Few words are more persuasive than 'woman-centred' care and 'midwifery-led' care to describe what should comprise the best of support for women in labour and birth. They are often used alongside the notion of 'choice in childbirth' and many of us believe that we can define the principal characteristics of all three terms.

However, as the cultural theorist Raymond Williams reminds us, definitions are crucially dependent on one's interpretive framework. In his important study, *Keywords: A Vocabulary of Culture and Society*, Williams described his puzzlement about the meanings of the word 'culture' in post-World War II Britain. He saw that the word was marked by a struggle between two broad but competing social groups: a bourgeois class who wanted to define the term to favour elitist interpretations only and thus to exclude all other meanings, and a working class that was anxious to valorize distinctive cultural practices that were far more wide-ranging and inclusive. Despite the contested ground between them, there was a sense that both sides understood what was meant by 'culture'. Williams observed that we all have a repertoire of such words that we use in an effort to establish meaning even when there is a struggle over how that meaning is applied.

'Keywords' comprise a

> general vocabulary ranging from strong, difficult, and persuasive words in everyday usage to words which, beginning in particular specialized contexts, have become quite common in descriptions of wider areas of thought and experience. This, significantly, is the vocabulary we share with others, often imperfectly, when we wish to discuss many of the central processes of our common life.
>
> (Williams 1983: 14)

The pattern Williams captures in this passage, words from specialized contexts that come to possess fundamental powers of persuasion and rightness and about which there appears to be a general, if imperfect, understanding, can also be seen in the current keywords used about birth and midwifery. We know there is a vigorous struggle about what constitutes 'choice' and 'woman-centred care' and about the context necessary to achieve these aims for women. As Sheila Kitzinger has observed (2006: 88, 158), the woman who 'chooses' an epidural or a Caesarean section is often not taking a decision so much as she is endeavouring to protect herself in a setting where her fears are going unaddressed and her support needs neglected, making this an enforced 'choice'. The term, active management of labour (AML), also presents us with a struggle about meaning. In the National Maternity Hospital, Dublin, where AML dominates maternity care, it is defined as 'midwifery-led' care (O'Driscoll *et al.* 2004: 1; Hunter 2010), a notion that would be hotly contested by midwives working in free-standing birth centres (Walsh 2006) or in independent group midwifery practices (Reed and Walton 2009) where women and midwives genuinely work in partnership particular to each woman's needs.

There is another group of keywords that is far less commonly used in debates on childbirth but which nonetheless bears examination for their impact on midwifery and our maternity services. 'Globalization', the 'modernizing state' and 'privatization' are three concepts working at a meta-level that are reshaping the location and control of maternity services. This shifting pattern is seen most readily in countries that heretofore have had a commitment to the welfare state. Many states have now moved decisively away from their work of providing core services and towards well-known tenets of 'neoliberalism', seen as a building block of market globalization. David Harvey (2005: 2, 3) has defined neoliberalism as an economic theory that prioritizes 'entrepreneurial freedoms . . . within [a state] institutional framework characterized by strong private property rights, free markets and free trade'. These objectives are promoted as the best route to maximizing widespread benefits for all by 'maximizing the reach and frequency of market transactions' (Harvey 2005). Despite the contention that all people are helped to a better way of life under this economic regime, the move to 'bring all human action into the domain of the market' (Harvey 2005) has led to the erosion of the state's commitment to a public health care system which, up to now, has been free at point of access and has been seen by ordinary citizens as a common social good (Bauman 1998a; Mishra 1999; Esping-Andersen 2002). The principal impetus for the move away from a state-supported and state-funded health structure is the increasing level of profit to be gained from the commodification of health (Shaffer and Brenner 2004: 86). Turning health services into a commodity to be bought and sold in some form or other is the cornerstone of the expanding 'global market' in health care that is conservatively valued at more than 3.5 trillion dollars (Bulard 2003). This commodification of health is primarily an American model, where since the 1970s, and the introduction of Health Maintenance Organization (HMO) legislation in 1973 (Gruber *et al.* 1988), ordinary people have had to pay into these private sector HMOs for health insurance cover. It has produced a vastly profitable business, with cripplingly high rates of insurance helping to inflate health care costs for individuals, while HMOs, along with the pharmaceutical and medical technology industries, have enjoyed record returns. Moreover, the creation of HMOs garnered extensive federal funding to help put in place what were seen as public-private partnerships, a term that we will return to below.

In relation to childbirth, turning it into an insurable commodity has led to a 'market share' in the United States that in 2000 entailed for every 100 live births, an estimated 84 applications of electronic foetal monitoring, 67 ultrasound screenings, 23 Caesarean sections, 20 inductions of labour, 18 accelerated labours, and seven vacuum or forceps extractions (Perkins 2004: 12). Based on figures from the Health Insurance Association of America, Perkins (2004: 13) estimates that by 1993 national expenditure on pregnancy, birth and post-natal care, largely channelled through HMOs, came to 40 billion dollars, with obstetrical interventions and neonatal intensive care accounting for the lion's share of these costs. Despite this, the rates of perinatal mortality worsened throughout this period (ibid.: 12) and by 2003 the United States stood at the bottom of perinatal rankings for 23 developed countries (Lane 2008: 30).

Pressure groups from the corporate health sector, anxious to increase the global scope of the health care market, have played on growing fears expressed by influential international organizations such as the International Monetary Fund (IMF) and the World Bank that national governments could not afford their 'social contract' to underwrite health and welfare costs if they were to remain internationally competitive (Mishra 1999: 7; Bulard 2003). In 1995, after the establishment of the World Trade Organization, the General Agreement on Trade in Services (GATS) extended international rules governing multilateral trade to include health as a tradeable commodity across national borders to the benefit of these corporate industry interests (Shaffer and Brenner 2004: 92). This move licensed the expansion for the corporate health sector in countries that had tried to maintain strong public commitment to health but which now privatized and outsourced aspects of care with accompanying steep rises in administration costs unconnected with frontline services (Shaffer and Brenner 2004: 86; Pollock 2004: 37; Burke 2009: 84–86).

Alongside other complex factors, this aspect of global trade has impacted adversely on health outcomes and made life more uncertain for many millions of people. For example, international improvements in the drop in infant mortality rates did not continue past the 1970s (Bezruchka and Mercer 2004: 15). Two countries that have managed to preserve their health services, and thus better health outcomes, are Sweden and Cuba (Bezruchka and Mercer ibid.: 16–17). However in neither country is there a particular emphasis on woman-centred care, and indeed in Cuba, home births are illegal (Sjöblom *et al.* 2006; Murphy 2008: 392).

I have sketched out a multi-layered scenario about birth and health that takes us away from the more specific contests about what constitutes woman-centred and midwifery-led care and points to the intricate frameworks within which our maternity services are located at the level of the state. In this chapter,

I will argue that it is crucial for our grasp of the depth of the struggles that are coalescing around how maternity services are developing to bring these terms about globalization, the modernizing state and privatization into our discussions. Examined as a group, they present us with profound challenges. I want to discuss the impact of these terms, using examples from current events and contexts of birth in Britain and Ireland. While the details are specific to those two settings, the underlying issues have resonance for women, birth activists and committed midwives across the world. I will conclude briefly with a word about activism that may prove helpful to movements working to protect health as a common social good internationally.

The big picture: globalization and the changing role of the state

There is a sizeable debate on the meanings and extent of globalization (Cameron and Palen 2004). Nonetheless, certain characteristics mark out this keyword that affects us all, although the impact is neither monolithic nor even. Yeates (2001: 4) offers the following as a 'basic' definition: 'an extensive network of economic, cultural, social and political interconnections and processes which routinely transcend national boundaries'. Bauman (1999: 28), following the arguments of Pierre Bourdieu (1998: 95) and Erving Goffman, adds that this is a 'strong' discourse, which favours one dominant form of economic relations, a particular notion of how 'free markets' should function, over others. These economic relations are often associated with offshore corporations with an international reach, that is, they are unconstrained by national boundaries. They have the capacity to operate in a flexible manner in the way they shift finance, technology and labour needs (often downsizing the latter) across the world while avoiding tax regimes that are seen to detract from their profitability for shareholders. It is the force of this offshore character-istic of flexibility that is especially troubling. Bauman (1998b) speaks of a global elite of corporate and international experts who routinely move untroubled across national boundaries. The notions coming from this elite of what reforms to national infrastructure will best contribute to increasing global economic growth are readily picked up by national governmental bodies. Cameron and Palen (2004: 7) speak about this version of globalization as a 'pervasive narrative' that assumes the status of an unassailable 'truth', which has altered dramatically what we think of as the work of the state.

This narrative (there could be others) has rewritten in concrete terms the 'technological, economic and institutional' processes we have seen as part of our society, while also rewriting the role that the state has held in trying to unify and prioritise our various needs and concerns (Cameron and Palen 2004: 7). This narrative asserts that there is a need to 'modernize' the state which, with little or no consultation of its citizens, appears to involve a reprioritization by the state of its core commitments. These need to be minimized or even dropped in order to help create a more flexible national space to support economic growth. The keyword 'privatization' comes to the fore here and is aided by moves towards 'liberalization' and 'deregulation' (Cameron and Palen 2004: 16) to help 'streamline', that is offload, the state's responsibilities. The argument is that these changes in tandem improve national competitive positions in an increasingly competitive international climate by opening up new markets and new possibilities. The work the state has done in the past, which we as ordinary citizens have welcomed in relation to health, education and welfare, has altered as a result, as has the way the state speaks of its responsibilities.

Coming from the top: changed priorities for maternity services

This shift is most jarring in relation to health. In Britain, the modernizing state has visited four major programmes of reform on the NHS in the last decade (Sennett 2008: 46–47), converting it into a version of the marketplace so that the health service might function as a more 'rational' distributor of what is now seen as its goods and services. As a result of these reforms, the health service from the top down has promoted notions of targeting, efficiency and cost control that come from the domain of corporate capitalism. We can no longer speak about a health service available to all on the basis of individual need, within which midwives, nurses and doctors can take pride in their work as a deeply respected set of skills, with truly able craftsmen who take time to learn, to practise and to deepen their judgment (Sennett 2008: 50–51). Sennett argues further that the base, which enables genuine skill to be developed and transmitted to new entrants to these professions, is under threat amidst a drift towards mediocrity due to the pressure to achieve performance targets. Sennett's analysis is seconded by Allyson Pollock (2004), who has examined the privatization of the NHS to the detriment of the general public who rely on it – creating hundreds of competing quasi-private companies in the form of trusts and foundation hospitals to tender for the provision of health services. This has led to poorer services, poorer outcomes, increasing health inequalities and the demoralization of health care workers. Pollock (2004: 4) pointedly observes that this marketization of the NHS, with its accompanying rhetoric around 'public-private partnerships', created a 'revolving door' so that the private sector businesses of finance, management and construction had direct access in shaping how planning and management functions of the NHS might be privatized. Despite that word 'partnership', public-private partnerships (PPPs) or private finance initiatives (PFIs) have given taxpayers no democratic say in the evolution of new hospitals, while the PPPs and PFIs have helped to create an unequal burden – ordinary citizens bear the direct and indirect costs of privatizing these functions, creating greater inequalities for many. While the private sector has benefited enormously from the profits of the restructured finance required by PFIs, people who must use hospitals and who work there must bear the reduction of annual care budgets, reductions in permanent staff numbers and beds, reduction in pay, and poor quality hospital plant to finance this most expensive form of funding with the high interest rates that PFIs entail (Pollock 2004: 97–98).

Midwives and midwifery have been under peculiar pressure within this welter of restructuring. On the one hand, birth support groups, supported by parliamentary review committee findings, along with the Royal College of Midwives and many dedicated practising and research-based midwives, have constituted a broad coalition to promote woman-centred care. The scope of this care has been refined in successive national policy documents in which the midwife is viewed as the lead professional working in partnership to support a woman to achieve what is best for her. The government mantra is 'choice'. On the other hand, the strains from a continually restructured and increasingly under-resourced health service, which is chasing paper efficiencies and throughput targets, come on top of the effort to change a midwifery culture that has been reluctant to embrace midwifery-led care. In too many instances, midwives feel unsupported and exhausted, leading to their burning out and leaving the profession (Deery 2005). In 2009, the Royal College of Midwives published the results of its survey carried out with heads of midwifery that showed some of the heavy costs of a commodified health service. Despite some recent additional government funding to deal with a shortage of 4,000 midwives, maternity services face an increasing birth rate, but a reduction in midwifery budgets, high long-term vacancy rates, ongoing problems of recruitment and retention, massive workloads, stress and burnout (Royal College of Midwives 2009).

Woman-centred midwifery care has fared no better in Britain's near neighbour, Ireland. This was an impoverished agrarian society dependent on emigration through the major portion of the twentieth century and lagging 25 years behind British society in challenging the public patriarchy of the state and of medicine (Kennedy and Murphy-Lawless 1998; Murphy-Lawless *et al.* 2004; Devane *et al.* 2007). In the mid-1990s as Ireland began to participate more completely in the globalized economy of transnational corporations, foreign direct investment and the financial services sector expanded employment after decades of underfunding in the health services led to a return of emigrants from Britain and elsewhere. This included midwives anxious to make changes and build alliances with midwives already in post to bring about that change. It should have been possible in a small country. Yet Irish women no sooner gained maternity services free at the point of use for all, than private health insurance-funded consultant obstetric care expanded its already considerable options. The same obstetricians who reinforced a rigid hierarchical culture, overseeing consultant-led policies, such as active management of labour in the major public hospitals, encouraged private antenatal care that provided them with a lucrative income in addition to their generous public contracts. The growth of private facilities contributed to an increase in interventions, seen clearly in relation to the steep rise in Caesarean sections (Cuidiú 2008; Brick and Layte 2009). That trend in the private sector continued to merge in subtle and not so subtle ways within the public sector, where committed midwives worried about their lack of skill in supporting normal birth while intervention rates rose (Murphy-Lawless 2002). By 2001, with a steep increase in birth rates, directors of midwifery expressed publicly concerns about overstretched resources with too few midwives in post (Haughey 2001). This picture was bucked in some part by a handful of pilot projects including direct entry midwifery teaching, 'domiciliary in and out' (DOMINO: continuity of care, but with the option of hospital as well as home birth) and home birth schemes and a tiny community midwives group backed by the voices of equally small birth support groups. A local political struggle over the closure of hospitals in 2001 led to the important work of setting up and evaluating the first midwifery-led units from 2003 (School of Nursing and Midwifery 2009). The official Domiciliary Births Group, convened in 2004 to consider domiciliary births, recommended more broad-ranging strategies, but the impact of the group's report was minuscule measured against the weight of the consultant system of care. There was no concerted national impetus from the top of government to review the problems and scope of maternity services across the country, nor to consider the need for midwifery-led care through the official policy-making process that begins with a White Paper.

In fact, the national Department of Health was preparing to shed many areas of direct executive decision-making and to ready the country for a new indirect and democratically less-accountable monolith, the Health Services Executive. A private management consultancy firm was awarded an audit of the health services and the findings, along with several other reports, led to the launch of a Health Services Reform Programme to 'modernize' the health services, introducing the notion of an internal market. There was an over-representation of private sector finance people on its new board (Burke 2009: 50–53, 55). While there was clear need to properly undertake new infrastructure and innovations within the public health system after decades of neglect, cutbacks and parochial decision-making, this reform strategy instead placed Ireland firmly on the road to expanded private health care consortia, including tie-ups with international corporations. The public sector continues to subsidise private beds in public hospitals, including maternity hospitals, while the growth of private for-profit hospitals has been actively supported by government, with generous tax incentives (Burke 2009).

The new Health Service Executive (HSE) in the meanwhile operates as a peculiar hybrid with salaries and perks that reflect top private-sector pay for its CEO, other management executives and its freelance management consultants and, as of 2009, deep cuts in pay and permanent embargoes on posts for frontline staff who have already lived with a series of temporary embargoes (Burke 2009: 87–88).

There has been chronic overcrowding in the four largest maternity hospitals over the last decade; one hospital hired nearby hotel rooms for patients needing daycare in 2007. Currently women in all these hospitals are told that they must book for antenatal appointments as soon as their pregnancy is confirmed, as they are otherwise unlikely to be seen for the first time until they are well into their second trimester (Ingle 2007; Donnellan 2009). The head obstetrician of one hospital has voiced concerns about patient safety and has sent internal reviews about the serious shortage of resources to the HSE with no response (Ingle 2007). Unsurprisingly, midwives and midwifery students are feeling the acute strain of working in such pressurized conditions, which makes woman-centred, midwifery-led care feel unobtainable. The average length of booking visits in hospital is thought to be often as little as 15 minutes.

A commissioned report for the HSE by the international management consultancy firm, KPMG, confirmed significant understaffing in the three Dublin maternity hospitals, as well as lack of privacy, too few delivery suites and too many Nightingale-style wards. Its solution, however, was to merge these standalone hospitals, centralizing their services within existing acute hospitals, citing the commercial value to the health services of selling off the vacated properties. While the report called for an expansion of community midwifery, nowhere did it articulate how this could be achieved given the embedded nature of private obstetric care (KPMG 2009). The latest National Health Service plan does not say anything specific about maternity services in any form (HSE 2010). It does, however, lay out performance indicators, targets and 'deliverables' all of which, according to the CEO of the HSE, need to be accomplished through greater effectiveness in how services are delivered within current pressures to reduce costs (Taylor 2010).

The contradictions: under-regulation and over-regulation

These brief overviews of maternity services in Britain and Ireland indicate the extent to which they have been permeated by the language and perspectives of states that have moved steadily towards a 'globalizing co-partnership' with private capital interests. In this relationship, the state becomes ever more 'market-oriented' (Wolin 2008: 238) and ever more distanced from and seemingly uncomprehending of its detrimental impact on the people whose health it was once meant to support. Where midwives, nurses and doctors might have aspired to a kind of generosity in working in the public health services, they are now reduced to the sum of their 'deliverables' under so-called efficient targeting, and the very notion of a public service is questioned. Even the King's Fund in Britain, an independent think-tank that recently explored the worrying issue of safety in English maternity units (O'Neill 2008) and that might have been expected to challenge this rhetoric, has fallen prey. Their annual conference in 2009 focused on how further change can deliver more efficiencies, greater productivity and, they argue, improved services.

Despite the rhetoric of improvement, there are only small pockets where this has been genuinely secured for women and midwives. Much of this is now under threat from the profound convulsions of the last two years. If before

2007–2008, one was unaware of any troubling implications of that keyword globalization, the sudden appearance of the 'global banking crisis' brought into sharp relief for countless people that corporate finance working on a global scale had seriously jeopardized their everyday well-being. The crisis of the unregulated corporate finance sector flowed remorselessly into the 'current economic crisis'. The connection for many was bank bail outs. State governments around the world began to cut back public expenditure on the core services of health, education and welfare, while unemployment and the burden of public debt grew. Health was a particular target. In the wake of taxpayer revenues being used to refinance the banking sector, the IMF warned Britain it must cut the NHS in order to deal with increased public debt (Elliott 2009). In Ireland alone, 80 billion Euros of tax revenues were targeted to shore up the banking system.

Slavoj Zizek (2009) argues that the extent of this crisis lets us see how deeply irrational the fantasies of globalized capitalism are and equally how swiftly governments move to act to protect what they see as their real interests and priorities, which are not the same as ours. The speed with which funds were taken from the public purse to accomplish the bank bail outs while health budgets suffered cuts is chilling. It also suggests a deeply anti-democratic bias in the way these decisions are made. The electorate has not been given the chance to make a choice between bank bail outs and swingeing cuts in government-financed services. The complex outcomes of this fantasy have done great damage to our health services, including our maternity services. As just one example, the award-winning Montrose Midwifery Unit in Scotland has had plans for a new purpose-built unit suspended indefinitely (Birth in Angus 2010). The proliferation of agencies the modernizing state has set up ostensibly to protect us actually creates less transparency and accountability (favoured words from that corporate world), while exerting control over areas where we most need to remain open and reflexive. Britain has made this concrete without a hint of irony, setting up 'Arm's Length Bodies' (ALBs) as a 'network' to 'manage' the NHS. These bodies have an association with and are government-funded. However, the state has now privatized expertise while intensifying its regulatory apparatus – ALBs are not directly democratically accountable to us through government though they speak of 'governance'. The state has fragmented and scattered its work so we are far less able to affect decisions and outcomes, even while it has more bodies to monitor us. Sadly, in Britain this movement has led to the demise of a crucial instrument for improving maternal health, The National Confidential Enquiry into Maternal Deaths, once a committee reporting directly to the Minister for Health and internationally respected for its rigorous work, this has become a private 'charity'. The Centre for Maternal and Child Enquiries (CMACE), funded only in part by an ALB known as the National Patient Safety Agency, needs to fundraise through open tenders elsewhere and can no longer practise within the scope and reach of its original work. These unaccountable networks confuse and disorientate even as they disempower ordinary citizens.

The under-regulation of the financial sector contrasts sharply with this over-regulation and monitoring of health, a pressing matter for midwifery in particular. Within what Bauman (1999: 173) terms the 'political economy of uncertainty', midwives who are working creatively and openly in partnership with women come under increasing and troubling scrutiny for standing outside a deeply questionable systematization of birth. Thus recent cases taken against independent community midwives (Beech 2009) and, above all, the enforced closure by King's College Hospital of the beacon Albany Midwifery Practice, aided in part by a report from CMACE (Reed 2010), signal an anxiety about any midwifery practice that cannot be monitored with the targeting strategy now in vogue to measure 'outcomes'. In the instance of the Albany, its outcomes working in an impoverished community have been second to none, yet its mode of work contests the direction that mainstream maternity services are taking within a modernized, privatizing state.

The Albany, Montrose, midwifery-led units in Britain and Ireland, independent community midwives – all have reached out to protect and nurture a space that the state as a whole is seeking to abandon in relation to birth, along with many other projects about the common good. In a curious way, this is helpful. The concerted campaign to save the Albany shares the same collective space that is increasingly seen in other crucial public campaigns where people fight for improved welfare services or housing or vital environmental measures. This space is using evidence and activism, identifying and analysing the keywords that are anti-democratic in their operations, retrieving a language that truly speaks for the perspectives that relate to ordinary people's lives, for where people are fighting to take back control of their lives. It helps us to see where we must make common cause.

References

Bauman, Z. (1998a) *Work, Consumerism and the New Poor*. Buckingham: Open University Press.

Bauman, Z. (1998b) *Globalization: The Human Consequences*. London: Polity Press.

Bauman, Z. (1999) *In Search of Politics*. London: Polity Press.

Beech, B. (2009) 'Midwifery – running down the drain', *AIMS Journal*, 21, 3: 3–5.

Bezruchka, S. and Mercer, M. A. (2004) 'The lethal divide: how economic inequality affects health', in M. Meredith, M. A. Mercer and O. Gish (eds), *Sickness and Wealth: The Corporate Assault on Global Health*. Cambridge, MA: South End Press.

Birth in Angus (2010) 'Montrose maternity plans scrapped, 25 January 2010'. Online. Available at: www.birthinangus.org.uk/index/news-app/story.137/title.montrose-maternity-plans-scrapped/menu.no/sec./home (accessed 23 March 2010).

Bourdieu, P. (1998) *Acts of Resistance: Against the New Myths of Our Time*. Cambridge: Polity Press.

Brick, A. and Layte, R. (2009) *Recent Trends in the Caesarean Section Rate in Ireland 1999–2006*. Dublin: Economic and Social Research Institute.

Bulard, M. (2003) 'France: health as a commodity', *Le Monde diplomatique*. December 2003. Online. Available at: http://mondediplo.com/2003/12/13socialsecurity (accessed 29 January, 2010).

Burke, S. (2009) *Irish Apartheid: Healthcare Inequality in Ireland*. Dublin: New Island Books.

Cameron, A. and Palan, R. (2004) *The Imagined Economies of Globalization*. London: Sage.

Cuidiú (2008) 'Cuidiú-ICT's Consumer Guide to Maternity Services in Ireland'. Online. Available at: www.cuidiu-ict.ie/frulcrum.html?ep=13&ad=22&to=0 (accessed 23 March 2010).

Deery, R. (2005) 'An action-research project exploring midwives' support needs and the affect of group supervision', *Midwifery*, 21, 2: 161–76.

Devane, D., Begley, C. and Murphy-Lawless, J. (2007) 'Childbirth policies and practices in Ireland and the journey towards midwifery-led care', *Midwifery: An International Journal*, 23, 1: 92–101.

Donnellan, E. (2009) 'Pregnant women face long delays at hospitals', *Irish Times*. 19 August 2009.

Elliott, L. (2009) 'Cut NHS costs to pay off debt, IMF warns Britain', *Guardian*. 1 October 2009. Online. Available at: www.guardian.co.uk/politics/2009/oct/01/nhs-debt-imf-britain (accessed 18 January 2010).

Esping-Andersen, G. (2002) *Why We Need a New Welfare State*. Oxford: Oxford University Press.

Gruber, L., Shadle, M. and Pollich, C. (1988) 'From movement to industry: the growth of HMOs', *Health Affairs*. 7, 3: 198–208.

Harvey, D. (2005) *A Brief History of Neoliberalism*, Oxford: Oxford University Press.

Haughey, N. (2001) 'Matrons tell Martin about "debilitating haemorrhage of midwives"', *The Irish Times*. 11 August 2001.

Health Service Executive (HSE) (2010) National Service Plan, 2010. Dublin: National Service Executive. Online. Available at: www.hse.ie/eng/services/Publications/corporate/National%20Service%20Plan%202010.pdf (accessed 22 March 2010).

Hunter, N. (2010) 'Holles Street cap on births to go ahead'. Online. Available at: www.irishhealth.com/article.html?level=4&id=6976 (accessed 18 January 2010).

Ingle, R. (2007) 'There is now a real concern for patient safety. We need more doctors, more midwives, more nurses', *Irish Times*. 22 September 2007.

Kennedy, P. and Murphy-Lawless, J. (1998) 'Risk and safety in childbirth: who should decide?' in P. Kennedy and J. Murphy-Lawless (eds), *Returning Birth to Women: Challenging Policies and Practices*. Dublin: CWS, TCD & WERRC.

Kitzinger, S. (2006) *Birth Crisis*. London: Routledge.

KPMG (2009) 'Independent review of maternity and gynaecology services in the Greater Dublin area'. Online. Available at: www.hse.ie/eng/services/Publications/services/Hospitals/Appendix_A-G.pdf (accessed 22 March 2010).

Lane, S. (2008) *Why Are our Babies Dying? Pregnancy, Birth and Death in America*. Boulder: Paradigm Publishers.

Mishra, R. (1999) *Globalization and the Welfare State*. Cheltenham: Edward Elgar.

Murphy, D. (2008) *The Island That Dared: Journeys in Cuba*. London: Eland.

Murphy-Lawless, J. (2002) 'Meeting the changing needs of women in childbirth'. Unpublished, School of Nursing and Midwifery: TCD.

Murphy-Lawless, J., Oaks, L. and Brady, C. (2004) *Understanding How Sexually Active Women Think About Fertility, Sex, and Motherhood*, Dublin: Crisis Pregnancy Agency.

O'Driscoll, K., Meagher, D. and Robson, M. (2004) *Active Management of Labour*, 4th edition. Edinburgh: Mosby.

O'Neill, O. (2008) *Safe Birth, Everybody's Business: An Independent Inquiry into the Safety of Maternity Services in England.* London: King's Fund.

Perkins, B. B. (2004) *The Medical Delivery Business.* New Brunswick, NJ: Rutgers University Press.

Pollock, A. (2004) *NHS Plc: The Privatisation of Our Health Care.* London: Verso.

Reed, B. (2010) 'Choices are not choices if you are not allowed to make them for yourself', *The Practising Midwife*, 13, 1: 4–5.

Reed, R. and Walton, C. (2009) 'The Albany midwifery practice', in R. Davis-Floyd, L. Barclay, B. A. Daviss and J. Tritten (eds), *Birth Models that Work.* Berkeley, CA: University of California Press.

Royal College of Midwives (2009) Press release on report, 'Results of the Royal College of Midwives Survey of Heads of Midwifery', September 2009. Online. Available at: www.rcm.org.uk/college/media-centre/press-releases/senior-midwives-report-falling-budgets/ (accessed 29 January 2010).

School of Nursing and Midwifery, Trinity College Dublin (2009) *An Evaluation of Midwifery-led Care: The Report of the MidU Study.* Dublin: HSE.

Sennett, R. (2008) *The Craftsman.* London: Allen Lane.

Shaffer, E. and Brenner, J. (2004) 'Trade and health care: corporatizing vital human services', in M. Fort, M. A. Mercer and O. Gish (eds), *Sickness and Wealth: The Corporate Assault on Global Health.* Cambridge, MA: South End Press.

Sjöblom, I., Nordström, B. and Edberg, A. K. (2006) 'A qualitative study of women's home birth experiences in Sweden', *Midwifery*, 22, 4: 348–55.

Taylor, C. (2010) 'HSE budget plan for 2010 published', *Irish Times*, 8 February 2010.

Walsh, D. (2006) *Improving Maternity Services: Small is Beautiful – Lessons from a Birth Centre.* Abingdon, Oxon: Radcliffe Publishing.

Williams, R. (1983) *Keywords: A Vocabulary of Culture and Society*, 2nd edition. Oxford: Oxford University Press.

Wolin, S. (2008) *Democracy Incorporated: Managed Democracy and the Spectre of Inverted Totalitarianism.* Princeton, NJ: Princeton University Press.

Yeates, N. (2001) *Globalization and Social Policy.* London: Sage.

Zizek, S. (2009) *First as Tragedy, Then as Farce.* London: Verso.

2 Sustaining midwifery in an ever changing world

Ina May Gaskin

'To sustain' means 'to keep in existence', 'to maintain' and 'to keep going'. In order to create a sustainable midwifery profession, educators, policymakers and activists must avoid short-term thinking and make ever greater efforts to consider how their words and actions – both individual or collective – will impact future generations of midwives and birthing women in all parts of the world.

It would make sense to begin this chapter by considering the obstacles that currently stand in the way of a sustainable midwifery profession around the globe. We know that it is possible for the profession – a profession so vital to the health and well-being of mothers, babies, families and society in general – to be marginalized, or even obliterated and erased from the memory of a particular culture. A century ago, this dramatic change is exactly what took place in North America, largely because the newly-established profession of obstetrics desperately wanted access to women for teaching material and because the professionalization of medicine itself was still in its infancy (Borst 1998). The US obstetric profession of the early twentieth century lacked the boundaries that existed in most European countries, where medical societies had historically developed codes of behaviour and scopes of practice that included an assumption that midwives were a necessary component of any rational system of maternity care (Radosh 1986). When significant numbers of births were beginning to occur in hospitals in the US, midwifery was being made illegal in some states. A virulent anti-midwife campaign managed to convince large numbers of people that hospital birth was a sign of upward social mobility (Barrett 1978). Midwives belonged primarily to the lower socio-economic classes, so no mother in her right mind, as a result of the message rather successfully promoted by the campaign, would choose the midwife if she could afford to pay a doctor to attend her birth.

In the twenty-first century, an almost entirely new set of obstacles are present to hamper the establishment of a sustainable midwifery profession. When countries in South America, such as Brazil, are reaching a Caesarean section rate of over 90 per cent in private hospitals (Hopkins 2000), we may assume the cooperation of governments, medical professional bodies and Ministries of Health. Such trends could lead quite quickly to the obliteration of the profession of midwifery in their countries. When women are no longer able to hear the birth stories of women who gave birth vaginally, most will eventually assume that the Caesarean, even when they are afraid of being subjected to one, is a less frightening and painful prospect than the experience of labour and vaginal birth. In a world in which profit-making entities (corporations) stand to benefit from ever-increasing Caesareans and other unnecessary interventions, the pressures against a sustainable form of midwifery grow to be even stronger.

I entered midwifery early enough to be unable to imagine that a large percentage of the population of women of childbearing age could become so frightened of their own bodies that they would readily choose scheduled Caesarean surgery rather than accept the opportunity to give birth vaginally. In 1970, when the Caesarean rate in the United States stood at only 5 per cent or so, few women knew anyone who had had a baby by Caesarean section. At that time it was recognized that a Caesarean section was major abdominal surgery and that it would therefore be accompanied by post-operative pain and a period of healing that would make caring for a newborn infant more difficult. Who could have guessed at that time that countless images of Caesareans would soon be aired on television daily, on series such as 'Birth Day'? Who would have guessed that a great number of childbearing women could be persuaded that a Caesarean section is the one form of abdominal surgery that is painless and without risk? Obviously, the films that are aired never involve anaesthetic complications or surgical errors and never portray the post-operative pain that surprises so many women during the days following the surgery. The Caesearean section rate in the United States has yet to reach the levels observed in urban areas of Brazil and Mexico, but the trajectory has been rising over the past decade and shows no signs yet of levelling off (Hamilton *et al.* 2007).

It is believed that many women throughout the world are subject to intense fear and are therefore susceptible to being manipulated through the mass media (Geissbuehler and Eberhard 2002). Women are also influenced via personal relationships with individuals (both medical and non-medical) into making choices that many will later have cause to regret (Geissbuehler and Eberhard 2002). This knowledge must surely place us in a better position to identify the components of a sustainable form of midwifery – one that might have roots strong enough to keep it anchored in the ground of common sense and the realities of nature, but also knowledge and understanding of appropriately used technology. Today, midwifery is in the most fragile state we have ever seen, because many women themselves are unable to understand its importance. Surely we know now that midwifery can only survive if enough women of succeeding generations continue to fight to sustain our survival, or if they have the courage and tenacity to reinvent it if it is once again destroyed. Birth is the feminist issue of the twenty-first century.

It is only during the last few decades that sizeable numbers of people have begun to grasp how various technological innovations, and the societal and attitudinal changes that accompany their use, can so drastically alter perceptions of women's bodies and birth that it becomes possible, even easy, to envision a world without midwives.

The laws of nature

For several centuries the medical profession has managed to convince the majority of the population, where Western medicine is the dominant ideology, that obstetrics is more scientific than any sort of folk medicine or indigenous midwifery. It is interesting that obstetrics has been able to maintain its appearance of being scientific even as it violated some of the most basic laws of nature and actually created new kinds of 'superstition'. A word limit won't permit me to make an exhaustive list, but I can provide a couple of examples that illustrate the point. During the mid-twentieth century the rate of forceps deliveries in the United States rose to 40 per cent or more (Devitt 1996). When obstetricians were pressed to explain the difference between the US forceps rate and that of various European countries (where it was far lower), they stated that the great variety of ethnic backgrounds and mixed ancestry of most US women had produced a nation of women with small pelvises (Walsh 2008). As a result they were producing babies with heads too large to fit through these pelvises. The fallacy of that particular superstition became apparent to me during the early years of midwifery practice in my community by learning, a birth at a time, how rare cephalo-pelvic disproportion really is in populations who are free from rickets.

Another superstition still present in many countries, which also masks itself as 'science', holds that placental blood suddenly becomes dangerous to the newborn baby as soon as the baby is outside the uterus. This belief has led to the fashion of immediate cord clamping and cutting. When it comes to changing such superstitious practices, the burden is now placed on those who advocate practices that assume that nature's design is usually right. *They* are the ones who must produce evidence that the still-pulsating cord doesn't represent a danger to the newborn, because they are too often functioning within a culture of medical assumptions that nature is nearly always wrong and must be improved upon when it comes to labour and birth.

It would appear that those who were the driving force in inventing technologies and formulating public policies in the area of birth forgot some of the most basic laws of nature. In many countries, for instance, the role that gravity plays in labour and birth seems rarely to have been considered by physicians who organized hospital maternity care, even in countries in which that care included midwives as part of the team. Dr George Engelmann, author of an ethnographic study, *Labor Among Primitive Peoples* (1883), provides some insight regarding this omission of what would have seemed, I suspect, obvious to most midwives of his time in the United States. He wrote that he only understood that 'there was a method in the instinctive movements of women in the last stage of labor' after he began studying the positions assumed by birthing women from diverse cultures in all parts of the world. 'I had seen them toss about, and sought to quiet them; I bade them have patience, and lie still upon their backs'; he wrote, 'but, since entering upon this study, I have learned to look upon their movements in a very different light. I have watched them with interest and profit, and believe that I have learned to understand them.' We should bear in mind that Dr Engelmann was one of the few who had any curiosity surrounding the subject of maternal posture or movement during labour and birth.

Unfortunately, Dr Engelmann and the physicians who contributed their observations and drawings to his book more than a century ago, were unable to persuade their colleagues that prolonged labours could often be resolved by allowing mothers to move into the positions they instinctively chose. However, his book is as relevant now as it was when first written. A curriculum in a sustainable midwifery programme should surely include his book – both for the knowledge and practices that it promotes and as a basis for the historical understanding of why his wise advice was ignored. Dr Engelmann's confessed inability to understand the movements of labouring women confined to bed, before his exposure to the birthing ways of 'uncivilized women', points to one of the central weaknesses of any training in obstetrics. That is exposure to essential components in physiological birth before being introduced to the potential pathologies and complications of labour. Even this man, who appears to have been more open-minded than many of his colleagues at the time, by learning from non-traditional sources, had trouble at first seeing the obvious. How much more difficult is it for someone who approaches medical education with a mind less flexible than Dr Engelmann's?

Love, kindness and other ways of knowing than those we were taught

Even though numerous studies that have produced evidence demonstrating that mothers' and babies' feelings *do* matter with regard to the optimum health and well-being of both, such studies tend to be ignored. The work of Newton (McCraw 1990) and Klaus and Kennell (2002) fits into this category. Clearly, a sustainable midwifery profession must produce more research in this area. I don't know if anyone yet has stated the need for mothers in labour to be treated with love and kindness as a law of nature, but if it hasn't, I suggest that the time has come. It does seem to be more widely understood that it is necessary for animal mothers to be treated with kindness and tenderness while they are in the process of giving birth and that human mothers and babies require the same consideration. No one seems to believe that animal mothers must be placed in unnatural positions or have their young separated from them just after birth.

Indigenous people (who, among our species, I consider to be the true experts on sustainability) understand very well that kindness, consideration and patience assist the process of birth. Mammals of all species, except for most civilized humans, also understand this truth. Human mothers have the same needs as those of other mammals. A midwifery that is sustainable accepts the importance of care that is tender and considerate and ensures that this knowledge is passed on to succeeding generations. In order for midwifery and medical students of the future to understand this, they need to be exposed to what undisturbed birth looks like. It would also be good if they could see examples of what this looks like when applied to a variety of species. Fortunately, we now have the technology to accomplish this. Youtube.com is already a source of some excellent videos showing various mammals giving birth in different environments. I like to show people an elephant birth that took place in Bali in September 2009 that can be accessed by typing in 'The Dramatic Struggle for Life' (Bratt and Hinds 2009). The elephant, labouring alone, births her baby onto a concrete floor (why was a pile of straw not provided?), and because the baby doesn't breathe spontaneously, has to stimulate her to breathe. She manages to do this, first, by gently kicking her newborn and finally by entwining her trunk around that of her little one and then lifting its head with a jerk just strong enough to get her calf to begin breathing. When I use this video for teaching, I point out that the mother managed to apply her intelligence, her feet and her trunk to the problem, without having read a book. Nature, apparently, can be a source of wisdom. Can we midwives learn to access this wisdom and teach the medical profession to respect it as well? I think we have to.

The challenge we are faced with is how to keep the benefits that technology can bring without erasing the wisdom and common sense that people – entire cultures even – used to maintain? First, we have to enhance our own ability to think critically. We have to recognize that there are other ways of knowing, than to accept – without question – only received medical authority on the subject of labour and birth, no matter how demonstrably false it may be at times.

We do have some humans on this earth who are experts on the subject of sustainability, whether we are speaking of the environment, about humans or other species of beings. I am referring especially to those indigenous people who still have their traditional midwives among them. I would suggest that midwifery educators begin to actively study both the philosophy and the methods of the traditional midwives of Central and Latin America, where there exist *comadronas*, *parteras* and *parteiras* who would be happy to teach what they know to midwives of cultures with less respect for nature. Traditional midwives are still numerous in at least three Mexican states; it is estimated that there are more than 35,000 still working in Guerrero, Chiapa and Oaxaca. Some *parteras* have been able to make alliances with childbirth educators and other midwifery activists and thus have been able to create video programmes, showing some of the ancestral methods that could easily be adopted in cultures in which ancestral ways have been completely erased. What we might call 'the technology of cloth' was well developed in Central America and is rather easily demonstrable. Videos have already been created that demonstrate how the *rebozo* – the long, woven shawl that can serve as a garment to provide warmth or a way to carry a newborn or toddler, leaving the mother's hands free – can also be used to prevent or correct a less than optimal fetal position or malpresentation. Such films and videos should be a required part of the curricula in midwifery or obstetrical education of the future.

I was taught a lifesaving technique for resolving shoulder dystocia from indigenous midwives of the highlands of Guatemala during my first decade of midwifery. As a result, I know that it is possible to bring such practical techniques into use in the most highly industrialized parts of the world. Pushing against the culture of medicine that has historically been resistant to accepting any knowledge that was not generated from within its own ranks by its most authoritative institutions is no easy task. Advocating such changes does take persistence and advocates do run the risk of being thought 'weird'. Nevertheless, these obstacles can and should be overcome. It is heartening to find that there are obstetricians all over the world who can be persuaded that there are other ways of knowing than those that western civilization has valorized over the last few centuries. We must do away with the currently accepted notion that knowledge only flows from hospital-based institutions where the latest forms of technology are available and that it can never flow from indigenous populations in which the written word was not the medium of communication primarily used to transmit midwifery knowledge. Cultures in which there are still large numbers of people who are not literate can and should be regarded as important sources of knowledge that can help to create a form of midwifery that can be sustained for future generations.

It is now possible to document and transmit such knowledge, using video cameras and the Internet and other modern technologies that can enable us to witness labours and births in private, protected settings that would have been otherwise inaccessible. Midwifery educators should make efforts to accelerate the flow of information from indigenous midwives, who still possess and use traditional methods, to the midwifery students whose education is taking place within institutions common in the industrialized world.

Midwifery educators must explore imaginative ways of making common cause with activists who work to reduce the irrational fears that are created in women who are exposed only to the cultural message that their bodies were badly designed for birth. How – if they are never given the chance to witness such labours and births – can women learn that giving birth in a way more similar to the ways their ancestors did does not mean undergoing torture, permanent injury or death (Gaskin 2008)?

Part of the problem confronting educators in this area is that so many midwifery students today have grown up within societies that are so disconnected from nature that they have never seen birth (Louv 2007). Comparatively few students will have grown up on family farms, which would have offered them a greater chance of exposure to the wisdom of nature that can be grasped by observing birth in other mammalian species. I am probably not the only midwife who has been able to notice that physicians possessing common sense are often those who came out of rural family backgrounds, in which it was possible to observe the workings of nature. Now that such settings are increasingly rare (at least in the part of the world where I live), educators and activists need to make extra efforts to widen perspectives and to encourage critical thinking skills where they are lacking.

In those countries where candidates for available spaces in midwifery schools are chosen according to criteria that make little sense, it would be good if midwifery educators could gain the latitude to make their own judgments as to which candidates seem to them to be the most likely to make the type of midwives necessary for maintaining a strong midwifery culture. I remember the Danish father who visited my community years ago and said that he thought his daughter would surely be a wonderful midwife when she grew up, because on several occasions she had, as a child, brought home motherless newborn animals or birds that would otherwise have died, and nursed them to health. His daughter was unable to enter midwifery school at that time, because her grades in Danish literature and history were not within the required percentile for admission. This restriction may no longer exist in Denmark, but I mention it as an example of the kind of thinking that may cramp the admissions process in some countries in ways that may be counterproductive.

It is also necessary, I believe, for midwifery educators to encourage their students to learn basic midwifery skills that were part of training before the use of electronic fetal monitoring and ultrasonagraphy became the norm. It is not just midwifery students, but young expectant parents as well, who can be surprised and delighted to learn that it is possible to hear the fetal heart with a Pinard or simply by pressing an ear against the pregnant mother's abdomen. This is just one simple way of awakening the mind to common sense. Medical students should be taught in this way as well; this is just one of the ways their education should teach respect for the practical ways that previous generations learned to check the vital signs of the baby during pregnancy and labour. The same goes for manual skills that once used to be part of midwifery and obstetrics curricula: the art of manually diagnosing babies' presentation, position and weight, as well as the inner dimensions of the maternal pelvis. Technology should not completely replace the skills of the past so that these fall into disuse.

Midwifery educators and activists must also take note of the way that Puritanism has manifested itself in modern times, and the effect this powerful force exerts around the world in creating fear and ignorance about human birth. Women of childbearing age who have access to television are now able to watch epidurals being placed, the scrubbing that precedes a Caesarean, the incisions being made, and the extraction of the baby – blood and all – but the sight that is absolutely prohibited is emergence of a baby from the mother's vagina. Because this is a sight that must be seen to be believed by people of cultures that have already lost a basic trust in nature, we have to find ways to teach that women's reproductive organs are adequate to the task. Exposure to videos of large animals successfully giving birth can be a great help in this area, especially when educators take the time to ask their students to examine the question: if every other mammal appears to be well designed for birth, how could it be that the human female was not?

There are other areas of the organization of midwifery in various countries that have profound effects on the sustainability of our profession. I mentioned earlier in this essay that midwives and medical students who will become obstetricians need to be taught respect for nature by witnessing, in whatever ways can be arranged, labour and birth taking place in mammalian mothers (hopefully including humans who have not been medicated or restricted in their movements). The late Dr Galbo Araujo of Brazil, formerly Professor of Obstetrics at the Assis Chateaubriand Maternity Hospital of the Federal University of Ceará, required his medical students during the mid-1970s to sit quietly in the corner of women's small huts in north-eastern Brazil, observing how women were able to safely give birth with the care of the indigenous midwives, whose ancestral skills were so respected by Dr Araujo. Some of those former medical students are trying to replicate some of this work in Brazil today, in order to reduce the alarming rates of Caesareans (Misago *et al.* 2001).

In conclusion, over my years in practice, it has surprised me how the US medicalized way of giving birth has been so successfully marketed and adopted in countless countries around the world. Even some nations whose maternal and newborn outcomes are superior to those achieved in the US have embraced what could be regarded as questionable practice and wisdom (Wagner 2006). Midwives in these countries need to recognize when this is happening and take collective action to halt and reverse this process. They will need to make this information available to their students, their respective medical professions and Ministries of Health. Midwives around the world need to educate themselves as to why it is unwise for obstetricians and midwives in countries other than the United States to depend upon US government institutions such as the Food and Drug Administration, for reliable information regarding the safety of medications, or the Centers for Disease Control, for the accurate counting of maternal mortality and morbidity. Even the medical literature produced in the United States (now heavily influenced by the power of the pharmaceutical industry) must be read with a critical eye and awareness of the precautionary principle. Adhering to this advice may help to achieve a major step towards achieving both sustainable ways of birthing and sustainable midwifery practices around the world.

References

Barrett, J. (1978) *American Midwives: 1860 to the Present.* Westport, CN: Greenwood Press.

Borst, C. G. (1998) 'Teaching obstetrics at home: medical schools and home delivery services in the first half of the twentieth century', *Bulletin of the History of Medicine,* 72, 2: 220–45.

Bratt, I. and Hinds, S. (2009) 'Elephant birth the dramatic struggle for life'. Online. Available at: www.youtube.com/watch?v=8LAmquL7MsA (accessed 14 December 2009).

Devitt, N. (1996) 'The transition from home to hospital birth in the United States, 1930–1960', in *Childbirth: Changing Ideas and Practices in Britain and America 1600 to the Present*. New York: Garland Publishing.

Engelmann, G. J. (1883) *Labor Among Primitive Peoples: Showing the Development of the Obstetric Science of Today: From the Natural and Instinctive Customs of All Races, Civilized and Savage, Past and Present*. St Louis, MO: J. H. Chambers.

Gaskin, I. M. (2008) 'Masking maternal mortality I', Online. Available at: www.inamay.com/?page_id=164 (accessed 2 February 2010).

Geissbuehler, V. and Eberhard, J. (2002) 'Fear of childbirth during pregnancy: a study of more than 8000 pregnant women', *Journal of Psychosomatic Obstetrics & Gynecology*, 23, 4: 229–35.

Hamilton, B. E., Martin, J. A. and Ventura, S. J. (2007) 'Births: preliminary data for 2006'. National Vital Statistics Reports Website. Online. Available at: www.cdc.gov/nchs/data/nvsr/nvsr56/nvsr56_07.pdf (accessed 14 November 2009).

Hopkins, K. (2000) 'Are Brazilian women really choosing to deliver by Cesarean?', *Social Science and Medicine*, 51: 725–40.

Klaus, P. and Kennell, J. (2002) *The Doula Book: How a Trained Labor Companion Can Help You Have a Shorter, Easier, and Healthier Birth*. New York: Da Capo Press.

Louv, R. (2007) *Last Child in the Woods*. New York: Alonquin.

McCraw, R. K. (1990) *Newton on Birth and Women: Selected Works of Niles Newton, Both Classic and Current*. Seattle, WA: Birth & Life Bookstore.

Misago C., Kendall C., Freitas P., Haneda, K., Silveira, D. *et al.* (2001) 'From 'culture of childbirth' to 'childbirth as a transformative experience': municipalities in northeast Brazil', *International Journal of Gynecology & Obstetrics*, 75: S67–S72.

Radosh, P. J. (1986) 'Midwives in the United States: past and present', *Population Research and Policy Review*, 5, 2: 129–46.

Wagner, M. (2006) *Born in the USA: How a Broken Maternity System Must Be Fixed to Put Women and Children First*. Berkeley, CA: University of California Press.

Walsh, J. (2008) 'Evolution and the Cesarean section rate', *The American Biology Teacher*. Online. Available at: www.bioone.org/doi/full/10.1662/0002–7685%282008%2970%5B401%3AETCSR%5D2.0.CO%3B2 (accessed 24 January 2010).

3 Costing birth as commodity or sustainable public good

Sally Tracy

Background

The subject of cost and sustainability within maternity services may lead the reader to believe the 'Mad Hatter' has made a comeback posing a riddle without an answer and at the same time trying to achieve the 'unachievable'.

> The resources available for health care are limited compared with demand, if not need, and all health care systems, regardless of their financing and organization, employ mechanisms to ration or prioritize finite health care resources

(Petrou and Wolstenholme 2000: 34)

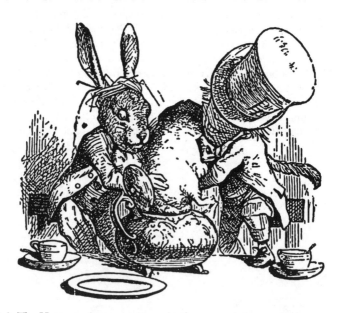

Figure 3.1 The Hatter trying to squeeze the dormouse into a teapot!

Source: *Alice's Adventures in Wonderland* by Lewis Carroll 1865 (Macmillan and Co., London.) Illustration by John Tenniel.

Decisions about the worth of services and who should receive the benefit of maternity service resources are made at many levels: government policy and funding level; local area or District Health Board or Area Health Service level; and finally at the level of the pregnant woman and her family. Before the worth of anything can be established, however, it is imperative to ascertain from whose perspective the cost will be calculated. For example, those directly involved with maternity services will weigh up the cost of the service from their own particular standpoint, which is also shaped by a wider political and economic context within which they live. This chapter explores the concept of the 'economic evaluation' of maternity in the context of our current economic crisis and the neoliberal forces that shape the 'health market', with a reference to ideas emerging from a feminist critique of economics and sustainability. It proposes a set of questions that should be considered in any economic evaluation of maternity care where 'sustainability' is the key.

Introduction

Mainstream economics is portrayed as scientific and rigorous. It is communicated through mathematically formalized theories, quantitative measurement and econometrics. It appeals to the logic and reasoning of policymakers and decision makers. However, modern feminist scholars have argued that classical and neo-classical economics are concerned largely with the nature and existence of 'economic man' and that:

> Economic, 'rational' and 'scientific man' are all manifestations of the dualisms that are central to western society and culture. These dualisms are not merely dichotomous; the economic as against the uneconomic, the rational as against the irrational, the scientist as against the untutored layperson, they are also judgmental, with the second half of the pair seen as inferior and subordinated to the first. Within these dichotomies women are generally assigned to the subordinate part alongside, and as members of, other marginalized and stigmatized groups.
>
> (Mellor 1997:129)

Standard economic evaluation methods generally focus on efficiency (i.e. the maximization of health gain) rather than on equity otherwise referred to as the 'distribution of health gain' (Drummond *et al.* 2007). (In fact the most common trends in economic evaluation today seek to establish minimum resource costs per unit of measured output.)

Studies in sustainability on the other hand deal with the way humans in all their complexity connect with and are embedded within the natural world. Evaluations in sustainability tend to focus on vision, ethics, care, responsibility and community, with an emphasis on connectedness and community (Nelson 2009).

In contrast to the mainstream view of economics, contemporary 'ecological economists' see an extremely urgent need for big changes in economic life, particularly concerning limits to through-put and consumption and the centrality of the 'market' (Nelson 2009).

In her article on 'Feminism, ecology and the philosophy of economics', Julie Nelson defines economics in the following way:

> The list of hierarchical dualisms that underlie much of western thought can be extended to include many characteristics that define contemporary economics. Mainstream economics as a profession privileges the public (market and government) over the private (family); agents over institutions; self-interest over other-interest; autonomy over dependence; mathematical analysis over verbal analysis; abstract models over concrete studies; 'positive' over 'normative'; and efficiency over equity.
>
> (Nelson 1997: 159)

Producing goods and services does not take place in isolation however. Outside the economists equation sits the very often invisible and unaccounted for network of services and contributions of households, nature and, of course, the work of invisible men and women. One of New Zealand's pioneering feminist economists claimed that in the current accounting system women are considered 'non-producers' and as such they cannot expect to gain from the distribution of benefits that flow from production. Issues like nuclear warfare, environmental conservation, and poverty are likewise excluded from the calculation of value in traditional economic theory. As a result, public policy, determined by these same accounting processes, inevitably overlooks the importance of the environment and half the world's population (Waring 1999):

> This qualitative distinction between counted (valuable) and unaccounted for (valueless) production promotes a focus on the production process itself, that is, an 'inside' focus. The 'outside', that is, the social and bio-physical context within which production takes place remains external to this focus ... Yet these contributions remain largely unaccounted for and unenumerated.
>
> (O'Hara 1997: 147)

It is claimed that women share similar treatment to the environment in neo-classical economics:

> They are, variously, invisible; pushed into the background; treated as a 'resource' for the satisfaction of male or human needs; considered to be part of a realm that 'takes care of itself'; thought of as self-regenerating (or reproductive, as opposed to productive); conceived of as passive; and/or considered to be subject to male or human authority . . . The bearing and

raising of children and the care of the aged and sick – traditionally women's responsibilities – are, like nature, too unimportant to mention.
(Nelson 1997: 156).

The treatment of both women and nature as passive, exploitable resources is not, however, just coincidental, or incidental to neoclassical analysis. 'Such thinking is part of a broader cultural way of viewing the world, with roots going far back in history' (Nelson 2009: 2).

The table below shows the dualisms that have strongly influenced the Western conception of the order of the world in economics. (It could also be argued that obstetrics and medicine would find a place on the left-hand side of this table in opposition to the art of midwifery on the right.) The following table is reproduced from Nelson (2009: 3).

The end of the 'golden years' – the crisis of capitalism

In recent times we have lived though tumultuous waves of change in global economic thinking and behaviour so that any evaluation of maternity services in terms of sustainability and cost should be viewed within the current broader economic and political context. In most resource-rich nations during the past 30 years the general shift towards a neoliberal market ideology in health has been coupled with deregulation and privatization, which have become central themes in debates over the restructuring of health and welfare.

Table 3.1 Splitting the world, genders and schemas in the neoclassical world of economics

Economics (hard)	*Not economics (soft)*
Definition	
Markets	Non-market
Mental choice	Bodily experience
Scarcity	Abundance
Model	
Individuality	Relatedness
Autonomy	Other interest
Self interest	Interdependence
Rationality	Emotion
Methods	
Quantitative	Qualitative
Formal	Verbal or intuitive
Positive	Normative
Objective	Subjective
General	Particular
Gender	
Masculine	Feminine

Prior to the 1970s, under the Keynesian model, governments' provision of goods and services to a national population was understood as a means of ensuring social well-being (Larner 2000). In the last three decades of the twentieth century world economies have collapsed and left in their wake a huge vacuum of uncertainty in terms of future economic trends. In addition to this, 'globalization' promoted by the World Bank, the International Monetary Fund, the World Health Organization and other international agencies, has further changed the role of national governments who embraced neoliberal policies (Navarro 2009).

Current observers of neoliberalism and globalization believe that what is happening today 'is not actually a reduction of state interventions but a change in the nature and character of those interventions' (Navarro 2009). Some claim that 'neoliberalism effected a major change in class (and race and gender) power relations in many countries which has caused the enormous health inequalities in the world today' (Navarro 2009: 423). Alliances were established between the dominant classes of developed and developing countries – a class alliance responsible for the promotion of its ideology, neoliberalism. This distribution of power in our societies benefits some classes at the expense of others.

Birth outcome as commodity

In its simplest terms the objective of conventional economic analysis is to demonstrate whether what we do is worthwhile, whether we have made the best use of resources and how this compares with alternative courses of action in terms of their costs and consequences. Health economics provides a way of thinking about health and health care resource use; introducing a thought process that recognizes scarcity, the need to make choices and, thus, that more is not always better if other things can be done with the same resources (Shiell *et al.* 2002: 85).

In technical terms economic evaluations aim to map out whether what we do is efficient (i.e. that we make the best use of resources) and this behaviour is effective (i.e. the findings can be applied in the real world with a wide variety of providers). To aid the universality of health economics, resource use is valued in monetary terms – for example, midwife/doctor time; transport drugs and hospital resource use can be measured in dollar terms. In other words, economic evaluations necessarily translate the outcomes of a service into a measurable commodity – or consequence. Although the different forms of economic evaluation consider the same categories of costs, they differ in the manner in which outcomes are measured and valued (Petrou *et al.* 2001) and in the type of question they can address. Conventional cost analyses use methods that are well described and adhere to set methodological principles. When we are dealing with a system operating within a finite budget, as public health systems do, an economic evaluation aims to not only weigh up the actual costs involved in undertaking the service, but to provide information regarding whether the best value was gained from doing things in the way they were done. Cost benefit analysis (CBA) determines the consequences (health outcomes) of the options in explicit monetary terms – in other words, both the costs and the consequences are measured in monetary units and as commodities they are assigned a dollar value (National Health and Medical Research Council 2001).

In cost-effectiveness analysis (CEA) the consequence is measured in 'natural' as opposed to monetary units – for example, the number of Caesarean sections avoided – and the question to be asked is 'what is the cost per Caesarean section avoided?' In this case the Caesarean section is the commodity that is weighed up as a cost-effective outcome or not.

Although the framework underlying classical economic evaluations centres on the importance of 'utility' as a desired outcome, there are other schools of thought, for example, the 'welfarists' who focus on the importance of health, and not utility, as the crucial outcome of health policy. Within this framework, allocation of resources is based on the 'need for health care' rather than individual demand (Hauck *et al.* 2003). In classical economic evaluations the word 'utility' refers to the measure of satisfaction or desirability people gain in consuming goods and services (Harrison *et al.* 2010). From these concepts we derive the notion of 'consumer choice', which is of course firmly based within the market model of health.

Without commodifying women's well-being following birth in complex obscure measures such as 'quality-adjusted life-years' or QALYs, it is difficult to know how to measure the economic worth of maternity services due to our inability to predict how different alternatives will develop into the future and affect not only cost effectiveness but also health policy (A QALY is derived from a formula that looks at the extent to which health treatment and care can generate both quantity and quality of life) (Petrou and Renton 1993). Take for example the emerging research into diabetes and asthma and their relationship to having been born by Caesarean section (Cardwell *et al.* 2008; Cardwell *et al.* 2010; Thavagnanam *et al.* 2008). Will economists ever be able to evaluate the well-being of the adult and relate this back to events that happened at birth? We are in fact limited in our ability to plan rationally for the future, with costing analyses or with any other method, if we take into account the inability to know the consequences of an action well into the future. As analyses are extended into the future, uncertainty naturally increases until we reach a point where prediction becomes meaningless. At the heart of this criticism is discomfort with the notion that health care interventions should be assessed and valued on the basis of the health outcomes and not the utility they generate.

Evaluating health from an economic perspective necessitates making choices and considering whether what is achieved is also what is most valued. The challenge lies not in measuring the outcomes of health interventions but in deciding what the objectives of the maternity system ought to be (Shiell 1997).

The 'cost' of maternity

Health care is one of our biggest industries and yet it expands largely unchecked both socially and environmentally. Contrary to the claims of neo-liberal theory, governments have not stopped public spending – there has not been a reduction in state interventions, but rather a change in the nature of these interventions.

The privatization of health services continues to grow – similarly, the private management of public services has been accompanied by an increased reliance on markets, co-payments and co-insurances, public and private investment in biomedical and genetics research, in pursuit of the biological bullet that will resolve today's major health problems. The main emphasis on the biomedical model – and all of this occurs under the auspices and guidance of the biomedical and pharmaceutical industry, clearly supported with tax money (Navarro 2009).

The most important reason for measuring the cost of maternity is to help guide the allocation of resources by providing cost-effectiveness information that values not only the cost of a commodity but places a value on the quality of the outcome for women and their families. In this instance we are trying to measure the quality of women's health as a 'state of health' following childbirth rather than simply measuring a health consequence or commodity. In judging how good or bad health states are, both individuals and policy-makers appropriately take into consideration a great deal besides the health states themselves. The physical, technological and social environment matters, too (Hausman 2009).

Maternity systems and women's health generally offer us a broad palette to illustrate the way free-market fundamentalism, or extreme capitalism, has manifested. The neoliberal world can be viewed as a giant supermarket. However, women within the maternity system are standing on the outside looking in. They are permitted to come in on the invitation of those in power and they 'consume' within the boundary of what is 'good' for them. The relationship is one of power – between the various participants of health care – based on individualistic policies (the power of the profession).

In a study that sought to analyse the phenomenon of rising Caesarean sections, by drawing on empirical qualitative data to describe the discourses used by midwives, obstetricians and women and their experiences of Caesarean birth, Bryant *et al.* (2007) revealed that the belief systems through which decisions about Caesarean birth are made are indeed shaped by the neoliberal discourse, which gives authority to women's choices. Although it emerged that women were limited in their ability to make choices that did not tally with those of their attending obstetrician or midwife, who deemed her situation to be 'medically unsafe', women were viewed as self-determining individuals who govern their bodies with the guidance of medical professionals. The privileging of individual autonomy and self-governance, and the positioning of medical professionals as guides or information/service providers, reflected the highly pervasive modern discourse of neoliberalism, which focuses on the individual rights as they operate within free-market principles (Bryant *et al.* 2007).

Costing maternity: what have we achieved?

To date the handful of published studies that have tried to untangle the economic complexity of costing in maternity systems have concentrated on one or two aspects of the maternity service. In the UK Dr Stavros Petrou, a health economist based at the National Perinatal Epidemiology Unit at the University of Oxford, has published studies on measurement (Asim and Petrou 2005); early post-natal discharge (Petrou *et al.* 2004); and the comparison of costs between Caesarean section and uncomplicated vaginal birth (Petrou *et al.* 2001), among others. Petrou *et al.* (2004) established that among women who gave birth to a full term baby following an uncomplicated pregnancy and labour, the policy of early post-natal discharge combined with home midwifery support is significantly less costly than traditional post-natal care without compromising the health and well-being of the mother and infant (Petrou *et al.* 2004). In 2002 his team from Oxford published a study estimating the economic costs attributed to three modes of birth following two months postpartum for a sample of over 1,000 women (Petrou and Glazener 2002). Using a combination of health surveys, medical case notes and computerized hospital discharge records, costs were collected on the extent and volume of all the resources used and a net cost per woman was calculated. The researchers found there were significant differences in initial hospitalization cost between spontaneous vaginal birth (£1,431), instrumental birth (£1,970) and Caesarean section (£2,924) at 1999–2000 UK prices. There were also significant differences in the cost of hospital readmissions, community midwifery care and general practitioner care in association with the three methods of giving birth. In terms of total health costs the study found significant differences. Women who had an instrumental birth cost 25 per cent more in total health care costs than those who gave birth vaginally. For women who had Caesarean sections the health care costs were almost double those who had an uncomplicated vaginal birth.

In Australia, in a modelling exercise to establish the incremental rise in units of cost when women who were otherwise healthy and gave birth at term had interventions in their labour (Tracy and Tracy 2003), found that the strongest association with a rise in cost per birth was the introduction of an epidural in labour. The researchers identified similar cost ratios to those in the UK studies. When the cost of a spontaneous vaginal birth was compared to an instrumental birth the ratio was 1:1.3 cost units; and the ratio of cost units between spontaneous vaginal birth compared to Caesarean section was 1:2.5. These cost ratios were based on the state costing data provided by each state health department as part of the case-mix funding formula that Australia now uses to fund hospital activity.

Usually without exception, the published economic research in this area values resources invested in the activity in terms of 'direct costs'. That is, the economic analysis establishes and measures the cost of all the resources associated with the provision of an intervention or treatment, such as rent, wages, running costs of equipment and the salaries and wages of midwives and doctors.

What is often missing from most economic equations are the indirect costs, which refer to the indirect consumption of resources such as the value of lost earnings by partners unable to work as a result of the birth of the child; child-minding or extended travel for visiting especially if the family have had to travel long distances to reach the nearest birth unit, or if the woman has undergone an operative birth and is not able to go home immediately. On the other side of the equation indirect costs such as losses in productivity, sick leave and loss of morale among midwives also need to be counted. By far the most invisible cost in economic analyses is the intangible costs such as pain or grief experienced by women and their families. In the market-based ideology governing economic analyses it remains controversial to value intangible costs in monetary terms as there is no real market in existence. To date there are no studies that set out to estimate the intangible costs in maternity care. Ignoring this important cost component could significantly underestimate the true costs related to giving birth, for example the pain and loss that remote Aboriginal women feel when they are required to leave their families and communities to give birth in large unfamiliar tertiary hospitals, or the woman required to give birth in hospital when a home birth was planned. Intangible costs may also show significant differences between those women who experience a high level of global well-being versus those who are homeless or otherwise not considered to have a high health status at the outset.

Where does the future lie?

Is it possible and timely to reverse the neoliberal metaphor of the consumer in the marketplace and replace it with the notion of community? A caring society protects and enhances human life and dignity. Health services can surely only achieve this through seeing themselves as promoting a public good and not a commodity market. Community is a concept based on the notion of a society unable to exist and progress without individuals expressing mutual obligations to each other and to the groups of which they are a part (Citrin 1998). Within communities people are intimately connected to each other and to nature in time and space. The commodification of health currently denies the quality of shared values or mutual obligations and is driven by the economics of producing a quality product at the lowest price that secures a maximum investment return and continued growth (Citrin 1998). Challenging the neoliberal mindset is a first step towards humanizing health care policy. The embrace of a neoliberal approach has affected the very nature and purpose of health care, for example, by making health care part of the free, competitive market, by commodifying health care, and by replacing the notions of the common good, social justice and public health care with an emphasis on the rational, self-interested consumer, individual responsibility and self-sufficiency (Ruthjersen 2007).

The economics of sustainability

With the crises before us, such as the global finance crisis and the prospect of climate change, losses in biodiversity and a lack of water on a global scale, there is a widespread and increasing feeling among both economists and society at large that economics should address issues of sustainability (Baumgärtner and Quaas 2010). From a total cost–benefit perspective, as we have already discussed where financial, environmental, emotional and other short- and long-term costs and benefits are adequately considered as indirect as well as intangible costs, it would be difficult to uphold the current medical maternity model as one that is either efficient or sustainable. Sustainability is a complex concept. The common thread of sustainability refers to

> those approaches that provide the best outcomes for the human and natural environments both now and into the indefinite future. Sustainability relates to the continuity of social, environmental, economic and institutional aspects of human society, as well as to all aspects of the non-human environment.
>
> (Verkerk 2009: 4)

Loss of primary-level maternity units is a clear example of the consequences of the lack of attention being given to the relationship between health care, sustainable communities and overall quality of life (Tracy *et al.* 2006). In the present climate of cost cutting and rationalizing services, maternity policy and decision makers are forced to consider whether low-volume maternity services are viable. In doing so, it is apparent that many of the relevant issues that tend to be overlooked include local community sustainability and community viability. Maternity services are a component of the socioeconomic capital of small rural communities, often central to their primary health infrastructure and serving as an entry point to further perinatal care (Nesbitt *et al.* 1997). In addition, they offer women the opportunity to give birth in their own communities without having to travel great distances. The results of the small units study in Australia (Tracy *et al.* 2006) are applicable to other countries where sophisticated obstetric and neonatal facilities are becoming increasingly centralized, and where local maternity care is being lost to women who have no known risk markers in pregnancy. There is a real need to address the issues of sustainability in the long-standing controversy of whether it is counterproductive to concentrate all maternity care in large units in major cities. The Australian study demonstrated that for normal weight babies and women with no identified risk markers in pregnancy small hospitals provided a safe and protective environment for birth. In an environment where sustainability is prioritized alongside safety, research is needed to assess the impact of the loss of maternity hospitals within communities struggling to retain community infrastructure in the face of health service consolidation. The comparative benefits and risks of regionalization versus centralization need to be evaluated from a system-wide perspective, taking into account the wider needs of communities and women. In indigenous communities different and profound risks emerge in the quest for sustainability. Cultural knowledge and practices are very often relegated to the background behind the authoritative foreground of the biomedical model.

The environmental costs of natural resource consumption in maternity care and the cost of environmental waste in maternity care have not been carefully studied. Consequently the degree to which the activities involved contribute to environmental deterioration is difficult to assess (Jameton and Pierce 2001).

In their essay titled 'What is sustainable economics?', Baumgärtner and Quaas (2010) claim that sustainable economics can be 'defined by four core attributes':

1   Subject focus on the relationship between humans and nature.
2   Orientation towards the long-term and inherently uncertain future.
3   Normative foundation in the idea of justice, between humans of present and future generations as well as between humans and nature.
4. Concern for economic efficiency, understood as non-wastefulness, in the allocation of natural goods and services as well as their human-made substitutes and complements.

(Baumgärtner and Quaas 2010: 445)

In operationalizing the economics of sustainability modern theorists appear to have settled on a combination of neoliberal and social democratic policies. Murphy (2000) identifies several aspects of ecological modernization theory that interlink business innovation with the role of government in raising environmental standards. Sustainability is promoted through market-based solutions rather than traditional forms of regulation. Community-based decision making replaces state-based policymaking and 'civil society' (non-governmental organizations and citizens' groups) is encouraged to achieve social consensus on environmental policymaking (Murphy 2000).

Conclusion

The sustained good health of populations depends on progressive and enlightened management and wise use of all the resources that surround us. In addressing both inequality and over-consumption there is an opportunity to redesign our maternity services in recognition that human survival is intimately connected to the balance in nature. In a world where the degradation of nature and the oppression of women are theoretically, symbolically and historically connected, (McMahon 1997) developing sustainable maternity services offers women a unique opportunity to lead the way in the redesign of sustainable health services.

References

Asim, O. and Petrou, S. (2005) 'Valuing a QALY: review of current controversies', *Expert Review of Pharmacoeconomics Outcomes Research*, 5, 6: 667–69

Baumgärtner, S. and Quaas, M. (2010) 'What is sustainability economics?', *Ecological Economics*, 69: 445–50.

Bryant, J., Porter, M., Tracy, S. K. and Sullivan, E. A. (2007) 'Caesarean birth: consumption, safety, order, and good mothering', *Social Science & Medicine*, 65, 6: 1192–201.

Cardwell, C. R., Stene, L. C., Joner, G., Cinek, O., Svensson, J. *et al.* (2008) 'Caesarean section is associated with an increased risk of childhood-onset type 1 diabetes mellitus: a meta-analysis of observational studies', *Diabetologia*, 51, 5: 726–35.

Cardwell, C. R., Stene, L. C., Joner, G., Davis, E. A., Cinek, O. *et al.* (2010), 'Birthweight and the risk of childhood-onset type 1 diabetes: a meta-analysis of observational studies using individual patient data', *Diabetologia*, 53, 4: 641–51.

Citrin, T. (1998) 'Topics for Our Times: Public Health-Community or Commodity? Reflections on Healthy Communities', *American Journal of Public Health*, 88, 3: 351–52.

Drummond, M. F., Weatherly H. L. A., Claxton, K. P., Cookson, R., Ferguson, B. and Godfrey, C. (2007) 'Assessing the challenges of applying the standard methods of economic evaluation to public health programmes'. York: Public Health Research Consortium.

Harrison, M. J., Lunt, M., Verstappen, S. M., Watson, K. D., Bansback, N. J. and Symmons, D. P. (2010) 'Exploring the validity of estimating EQ-5D and SF-6D utility values from the health assessment questionnaire in patients with inflammatory arthritis', *Health & Quality of Life Outcomes*, 8: 21.

Hauck, K., Smith, P. C. and Goddard, M. (2003) 'The economics of priority setting for health care, health, nutrition, and population family (HNP) of the World Bank's Human Development Network', Washington, DC.

Hausman, D. (2009) 'Valuing health: a new proposal', *Health Economics*, 19, 3: 280–96.

Jameton, A. and Pierce J. (2001) 'Environment and health: 8. Sustainable health care and emerging ethical responsibilities', *Canadian Medical Association Journal*, 164, 3: 365–69.

Larner, W. (2000) 'Neo-liberalism: policy, ideology, governmentality', *Studies in Political Economy*, 63: 5–25.

Lewis Carroll (1865) *Alice's Adventures in Wonderland*. London: Macmillan & Co.

McMahon, M. (1997) 'From the ground up: ecofeminism and ecological economics', *Ecological Economics*, 20, 163–73.

Mellor, M. (1997) 'Women, nature and the social construction of "economic man"', *Ecological Economics*, 20, 129–40.

Murphy, J. (2000) 'Ecological modernisation', *Geoforum*, 31: 1–8.

National Health and Medical Research Council (2001) *How to Compare the Costs and Benefits: Evaluation of the Economic Evidence*. Commonwealth of Australia, Canberra NHMRC.

Navarro, V. (2009) 'What we mean by social determinants of health', *International Journal of Health Services*, 39, 3: 423–41.

Nelson, J. A. (1997) 'Feminism, ecology and the philosophy of economics', *Ecological Economics*, 20: 155–62.

Nelson, J. A. (2009) 'Between a rock and a soft place: ecological and feminist economics in policy debates', *Ecological Economics*, 69: 1–8.

Nesbitt, T. S., Larson, E. H., Rosenblatt, R. A. and Hart, L. G. (1997) 'Access to maternity care in rural Washington: its effect on neonatal outcomes and resource use', *American Journal of Public Health*, 87, 1: 85–90.

O'Hara, S. U. (1997) 'Toward a sustaining production theory', *Ecological Economics*, 20: 141–54.

Petrou, S. and Glazener, C. (2002) 'The economic costs of alternative modes of delivery during the first two months postpartum: results from a Scottish observational study', *British Journal of Obstetrics & Gynaecology*, 109, 2: 214–17.

Petrou, S. and Renton, A. (1993) 'The QALY: a guide for the public health physician', *Public Health*, 107, 5: 327–36.

Petrou, S. and Wolstenholme, J. (2000) 'A review of alternative approaches to healthcare resource allocation', *Pharmacoeconomics*, 18, 1: 33–43.

Petrou, S., Henderson, J. and Glazener, C. (2001) 'Economic aspects of caesarean section and alternative modes of delivery', *Best Practice & Research Clinical Obstetrics Gynaecology*, 15, (1) 145–63.

Petrou, S., Boulvain, M., Simon, J., Maricot, P., Borst, F. *et al.* (2004) 'Home-based care after a shortened hospital stay versus hospital-based care postpartum: an economic evaluation', *British Journal of Obstetrics & Gynaecology*, 111, 8: 800–6.

Ruthjersen, A. L. (2007) *Neoliberalism and Healthcare*, Brisbane: University of Technology.

Shiell, A. (1997) 'Health outcomes are about choices and values: an economic perspective on the health outcomes movement', *Health Policy*, 39, 1: 5–15.

Shiell, A., Donaldson, C., Mitton, C. and Currie, G. (2002) 'Health economic evaluation', *Journal Epidemiolology & Community Health*, 56, 2: 85–88.

Thavagnanam, S., Fleming, J., Bromley, A., Shields, M. D. and Cardwell, C. R. (2008) 'A meta-analysis of the association between Caesarean section and childhood asthma', *Clinical & Experimental Allergy*, 38, 4: 629–33

Tracy, S. K., Sullivan, E., Dahlen, H., Black, D., Wang, Y. A. *et al.* (2006) 'Does size matter? A population-based study of birth in lower volume maternity hospitals for low risk women', *British Journal of Obstetrics & Gynaecology*, 113, 1: 86–96.

Tracy, S. K. and Tracy, M. B. (2003) 'Costing the cascade: estimating the cost of increased obstetric intervention in childbirth using population data', *British Journal of Obstetrics & Gynaecology*, 110, 8: 717–24.

Verkerk, R. (2009) 'Can the failing western medical paradigm be shifted using the principle of sustainability?' *Australian College of Nutritional & Environmental Medicine Journal*, 28, 3: 4–10.

Waring, M. (1999) *Counting for Nothing: What Men Value and What Women Are Worth*. Toronto: University of Toronto Press.

4 'Choice' and justice

Motherhood in a global context

Zoë Meleo-Erwin and Barbara Katz-Rothman

In November of 2008, an Israeli gay male couple made headlines by becoming parents through the assistance of a surrogate woman in India. Because Israel heavily regulates the practice and bars gay couples from entering into surrogacy agreements, Yonatan and Omer Gher looked to the international market. The couple first considered the United States, which allows same-sex couples to hire surrogates, and children born in the US to Israeli couples are automatically afforded Israeli citizenship. However, the Ghers soon turned to India. Although India criminalizes homosexuality for citizens under Section 377 of Indian Law, the country nevertheless allows foreign gay and lesbian couples to legally obtain surrogacy services. And given the lax regulatory climate and relative affordability, India has become a top destination for gay and straight couples from around the world seeking assisted reproductive technologies (ART) and surrogacy.[1] Thus, in the end, the Ghers decided upon the Rotunda Fertility Clinic[2] located in Bandra, despite their displeasure over Section 377.

While the particularities of surrogacy in India and the ironies and complexities of the Ghers' decision are not the subjects of this work, their story does provide a useful entry point in examining the state of contemporary reproduction in the United States under the ideology of patriarchy, the proliferation of assisted reproductive technologies and international circulations of bio-capitalism. In thinking about American birth and birthing practices in this context and as related to international concerns about sustainability, we consider what *social relations* such practices engender and we explore their *social sustainability*.

The medicalization of pregnancy and birth

Before pregnancy and birth could move into the world of consumer products, they first had to go through the process of medicalization, moving them outside of the world of family and intimate life. By 'medicalization' we mean the social and historical process by which non-medical problems become defined and treated as medical ones. As this occurs, the source of a given problem is held to be within individual rather than the larger social environment and thus medical intervention instead of social action is seen as the solution (Conrad 2007). Medicine has long been involved in the production of certain epistemologies and the governance and shaping of populations and selves. However, within the contemporary neoliberal climate of reduced government spending, medical self-evaluation and improvement as strategies to preemptively avoid risk have increasingly become obligations (Rose 2006). Discourses of medicine and health, and practices designed to avoid risk and promote health can be seen as central to many people's lives today.

Key to the medicalization of pregnancy was its increasing definition as pathological over the course of the eighteenth century. By defining pregnancy as an abnormal state of the body, physicians, most particularly American doctors, held that birth and birthing practices rightly fell under their purview, essentially eradicating midwifery as a practice until its resurgence in the 1970s. By the twentieth century, a proper pregnancy in the United States was one managed by obstetrical prenatal care with a focus on searching for pathology. Medicine attempted to maintain the normalcy of the mother throughout the stress of pregnancy, viewing any deviation from a normal (non-pregnant) status as a symptom of disease that, in turn, justified medical treatment. Common physiological changes during pregnancy, such as changes in haemoglobin, blood pressure, blood sugar, fluid retention or weight gain, were seen by obstetricians as indicative of pathology.

Over the last several decades, discursive representations of pregnancy as abnormal have waned. However, as late as 1980, the medical textbook *Williams Obstetrics* noted that while pregnancy was a normal state, 'the complexity of the functional and anatomic changes that accompany gestation tends to stigmatize normal pregnancy as a disease process' (Prichard and Macdonald 1980: 303). Later editions of *Williams*, though they moved away from a pregnancy-as-disease framing, continued to contrast the changes brought about by pregnancy with the 'normal' status of the body, belying an ongoing view of pregnancy as pathological.

A significant factor in the continued medicalization of birthing practices is the subsumption of an increasing number of pregnancies under the category of 'risk'. Contemporary medicine distinguishes between 'low-risk' and 'high-risk' pregnancies – always maintaining the focus on risk. Some of the risk factors are engendered by changes brought about by the pregnancy itself, such as 'preclinical diabetes' or 'mild pre-eclampsia'. Others are natural categories of the woman, such as parity (number of previous pregnancies) and age. Since the introduction of the 'risk' approach to pregnancy, the 'high-risk' category has broadened through such practices as steadily lowering the age for prenatal testing for genetic and other disorders and conditions, and redefining 'grand multipara' from five previous births to the contemporary number of three, a shift that reflects larger trends in smaller family size. With obstetrical management focused on preventing, assessing and treating risk, pregnancy has become increasingly surveilled. In the medical regimen, a pregnant woman is expected to see an obstetrician each month during the first two trimesters, twice a month for the seventh and eighth months and then weekly during the final month. Evidence that such prenatal care actually leads to improved birth outcomes is lacking (Fiscella 1995: 468). Beyond regular prenatal care visits, the pregnant woman is encouraged to self-monitor to ensure she is providing the best environment for the fetus.

As with pregnancy, the field of medicine increasingly shapes and controls the birthing process. The medical literature defines childbirth as a process occurring in three stages. In the first stage, 'labour', the cervix dilates from nearly closed to its fullest dimension of approximately 10 centimetres. During the second stage, the baby is pushed through the opened cervix and through the birth canal and out of the woman's body. This is the 'delivery'. Finally, during the third stage, the placenta is expelled. Labour is defined as a situation necessitating hospitalization and generally a dilation of 3 centimetres is a criterion of admittance. Within the medical view of birth, labour is largely managed by hospital staff. Thus, labour is something that *happens to* a pregnant woman, not something she *does*. With a focus on attending to the needs of the *fetal patient*, with the introduction of electronic fetal monitoring, and by focusing on the length of labour, inductions and Caesarean sections have become increasingly commonplace. There is no data to show that continuous electronic fetal monitoring improves fetal outcome, but it does dramatically increase the incidence of Caesarean section. In more and more US hospitals the Caesarean section rate has surpassed 50 per cent, and in at least some cities (i.e. Monterrey, Mexico) the rate of Caesarean sections is now 90 per cent.

The focus on the control of the length of labour can be traced back to the development of the standard obstetrical model of labour as represented by 'Friedman's curve', a 'graphicostatistical analysis' of labour, which breaks the process into separate phases and computes the average length for each phase. The adoption of this model within obstetrics has resulted in the establishment of strict time limits for each phase of the birthing process, which, in turn, defines labour that falls outside the realm of statistical normality as necessitating medical intervention. That birth occurs in hospitals furthers this process, as births need to be meshed together to form an overarching institutional setting. Changes in what is considered an average first stage reflect this institutional speeding up of labour: the 1948 edition of *Williams* defines the first stage of labour as occurring over 12.5 hours and 10.5 hours for first and second/subsequent births, respectively. By the 1980 edition these numbers had dropped to 7.3 hours and 5 hours. While this speeding up of labour reflects institutional needs to rationally and predictably manage labour, the focus on medically intervening in those pregnancies defined as abnormal is justified as protecting the health and well-being of the fetal 'patient'.

The view of the fetus as a separate 'patient' with needs that may or may not be congruous with those of the pregnant woman is a relatively recent development. As a surgical practice, the work of obstetrics was to separate the fetus from the pregnant woman, to 'rescue' the entrapped fetus from a woman whose active participation in the birth was essentially made nil through the use of sedation and anesthesia. With the widespread acceptance of ultrasound, the medical industry began to share its image of the fetus as a patient trapped in a maternal environment. Today's birthing practices reflect this view, focusing first and foremost on visualizing, testing, treating and removing fetuses as the pregnant woman slips into the background.

Regardless of whether or not a woman is awake during her labour and birth, and even if kindly and humanly treated, within the medical model the baby is the product of the doctor's services. Contemporary medical knowledge and technologies not only monitor the needs of the fetus as separate from those of the mother, but also suggest that she cannot be relied upon to provide a protective uterine environment. As a highly politicized entity, the fetus has now acquired rights: rights to be genetically free of defect, rights to be free of 'abuse' by pregnant women and rights to medical treatment. The outcome of this framing is that women may become alienated from babies, their own bodies and the process of birth.

Framing medicalization in Western ideology

Just as pregnancy and birth have been shaped by their incorporation into the medical realm, their medicalization may be seen as having been formed through the processes of larger social phenomena. While certainly there are other routes to medicalization, we briefly review the ways in which the ideologies of patriarchy, technology and bio-capitalism have been particular influences.

The core definition of patriarchy is the idea that paternity is a central social relationship and that women's reproductive lives must be controlled in order to ensure it. While modern American kinship is bilateral (individuals are considered to be equally related to their mother's and father's sides of the family), ideas about abortion, 'illegitimacy', and women's sexual and pro-creative freedom reflect patriarchal concerns for maintaining paternity. In many ways, motherhood continues to be defined in terms of what women and babies signify to men. For women this can mean increasing or reducing the number of desired pregnancies; 'trying again' for a son; covering up male infertility through the use of donor insemination; not having access or full access to birth control and abortions, and being pressured into having an abortion. Further, the conceptual separation of woman and fetus, which is enacted through various visualizing technologies and the medical management of fetus and mother as separate patients, has its origins in a patriarchal understanding of pregnancy and birth. Finally, the focus on genetic con-nections as the indication of true parenthood can be seen as an extension of the patriarchal focus on seed. Within a patriarchal system, the genetic tie becomes a determining social and legal connection while relationships based on parenting and nurturance receive less weight. Thus women can hire other women to carry their seed – seed now understood to include egg as well as sperm – placing women in much the same position men have historically held, as owning and controlling babies that grow in the bodies of less-powerful women.

Reproductive technologies are based on this patriarchal focus on the seed as well as the industrial and post-industrial desire for efficiency. In the application of ideas about machines to human bodies, such bodies are asked to be more efficient. A focus on efficiency requires organizing life into component parts, systematizing and rationalizing them to better harness productivity. Not only does technological control frame the body in an object-ified way, it lends toward the conceptualization of aspects of mothering as commodifiable and aspects of reproduction as interchangeable. The substitu-tion of aspects of mothering has a long history, always with the same patterns: upper-class men and now women have bought the services of lower-class women to meet the needs of their children. With contemporary reproductive technologies, the situation remains the same as wealthy or relatively wealthy individuals purchase the reproductive materials of some and hire the surrogate services of others.

Although artificial insemination with donor sperm has been used for over 100 years, it was shrouded in silence. Today, assisted reproductive tech-nologies are a full-fledged industry. Despite the focus on altruism that allegedly guides the decision to 'donate' egg and sperm or to 'rent' ones womb, economic incentive is clearly a driving factor. With this said, reproductive technology websites that feature information about both egg and sperm donors and surrogates make clear the split between what is considered desirable and important in each.

The most prized egg and sperm donors are those who are only temporarily economically disadvantaged but otherwise share characteristics in common with reproductive technology patrons. Beyond the desire for a match along racial and/or ethnic lines, the reproductive technology industry heavily markets the idea that that some traits (both social and physical) are more desirable than others. Moreover, the idea that such traits reside in the genetic material of the donated egg and sperm, irrespective of the biological contributions of the gestating mother or the social and cultural environment in which the child is raised, is a key selling point (Tober 2002). Egg and sperm donors are thus screened for traits that are both truly genetic in nature as well as those that are not but are purported to be. Sperm donation does not garner a high monetary payment because of the ease through which it is acquired. However, men may repeatedly donate and, in fact, many clinics prefer to build a partnership with donors (Tober 2002). Conversely, egg donation, particularly by white, college-educated young women who approximate mainstream beauty ideals (tall, thin), is relatively highly remunerated, paying up to $10,000.[3] Although a woman may 'donate' eggs more than once, each donation is with risk to her own health and fertility because of the use of fertility drugs and surgical removal of the eggs.

In the case of surrogacy, women who are generally of poor or working-class status are paid for the temporary 'use of their bodies'. Commercial surrogacy entered the scene in the 1980s, when surrogacy brokers began assuring couples that there was still a way for the male partner to have his own baby when the female partner was infertile. Surrogate motherhood was sold as a solution to the tragedy of infertility and a way of resolving women's guilt at their own fertility. Today, in cases where the female partner is infertile, couples turn to in-vitro surrogacy wherein the implanted embryo is the result of the male partner's sperm and a donated egg. In other cases both the egg and sperm are purchased or donated. In such forms of surrogacy, the surrogate mother must only be screened to ensure that she is responsible and will provide a good 'environment' for the child that she has been paid to carry and deliver. To ensure the 'quality' of the child, contractual surrogacy agreements often dictate that a surrogate mother must undergo prenatal testing, including ultrasound and amniocentesis. Any action that is considered to be dangerous to the developing fetus is generally considered grounds for breaking the contract, causing her to forfeit payment and potentially opening her to legal action.

Surrogacy agreements are both uncompensated (with payments covering only the medical and legal costs associated with the surrogate pregnancy) and compensated (with additional payments made to the surrogate woman for her services). The total cost of surrogacy varies by state, by fertility clinic, whether or not egg donation is used and whether or not the surrogate woman has previous experience. Circle Surrogacy[4] estimates the price of surrogacy in the United States as being between \$55,000–\$65,0000, noting total programme costs can range as high as \$120,000. Of this, only approximately \$20–23K is paid to a first-time surrogate, with greater sums being commanded by second- and third-time surrogates.[5] By way of contrast, Yonatan and Omer Gher paid the Rotunda Fertility Clinic \$30K for both surrogacy and egg donation, and of this their surrogate was paid \$7,500 (*The New York Times* 3/10/08).

Most Western nations have banned the practice of surrogacy, however, it is both a legal and unregulated practice in the United States and laws on surrogacy vary state-by-state. While one might locate this reason for this difference in the deep-seated culture of market ideology held in the United States (Kimbrell 1993), in a globalized economy wherein Israeli, British and other well-off couples from the global north are increasingly seeking out ART and surrogacy services in the global south, a broader analysis is required.

The ART industry commonly represents egg and sperm donation and surrogacy as based in altruism.[6] The gift/commodity distinction has a long history that is well covered elsewhere (see Walby and Mitchell 2007), however, it is notable that despite the entanglement of gifts and commodities, the ART industry continues to frame 'reproductive work' (Tober 2002) in terms of the gift. This split between the reality of reproductive work and its discursive representation reflects not only an attempt to imbue it with meaning and differentiate it from what is clearly also a market transaction (Tober 2002), but also the tension between conceiving of children as precious and treating them as products at the same time. Based in the ideologies of patriarchy, technology and capitalism, ART increasingly shifts the focus from parenthood and motherhood to the creation of the commodity of a baby. Prices are negotiated for body parts, bodily fluids, human services and energy with caring and nurturing removed from the equation.

Assisted reproductive technologies need to be placed in a larger context of biomedical technologies, which involve 'a reorganization of the boundaries and elements of the human body' (Walby and Mitchell 2006). These novel forms of exchangeable body-part components circulate in lucrative bio-economies, or 'tissue economies' as Walby and Mitchell refer to them. A tissue economy, they state, can be seen as a system that maximizes the productive capacities of human tissues through their diversification, leverage, circulation and recuperation. Investment in and development of these bodily components guides much of current biomedical technology. Technicity, or the interaction between the tissues themselves and the technological means that harness, potentiate, store and circulate them, is key to the speculative nature of these economies.

For our purposes we take particular note of Walby and Mitchell's contention that 'the forms of circulation characteristic of any particular tissue economy both presuppose and constitute certain kinds of social relations, and indeed power relations' (2006: 33). Tissue economies, in this sense, must be seen as political economies. Scheper-Hughes (2002a) argues that bioeconomies have allowed the world to become bifurcated into two populations: those who are medically included and those who are medically excluded. The former, recognized as moral subjects who are believed to be suffering, desire the vitality of the latter, who are largely unseen aside from being suppliers of spare parts. While there are exceptions, especially at the local level, in general, the flows within bioeconomies, as with other forms of capital, are from south to north, economically disadvantaged to economically privileged, of colour to white.

The commodification of bodies, or the 'capitalized economic relations between humans in which human bodies are the token of economic exchanges', is masked by brokers and recipients in terms of the gift (Scheper-Hughes 2002a: 2). Those who sell their own reproductive and anatomical power often do so as a means of last resort. However, brokers and recipients commonly describe this sacrifice in terms of altruism and kindness. In the case of surrogacy, brokers describe the generosity of surrogates as that which helps couples 'realize their dreams' of having a precious child. Despite such discursive representations, the financial motivation behind the act of surrogacy is hardly veiled. In fact, in their March 2008 interview with *The New York Times*, the Ghers described the arrangement between themselves and their surrogate as 'mutually beneficial' and noted that their motivation to use an Indian surrogate was partly based on the desire to 'help someone in India', given the vast differences between Indian poverty and Western wealth.

What do we make of a case wherein fertility brokers frame the actions of surrogates as based largely in altruism while the patrons of the fertility clinic themselves see the act as one that is based in mutual generosity? Moreover, how can we understand the Ghers' assertion that it is the very act of remuneration that makes surrogacy ethical? It is our assertion that such a framing needs to be understood in terms of the focus on autonomy and choice in liberal, free-market philosophy. Within this framework, the vitality of the body is a resource to be used and even sold so long as this is undertaken in a way that is 'freely chosen'. Thus 'informed consent' becomes a key concept: if one consents or agrees to undertake such an action rationally, then one accepts the consequences of ones actions and coercion cannot be seen to have been a factor. However, such thinking fails to understand, or perhaps refuses to understand, that such 'choices' are often motivated by poverty and need and thus must be understood within a more complex view of power relations.

Scheper-Hughes noted that for the excluded, their

> only *real* sense of power and control in their lives derives from a certain kind of command and ownership of their bodies—the very grounds of their existence—which they express, paradoxically, by selling it off in parts or in its entirety, a modern-day tragedy of decidedly heroic proportions.
>
> (2002a: 8, emphasis in the original)

We might understand Indian surrogacy in this light. The Rotunda does not release the names of their surrogates or allow them to be interviewed, however the same *The New York Times* March 2008 article on the Ghers featured a quote from another Indian surrogate. Although Indian women who work as surrogates do so, in part, for reasons that are very personal, and local, we explore this woman's story as illustrative of some of the structural issues that do affect all Indian surrogates, despite individual variability. This woman, residing in Dehli, turned to surrogacy because her salary of 2,800 rupees, or approximately $69 a month as a midwife, did not cover the expenses of raising her son as a single mother. With the money she earned as a first-time surrogate, she was able to purchase a house. She told *The New York Times* that with the earnings from her second surrogate pregnancy, she intended to pay for her son's education.

While a liberal reading of this woman's story would suggest her to be a model of both the opportunities and choice available to even the most marginalized within a free-market system, a more critical reading makes clear the dynamics of which Scheper-Hughes speaks. Committed to a women-centered form of birth and pregnancy, this surrogate was nevertheless unable to make a living working as a midwife and thus sold the reproductive power of her own body. Her reproductive power was sold to a fertility clinic committed to a highly technological and lucrative medical model of pregnancy and birth. She gave birth to a child that was likely the product of either donor egg or sperm or both. While these reproductive materials were chosen based on how closely the donor or donors approximated traits (both truly genetic and nature and those purported to be) desired by the clients,[7] this woman was selected for her ability to provide a proper gestational environment and because of the relative affordability of her labour. The clients, who received the child she birthed, took the infant back to what was undoubtedly a middle-class or higher life in the global North. And with the funds the surrogate woman received, a fraction of that garnered by the clinic that brokered the deal and marketed her labour as an act of altruism, she was able to invest the future of the child to whom she is mother. Her case is not one of unencumbered free will or altruism but rather 'a modern-day tragedy of decidedly heroic proportions', indeed (Scheper-Hughes 2002a: 8).

While there is enormous pressure within liberal capitalist society to think of family formation in purely individual and psychological terms, as a series of individual choices, it is important to understand that these choices occur in a global environment, in ways that link all of humanity together. This is, perhaps, the single greatest lesson of the current century: catastrophic social and environmental changes occur at larger structural levels while people are pressured to understand what is happening as a series of individual consumer choices.

The global context: rethinking 'sustainability in terms of justice

In September 2009, nearly 100 world leaders attended the Summit on Climate Change in New York City. In his opening address, UN Secretary-General Ban Ki-moon urged leaders to work together at the upcoming United Nations Climate Change Conference in Copenhagen. At that time, leaders will attempt to create a global climate change agreement to begin in 2012 when the first commitment period under the Kyoto Protocol expires. In his closing statement he remarked: 'There is little time left. The opportunity and responsibility to avoid catastrophic climate change is in your hands.' With Copenhagen quickly approaching, warnings about the ramifications of refusing to think about long-term environmental sustainability are being sounded with alarm – from Ki-moon's address to the Yes Men's direct action[8] on the streets in New York during the Summit wherein activists distributed faux copies of *The New York Post* featuring the headline 'We're Screwed!' and 32 pages of articles warning New Yorkers of the lethal effects that climate change would have on the city.

In keeping with the theme of this anthology, we take 'sustainability' to mean, 'meets the needs of the present without compromising the ability of future generations to meet their own needs', as defined by the 1987 Bruntdland Report.[9] The Bruntdland Report stresses the imperative of considering: 1) the world's needs, particularly those of the poor, which should be prioritized, and 2) the interaction between the contemporary state of technology and social organization and the ability of the natural environment to meet both present and future needs. With a focus on *social* sustainability, we wish to consider ART and surrogacy practices in light of this definition and these key points.

Feminist philosophers Mies and Shiva noted, 'It is a historical fact that technological innovations within exploitative and unequal relationships lead to an intensification, not attenuation, of inequality, and to further exploitation of the groups concerned' (1993: 175). As soon as one concedes that technology is for something, one can no longer claim it to be a neutral tool that can be put to various uses:

> In fact, no particular technology, construed as a technological object, gadget, process or system, or even as an isolated bit of technological knowledge or know-how can be morally neutral. It was designed or conceived for some purpose, and any such purpose is subject to moral or ethical evaluation.
>
> (Durbin 1980)

It is not just that a given technology or practice, such as egg donation or surrogacy, may empower some at the expense of others, allowing one woman or couple to have a child while another woman faces physical and emotional risks for a fee. It is also that biomedical technologies, within a system of global capitalism, have unleashed an insatiable appetite for the vitality of 'the other' whose body is worth more as a 'reservoir of spare parts' than as a human being and that this exploitation, of an already objectified population, is disguised as altruism (Scheper-Hughes 2002b). The issue is power, not technology per se. And the consequences occur for all pregnant women, not just those who are most overtly selling their 'service.' Pregnancy itself is objectified, devalued and understood as 'cheap labour'.

The commodification of procreation perpetuates and intensifies disparities along lines of race, class, sex and nation. The maximization and circulation of diversified, leveraged and recuperated body parts may be lucrative for bioeconomies, but in a larger environment of great social and economic disparities wherein 'need' and 'choice' are fundamentally entangled, such practices are unjust. Whereas these technologies are both predicated upon and constitute forms of social organization and power relations that are exploitative and based in domination, we must consider them wholly unsustainable.

Thus far we have spoken of the ways in which the circulation of reproductive body parts and surrogacy practices within bioeconomies furthers exploitative power between *adults*. We now briefly turn to what we believe to be their effects on relations between mothers and babies and on mothering as a practice of care. The relationship between mothers and babies may be seen as both biological and social: pregnancy is a biological condition that occurs in a larger social context and a social connection that occurs in larger biological environment. Reproductive technologies, particularly imaging technologies, have encouraged the view of the fetus and mother as separate patients, with the priority being the fetus. In this process, pregnant women have been relegated to the role of unskilled workers on a reproductive assembly line, subject to quality control, regardless of whether they are birthing their own baby or one purchased by another couple. The fetus is imagined and shown to be trapped in a potentially hazardous gestational environment, and the role of obstetrics is to rescue the highest possible quality infant. And as babies and children have become products and mothers unskilled workers, reproductive technologies and practices have focused our attention on services and procedures rather than relationships.

Mothers are not the only individuals who can raise babies. Rather, defined broadly, mothering can be seen as an intimate kind of caring that has as its goal the creation of capable members of a larger community. The parent-child relationship is based not on genetics but on love and caring – social rather than physical characteristics. We therefore reject language, practices and technologies that reduce relations of care to relations of commodifcation, production and exploitation. A sustainable vision of mothering and reproduction at large is one based on nurturance and care.

Liberal feminism was not misguided in working to critique the definition of motherhood as a master status. However, the response of this form of feminism has been to frame everything, from home birth to surrogacy contracts to IVF and other assisted reproductive technologies, as 'choice.' And while choice may have been a necessary argument, all things considered, it was only a start. Questions of social justice provide the context in which issues of choice unfold and we argue that whether they derive from liberal feminists, mainstream LGBTQ (lesbian, gay, bisexual and transgender people) parenting rights organizations or fertility clinics, 'choice' masks not only exploitative power relations between privileged and marginalized populations but the further commodification of relations of care.

Roberts draws a related distinction between liberty and justice as ethical frameworks when she states:

> The dominant view of liberty reserves most of its protection for the most privileged members of society. This approach superimposes liberty on an already unjust social structure, which it seeks to preserve against unwarranted government interference. Liberty protects all citizens' choices from the most direct and egregious abuses of government power, but it does nothing to dismantle social arrangements that make it impossible for some people to make a choice in the first place. Liberty guards against government intrusion; it does nothing to guarantee social justice.
>
> (1997: 294)

We must go beyond concerns of liberty and choice and address issues of social justice. Reproductive decision making – from the decision to have an abortion to the decision to have a child to selling ones reproductive materials to using the reproductive power of ones womb – does not occur in a vacuum. We must place these practices and the assisted reproductive technologies that harness, potentiate and circulate bodily materials in a larger social, economic and political context while not losing sight of the very specific, grounded and local nature of individual decision making.

Conclusion: imagining a praxis of justice through midwifery

A fundamental insight within the social sciences is that knowledge comes from somewhere and that the 'who, what, where, why and how' of knowledge, as well as what must be forgotten for conceptual models to have ontological significance, is political. Thinking and doing are dynamically related to each other and to the larger social environment in which they occur. With this said, we suggest that midwifery is a feminist praxis. It offers not just different 'attitudes' toward birth but is fundamentally different from the biomedical approach. While midwifery is not our focus in this work and has been well covered elsewhere (Katz-Rothman 2000; Katz-Rothman and Simonds 2007), we argue that midwifery offers as an alternative ideological base, and consequentially the potential for developing an alternative and sustainable body of knowledge and practices about procreation. Midwifery works with the labour of the pregnant woman to transform and to create the birth experience to meet her own needs. It is a social, political activity, dialectically linking biology and society, the physical and the social experiences of motherhood. The very word midwife means 'with woman'. This is more than a physical location; it is an ideological and political stance. Midwifery, we argue, represents a rejection of the artificial dualisms inherent in patriarchy, biomedical technologies and capitalism-dualisms between baby and mother and between visible, moral subjects and invisible, excluded individuals who are valued more as parts than as human beings. More than rejecting dualisms, midwifery sees unity.

Within midwifery, a sustainable model of both reproduction and human interaction is one that sees a fundamental biological and social relationship between mothers and babies; that recognizes that a good and just world is one that provides all people with opportunities to nurture if that is what they want to do and provides women with genuine choices around pregnancy; that focuses not on the investment in and the proliferation of the circulation of body tissues and bodily capacities but addresses the underlying social and political disparities that shape the 'choices' of individuals to sell off the anatomical and reproductive power of their bodies; that prioritizes investigations into how environmental and social conditions affect and may be increasing infertility[10] and takes measures to halt these contributing factors; that opposes neo-Darwinist notions of genetics; that rejects the reduction of relations of care to relations of production; that highlights the enormous percentage of children in the United States within foster and institutional care and challenges the idea that some children are socially precious while others are 'socially dead';[11] and, among other basic human rights, demands free and unfettered access to quality health care, childcare and education.

What we take from the praxis of midwifery is a focus on social, biological and natural environments as a deeply connected *whole* rather than a series of commodifiable, interchangeable, circulatable parts. If we truly wish to consider a sustainable future, we must be clear about the real challenges we face and yet understand the dynamic relation between current practices and future outcomes. We must see a sustainable future as a dialectical, indeterminate, ever-receding horizon and work toward it nonetheless. At the very least, we must understand that 'choice' without social justice is wholly unsustainable at any level.

Notes

1 A May of 2009 *Thaindian News* report noting that a British child is born by an Indian surrogate every 48 hours. See http://www.thaindian.com/newsportal/world-news/surrogate-baby-is-born-in-india-to-a-british-couple-every-48-hours_100195492.html.

2 The Rotunda's website, http://www.iwannagetpregnant.com, offers information to potential clients in both English and Hebrew and features the words 'LGBT friendly' as well as several highly recognizable gay pride symbols.

3 Women whose eggs are considered highly desirable, such as those who are Ivy League educated with high standardized test scores, often advertise in newspapers commanding prices as high as $50k.

4 www.circlesurrogacy.com/.

5 See the Center for Surrogate Parenting, http://www.creatingfamilies.com/.

6 In the case of sperm donors, those who cite altruistic reasons for donation are more likely to pass donor screening (Tober 2002).

7 Of the egg donors they perused, the Ghers note, 'We picked the one with the highest level of education' (*The New York Times*, 3/10/08).

8 See http://www.theyesmen.org/blog/screwed.

9 See http://www.worldinbalance.net/agreements/1987-brundtland.php.

10 When infertility treatments became available, infertility changed from a stigmatizing social condition to a treatable medical condition, although one with low success rates of 'cure'. Thus, while we can say that infertility does most assuredly exist, it is also the product of invention: the conditions we define as infertility are socially constructed and socially legitimated. Involuntary childlessness has been medicalized.

11 Lock (2002) notes that though the Anatomy Act, 1831 in the UK prohibited sale of dead bodies, institutions such as hospitals and workhouses were considered to be in lawful possession of the bodies of the poor when they were unclaimed or when no money was available for a funeral. Given this, such institutions had full license to sell their bodies to medical researchers. 'In the interests of medicine, then, the poor were effectively defined as socially dead, their commoditized bodies not due the respect given to those of the rest of society' (67).

References

Conrad, P. (2007) *The Medicalization of Society: On the Transformation of Human Conditions into Treatable Disorders*. Baltimore: Johns Hopkins University Press.

Durbin, P. T. (1980) *A Guide to the Culture of Science, Technology and Medicine*. New York: Free Press.

Fiscella, K. (1995) 'Does prenatal care improve birth outcomes? A critical review', *Obstetrics and Gynecology*, 85, 3: 468–79.

Gentleman, A. (10 March 2008) 'India nurtures business of surrogate motherhood', *The New York Times*. Online. Available at: www.nytimes.com/2008/03/10/world/asia/10surrogate.html?_r=1&pagewanted=1 (accessed 11 October 2009).

Katz-Rothman, B. (2000 [1989]) *Recreating Motherhood*. New Brunswick, NJ: Rutgers University Press.

Katz-Rothman, B. and Simonds, W. (2007) *Laboring On*, New York: Routledge.

Kimbrell, A. (1993) *The Human Body Shop: The Engineering and Marketing of Life*. San Francisco: Harper San Francisco.

Mies, M. and Shiva, V. (1993) *Ecofeminism*. London: Zed Books.

Prichard, J. A. and Macdonald, P. C. (1980) *Williams Obstetrics*, 16th Edition. New York: Appleton Century Crofts.

Roberts, D. (1997) *Killing the Black Body: Race, Reproduction and the Meaning of Liberty*. New York: Pantheon.

Rose, N. (2006) *The Politics of Life Itself: Biomedicine, Power and Subjectivity in the Twenty-First Century*. Princeton, NJ: Princeton University Press.

Scheper-Hughes, N. (2002a) 'Bodies for sale – whole or in parts', in N. Scheper-Hughes and L. Wacquant, L. (eds), *Commodifying Bodies*. Los Angeles: Sage Publications.

Scheper-Hughes, N. (2002b) 'Commodity fetishism in organs trafficking', in N. Scheper-Hughes and L. Wacquant (eds), *Commodifying Bodies*. Los Angeles: Sage Publications.

Tober, D. M. (2002) 'Semen as gift, semen as goods: reproductive workers and the market in altruism', in N. Scheper-Hughes and L. Wacquant (eds), *Commodifying Bodies*. Los Angeles: Sage Publications.

Walby C. and Mitchell, R. (2007) *Tissue Economies: Blood, Organs and Cell Lines in Late Capitalism*. Durham, NC: Duke University Press.

Section two

Midwifery as a sustainable health care practice

5 'Relationships – the glue that holds it all together'

Midwifery continuity of care and sustainability

Nicky Leap, Hannah Dahlen, Pat Brodie, Sally Tracy and Juliet Thorpe

Introduction

In late December 2009, four midwifery leaders sat around a kitchen table in Sydney and audio-recorded a conversation about experiences of developing midwifery models of care. With this chapter in mind, we focussed on what we saw as features of sustainable models that enable women to develop a trusting relationship with their midwives through pregnancy, labour and the early weeks of new motherhood. Mostly we reflected on our experiences of setting up midwifery group practices in the Australian public health system where midwives are employed, but some of us also drew on our experiences in the United Kingdom (UK) and New Zealand (NZ); this included our involvement in models where midwives are self-employed and working either privately or as part of the public health system.

An analysis of the transcript of our conversation enabled us to identify several themes that emerged within an overarching theme that relationships are the most crucial elements of sustainability – relationships with women, between midwives who work together and supportive relationships within the maternity care system. We also identified some features of midwifery group practices that enhance the potential for these relationships to flourish. This chapter addresses these themes using direct quotes to preserve the flavour of the conversation with the hope that this will stimulate readers to engage in similar discussions and make comparisons with their own experiences and intentions.

We will use the term 'midwifery group practice' since, in our discussion, we were talking about models in publicly-funded health services where between two and eight midwives who are employed in a maternity service work in a 'caseload practice' or 'continuity of carer' model. In such models, each woman has a primary midwife who is her first point of reference and who takes responsibility for her individualized care through pregnancy, labour and birth and the early weeks of new motherhood (Homer *et al.* 2008a). Midwives practising in this way rely on backup from other midwives and referral and consultation with other practitioners and agencies according to the woman's individual needs and wishes. This is the primary care model that is funded in countries such as New Zealand, Canada and many European countries; it is also akin to the way in which self-employed midwives – sometimes referred to as 'independent' or 'privately practising' midwives – organise their working lives across the Western world. Some would say that this way of practising *is* midwifery and that it is counterproductive to talk about midwifery 'models', some of which may not include 'relational continuity of care' – a relationship built over time, involving trust and responsibility (Saultz 2003).

Discussions about definitions and nomenclature are important, particularly in debates where the necessity for an intrapartum component of midwifery continuity of care is challenged (Carolan and Hodnett 2007; Green *et al.* 1998). For the purposes of this chapter we take the position that intrapartum care is a vital component of midwifery continuity of care for both women and their midwives in terms of positive experiences and sustainability (Leap and Edwards 2006; McCourt and Stevens 2005; Page *et al.* 2006). We are also mindful that intrapartum care was an essential requirement for inclusion in a Cochrane systematic review, which concluded that all women should have access to the benefits of 'midwifery led care' (Hatem *et al.* 2008). In acknowledging the contribution that midwifery continuity of care can make to safeguarding the health and well-being of women and their families, we nevertheless hope that the principles discussed in this chapter can be considered in relation to the many ways in which midwives practise.

Our experience is that, where the funding of maternity services does not enable women to access continuity of care from a midwife or midwifery group practice of their choice, the system tends to perpetuate unpredictable, fragmented care for women from a range of unknown practitioners. The development and sustainability of midwifery group practices within publicly-funded maternity services is often down to local vision and determination: '*It is against the odds that they do get up*'. Our discussion kept returning to the barriers and difficulties faced in Australia – and to a lesser extent in the United Kingdom – in attempts to reorganize maternity services so that all women receive midwifery continuity of carer. We have therefore finished this chapter with an uplifting vignette written by Juliet Thorpe from New Zealand, where health service funding enables pregnant women to choose a midwife as their primary carer through pregnancy, labour and birth and the post-natal period, and where remuneration for midwifery services is not tied to maternity service provision.

Relationships: 'the glue that holds it all together'

The central theme of both our discussion and the vignette from New Zealand is that building strong, positive relationships is the most important element of sustainability when midwives provide continuity of care. A similar conclusion was identified in research carried out by Jane Sandall (1997) in

---

Box 5.1   Factors that should be in place to avoid burn out in midwifery continuity of care

Adapted from J. Sandall (1997) 'Midwives' burnout and continuity of care', *British Journal of Midwifery*, 5, 2: 106–111:

- The ability for midwives to develop meaningful relationships with women through continuity of carer.

- Positive working relationships and occupational autonomy: midwives being able to organize their working lives with maximum flexibility through negotiation.

- Supportive relationships at work and at home.

---

the UK over a decade ago. Her model of what needs to be in place to avoid midwives suffering from 'burn out' still stands as a framework to guide the development of sustainable midwifery group practices.

Meaningful relationships with women

Providing continuity of care can have a profound effect on the professional and personal development of midwives as they engage with women in a process of developing reciprocal trust and shared learning in the face of uncertainty (Downe and McCourt 2008; Leap 2010). The relationship requires maturity, self-awareness and the ability to share of oneself in a way that can be challenging for midwives as they take on new roles (Homer *et al.* 2008b; Leap and Pairman 2010). It is, however, the meaningful nature and quality of this relationship, the 'emotional work' and reciprocity, that midwives describe as the force that sustains them (Hunter *et al.* 2008; Sandall *et al.* 2008; McCourt and Stevens 2009):

> We repeatedly hear midwives talking about how working in a group practice has transformed their lives. That shift of moving from being 'with institution' to being 'with woman'. . . . Sure it can be hard at times but the joy and pleasure of 'going on the journey to new motherhood' with a woman and her family is deeply satisfying.

Setting up healthy boundaries

It can take time for midwives to work out how to negotiate the relationship in a way that optimises the potential for the woman to feel more powerful as a result of her experience of childbirth (Leap 2010; Leap and Pairman 2010):

It's about having the confidence to know the boundaries of your practice and boundaries of the relationship building with the woman and if it truly is woman centred then you are hopefully developing a philosophy and a model that has the woman feeling completely in control and independent of the midwife. But it can take time to get that when you've come from a fragmented model of care. You sort of almost swing the pendulum to the other extreme and think that you've got to be all things to women at first. That's where honest discussions with other midwives in the group can help you develop a sustainable way of working.

Relationships with midwifery colleagues in group practices

Midwives across the world who work in group practices report the importance of the interpersonal dynamics with their midwifery colleagues. Meeting and talking on the phone regularly are pivotal factors for support, connection and learning from each other. The following quotations describe our experiences of this:

Looking after ourselves and each other

We talk so much about giving women our best, woman-centred care and trying to be part of helping women have optimal experiences. I think if we don't look after each other and ourselves as well as we look after women, then we will not end up being able to look after women as well as we should. And knowing when to say: 'I actually can't do this, this week.' Sometimes you have to protect yourself and in caseload practice there are weeks where you need other people to help take up your slack.

Checking in on each other

The weekly group meetings are so important in terms of learning from each other and problem solving – putting our heads together – but they're also important in terms of understanding what is going on in each other's lives. Each meeting always starts with a round of, 'How are we?' Just a few minutes, checking out with each person. That is such an important precedent. For the 'how are we' session, if we have students or visitors, they will be asked to go and get a cup of tea and come back later because that's our time to make sure that we're all alright.

You know some people in the public health system can work quite closely with their colleagues and not know anything about what is going on for them at home. If someone is being negative about everything we can be really quick to say, 'that person's really negative, I don't like working with them'. And that's when divisions can start. Whereas if you know that they're having a really hard time at home, for example with their kids playing up, you can filter their negativity with the knowledge that they are having a really hard time in their life.

Good will and generosity of spirit

Good will and generosity of spirit form the glue that holds it all together. It's a willingness to give and take in ways that midwives would never have done in more traditional roles. The classic example is covering each other for functions – such as a meeting at your kid's school or a concert – for a few hours here and there: that willingness to be generous and flexible and not be boxed into a rule bound system.

Trusting each other

Trust between members of the group practice enables midwives to hand over to each other with confidence. For example, if you've got a midwife who has been really busy, you know that she is not going to relax and be off call if she can't actually hand over to a colleague – however complex the situation – and absolutely know and trust that that midwife is going to do it properly or how she would.

Feeling connected

So maybe for sustainability, every single one has to feel a sense of connection to the group and possibly to each other. There can be a lot of cultural issues there. One or two midwives in the past have said to me: 'I just didn't click. There were five of them that had their own way of being in the world and practising and it wasn't my cup of tea. I couldn't connect.'

Getting outside support

There are times when there needs to be some opportunity for outside supervision because you may not be able to talk about everything within your group and you may need to go outside to have an opportunity to reflect or you may need to bring someone in as a facilitator if you are having difficulties.

Collaborative relationships with medical colleagues

Effective collaboration is the cornerstone of providing safe midwifery care for women and their families who need to access medical care or advice (Brodie *et al.* 2008). The concepts of 'autonomous midwifery' and 'collaboration' can often be contentious where midwives are employed in public health systems that thrive on hierarchical control and a focus on 'risk management' strategies.

Collaboration is not a straightforward process of sharing; it requires those in powerful positions to relinquish power to those who have traditionally not been able to access it. This can only happen where there are sophisticated understandings of identity, power relationships and the importance of inter-professional learning (Brodie *et al.* 2008; Brodie and Leap 2008; Ford and Iliffe 1996; Freeth and Reeves 2004; Sandall *et al.* 2001):

> Midwives have to have that ongoing finger on the pulse. It is about maintaining an integrity of practice in terms of autonomy and collabora-tion. You have to work out acceptable ways of staying connected with the system if you are going to take women into it and particularly if you are going to be employed in it.

Harnessing strong medical support

In reflecting on our experiences of introducing midwifery models of care, we acknowledged that there had always been at least one obstetrician who understood the importance of midwifery continuity of care and was prepared to confront colleagues who were less amenable to developments:

> What we had in the early days was a senior medico in a strategic leadership position who was a shield. He basically kept the wild horses back and said to the doctors who were opposed, 'No, this is important for our service and it's going to happen.'

Relationships with managers

Strong managers or midwifery leaders can also play an important role in over-coming hurdles in the development of midwifery group practices. From the early days in the life of a group practice, a two-way relationship of trust can mean managers stepping back and letting the group sort out challenging dynamics as they arise:

> I think managers have to learn to give the group as much power as possible so that the midwives address things like, for example, somebody who is creating dependencies and isn't sharing their women because they think they're the only person that can care for that woman.

Enabling midwives in group practices to determine the nature of how they plan their service can be a challenge for managers, particularly as it can take some time for midwives who are new to caseload practice to find ways of working that suit them:

> In my experience in many different settings, it can take at least a year of trying different on-call arrangements, of settling in, before a group says,

'This is how it's actually going to work for us.' The joy of group practice is that it does allow for that maximum flexibility and ultimately that makes for better relationships all round.

The thing we've got to bite our tongue over is realising that these midwives have never had the opportunity to be autonomous and to be self-managing so of course they're going to make mistakes and fall over. We have to sort of go with it and offer support while they learn how to manage their practices and relationships.

Another challenge for managers in the public health system is designing recruitment systems that enable midwives in group practices to have some choice about who they work with. In our experience, this can be done without compromising equal opportunity recruitment principles, for example, through processes that include group interviews where potential candidates and existing group practice midwives engage in reflection and case review.

I do think there is something about midwives in group practices having some choice over who they work with that helps to develop the trust that midwives need to work closely in a relationship with the midwives in their group practice. Where they have some say in who they work with, then practices are set up to be more sustainable than if people get thrown together and don't necessarily like each other.

It's a different kind of leadership

While managers and midwifery leaders can play an important role in developing midwifery group practices within maternity services, their role in the long term is a source of debate:

I don't think every group practice needs a team leader or a manager. In terms of big systems, the system has to be strong enough and robust enough that the midwives know where they can go to get support.

I still think there is a need for very thoughtful and somewhat self-reflective leadership and a leadership style that ensures not necessarily a direct line management but a facilitation of the midwives' professional development, interpersonal confidence and skills, assistance with debriefing or reflection.

Relationships with students and new graduates

Nurturing students and new graduates within midwifery group practices is a key element of sustainability.

If you think about it from a sustainability perspective, from an environmental standpoint, you have to begin with the young. The young are the
future. If we care about our future, we care about our young. That first
year out is critical and the last thing we should be saying is, 'You can't
go out there and do continuity of care until you've been on labour ward
for at least a year or two.'

Having students with you should be core business

It should be absolutely automatic that every midwife working in a
continuity of care model sees it as part of their job to nurture students
and take them along with them. It shouldn't be seen as a choice to have
a student – its critical to the future sustainability of group practices that
they experience it first hand.

Features of midwifery group practices that enhance sustainability

Attention to a number of practical considerations enhance the development
of sustainable group practices in the public health system (Homer *et al.* 2008a),
beginning with the conditions under which midwives are employed:

Salary and employment

The annualised salary is absolutely pivotal. Everything else takes its
lead from that because once midwives are no longer being paid to do
'shifts' it gives them permission to begin to think about managing care,
managing their time, managing everything around work.

Premises: having a 'home'

Midwives in a group practice need a place that they can call 'home',
somewhere they can decorate and furnish that enhances their sense of
identity: 'This is who we are, this is where we come together – with
women and with each other; this is where we run groups and invite people
to meetings.'

As set out in the groundbreaking 'Vision' crafted by the Association of
Radical Midwives (ARM, 1986) midwives should ideally have premises in
the community in order to increase accessibility for women and foster
community development initiatives (Leap 2010). In our discussion we shared
experiences of organizing 'homes' for midwifery group practices in a range of
settings including: cottages, child health centres, youth and community work
projects, women's health centres, shopping centres, GPs' surgeries, playgroups
and leisure centres:

Flexibility in working arrangements

> Midwives need the potential to weave in and out . . . For some, there is a period of going back to being a core midwife for a while if they find themselves in a situation where they are struggling with a baby or they have a relationship breakdown and they have no childcare.

It is not inevitable, though, that midwives have to stop working in a group practice in such circumstances. The degree of occupational autonomy of midwives in group practices can determine how possible it is for them to support and accommodate the individual circumstances of their colleagues:

> In a group practice I worked in, at different times we had huge support-ive arrangements for midwives who had small children, unsupportive partners, bereavement or difficult personal circumstances. We looked after each other and it was 'swings and roundabouts'. As your kids grew up you put in more effort for those with small children in the way that others did previously for you. Sometimes, it might be that for a while you are not on call for births because of your circumstances but the group needs to be able to negotiate that and work out how to cover your work.

Sustainable change in maternity services

Changes to maternity services that enable sustainable midwifery continuity of care tend to occur when a series of factors and people coincide in one place with a willingness to work together to make change happen. This usually means strong midwifery and medical leadership and the involvement of more than a few token childbirth activists – *the right people in the right place at the right time*. The concern in such situations is the almost haphazard way in which those changes can fall apart when certain personnel leave a project:

> What needs to be in place is more than just those dynamic people. We need to put down foundations so that when those people are not there, it continues uninterrupted.

New ways of working and old ways of functioning

While we talk about developing 'woman-centred' care, most maternity services are 'system centred', which presents real challenges:

> We have our old way of functioning and we're trying to fit into it a new way of working and being. So we constantly stop ourselves developing what we know is ideal because we're trying to shove it into this old way of functioning.

We have the system on our shoulder with everything we do and it dominates. The more we can disconnect from the lumbering machine and get midwives to find their power, their autonomy, their pride and their resourcefulness – the more we build up enormous strength.

Making midwifery continuity of care the mainstream option

In a health system like Australia's, midwifery leaders constantly have to argue that midwifery continuity of care should be built into mainstream maternity service provision because it is cost effective, enables midwives to practise according to their full role and scope of practice and can improve outcomes for women, including when they have complicated pregnancies (Cornwell *et al.* 2008):

> It's not advanced practice and it shouldn't be attracting huge amounts of extra money – that's a nursing model where you've got some sort of ladder and you get paid more for taking on more responsibility. Midwifery isn't like that. When we're working to the full scope of practice that is midwifery and that is what we need to have funded flexibly and well.

> We still consider caseload practice this boutique little thing. So until it becomes the major way that maternity care is provided, it is always going to suffer these issues of being vulnerable but also being seen as somehow elite and different.

Concluding with the big question

We conclude this chapter by posing the question that we kept returning to in our discussion: is it possible to develop and sustain midwifery continuity of care – including the option of home birth – as the norm in publicly-funded maternity care systems where midwives are employed:

> Wherever you have strong sustainable midwifery group practices like in New Zealand, Holland and Canada, their systems have developed so that midwives can be self-employed, self-managing, running their own businesses, contracting in, linked completely to the system. So in a way maybe all the things we've talked about today, all the barriers and difficulties, a lot of them go back to having employment situations where midwives are part of a hierarchical structure where they can't be fully autonomous because there's all these things getting in the way.

This question will no doubt continue to be debated hotly. We are, however, clear that whatever the context, midwifery continuity of care enhances the potential for positive relationships and that sustainability depends on partnerships with women and their communities through ongoing cycles of planning, implementation and evaluation.

We should keep remembering that the community believes in midwifery continuity of care and that becomes the power base for all our efforts to improve services.

The vignette provided for us by Juliet Thorpe is a fitting conclusion to this chapter.[1]

Sustainability in a home birth midwifery practice in New Zealand

In 1993 I joined a midwifery practice providing a fully government-funded home birth service to the women in our city. This involved providing all maternity care to women throughout the antenatal, labour and post-natal period. Approximately 100 women per year use the practice and 91 per cent will have a normal physiological birth with the remaining 9 per cent requiring secondary care at Christchurch Women's Hospital (Anderson 2006). Seventeen years later I am still energized and passionate about midwifery and assisting women and their families to birth at home.

In 2005 I completed my Master's degree in Midwifery where I investigated how our particular group of midwives had maintained a sustainable model of care (Thorpe 2005). What was it about our way of working that had enabled us to work closely together in such a challenging profession for over 12 years without any signs of burnout or disharmony? After analysing the interviews I conducted with my colleagues I came up with three clear themes and I believe these themes, and the attached quotes, accurately describe our particular way of working:

- We work with people we like and who share the same philosophical beliefs about birth. We will be there for each other and will come when called, no matter when, no matter what. This directly impacts on the experiences of our clients. Whatever birth plan we create with our clients they know it will be respected no matter who comes to them in labour. Taking time off is much easier to do when you know your clients will receive the same care you would provide.

Jacqui: 'It's that generosity of spirit thing. It is about being generous to each other. If you're not doing that then how can you be generous to your clients? If we are not actually mirroring or using as an example our own relationships then how can we talk about building healthy alliances with our clients? How do you listen to them and value their point of view and respect what's important to them if you can't do that for yourself and each other':

- Talk, talk, talk. Obvious but true. Daily phone contact with colleagues means that we rarely feel isolated when working alone in the community. A day does not go by when we have not made contact with at least one member of the group for advice, support or just to maintain that connection. We meet weekly and make that meeting a ritual. Our practice meetings provide a regular venue for support both professionally and emotionally. The putting aside of four hours a week to devote to talk may seem to some as indulgent and even excessive but illustrates the most beneficial tool used by the practice in ensuring its sustainability. There would be few work settings that allow for this open communication, which has no limits or boundaries. Everyone talks until they have finished and everyone listens. There is always feedback, both positive and negative, and a pledge to finding compromise and solutions to any disagreements or problems.

Julie: 'I think for me it's that I can offload. I am with these people who I can trust who will hear me until I have finished speaking and that if it is important for me to bring here they will listen. It's being able to chew the fat really, I trust the reflections that come back and the opinions':

• Longevity creates a collective identity. Over time our group has become known as 'THE home birth midwives'. Along with this identity comes pride in each other's work and a sense of ownership. We are acknowledged by our peers and the obstetric community as having a specific way of working that involves strong advocacy for our clients in the hospital setting. We always have two midwives at a birth no matter where it takes place. Strength in numbers means that we support each other and our clients when birth plans change or when there are challenges to our philosophical beliefs. We place a lot of emphasis on looking after each other, thereby ensuring that we have the energy to honour the woman's birth plan.

Michelle: 'It's the core of what we do. When you end up going into the hospital, you have often done a long haul, you're energy is down and your energy for the woman is down as well and you know that that second midwife is going to come in and 'midwife' me as well as midwife the whole situation. I just love that, it is such a relief':

Home birth in New Zealand is still considered a radical birthing choice and it appears that women are, at times, actively discouraged from home birth by both medical practitioners and other midwives. As a home birth practice we have needed to constantly justify our existence and be clear about our purpose and philosophy. A commitment to meeting, talking and sharing is vital to the sustainability of the group and its identity. We consciously work at it on a day-to-day basis and unanimously agree that this midwifery work feeds our souls.

Note

1 It is noteworthy that we highlighted very similar issues before we had the opportunity to read each other's contributions.

References

Anderson, J. (2006) 'Outcomes for women who planned to birth with an established home birth practice in New Zealand', unpublished Master's degree thesis. Otago Polytechnic, New Zealand.

ARM (1986) *The Vision: Proposals for the Future of the Maternity Services.* Ormskirk, Lancashire: Association of Radical Midwives (ARM).

Brodie, P., Davis, G. and Homer, C. (2008) 'Effective collaboration with medical colleagues – making it happen', in C. Homer, P. Brodie and N. Leap (eds), *Midwifery Continuity of Care: A Practical Guide.* Sydney: Churchill Livingstone/ Elsevier.

Brodie, P. and Leap, N. (2008) 'From ideal to real: the interface between birth territory and the maternity service organisation', in K. Fahy, M. Foureur and C. Hastie (eds), *Birth Territory and Midwifery Guardianship: Theory for Practice, Education and Research.* Edinburgh: Butterworth Heinemann/Elsevier.

Carolan, M. and Hodnett, E. D. (2007) '"With woman" philosophy: examining the evidence, answering the questions', *Nursing Inquiry*, 14, 2: 140–52.

Cornwell, C., Donnellan-Fernandez, R. and Nixon, A. (2008) 'Planning and implementing mainstream midwifery group practices in a tertiary setting', in C. Homer, P. Brodie and N. Leap (eds), *Midwifery Continuity of Care: A Practical Guide.* Sydney: Churchill Livingstone/Elsevier.

Downe, S. and McCourt, C. (2008) 'From being to becoming: reconstructing childbirth knowledges', in S. Downe (ed.) *Normal Childbirth: Evidence and Debate.* 2nd Edition. Edinburgh: Churchill Livingstone/Elsevier.

Ford, C. and Iliffe, S. (1996) 'An interprofessional approach to care: lessons from general practice', in D. Kroll (ed.), *Midwifery Care for the Future: Meeting the Challenge.* London: Bailliere-Tindall.

Freeth, D. and Reeves, S. (2004) 'Learning to work together: using the presage, process, product (3P) model to highlight decisions and possibilities', *Journal of Interprofessional Care*, 18, 1: 43–56.

Green, J. M., Curtis, P. A., Price, H. and Renfew, M. (1998) *Continuing to Care. The Organisation of Midwifery Services in the UK: A Structured Review of the Evidence.* Hale: Books for Midwives Press.

Hatem, M., Sandall, J., Devane, D., Soltani, H. and Gates, S. (2008) 'Midwife-led versus other models of care for childbearing women', Cochrane Database of Systematic Reviews, Issue 4. Online: Available at: http://mrw.interscience.wiley. com/cochrane/clsysrev/articles/CD004667/frame.html (accessed 22 March 2010).

Homer, C., Brodie, P. and Leap, N. (2008a) 'Getting started: what is midwifery continuity of care', in C. Homer, P. Brodie and N. Leap (eds), *Midwifery Continuity of Care: A Practical Guide.* Sydney: Churchill Livingstone/Elsevier.

Homer, C., Brodie, P. and Leap, N. (2008b) 'Building blocks for success', in C. Homer, P. Brodie and N. Leap (eds), *Midwifery Continuity of Care: A Practical Guide.* Sydney: Churchill Livingstone/Elsevier.

Hunter, B., Berg, M., Lundgren, I., Olafsdottir, O. A. and Kirkham, M. (2008) 'Relationships: the hidden threads in the tapestry of maternity care', *Midwifery*, 24: 132–37.

Leap, N. (2010) 'The less we do, the more we give', in M. Kirkham (ed.) *The Midwife–Mother Relationship*, 2nd Edition. Basingstoke: Macmillan Press.

Leap, N. and Edwards, N. (2006) 'The politics of involving women in decision making', in L. A. Page and R. Campbell (eds), *The New Midwifery: Science and Sensitivity in Practice*, 2nd Edition. London: Churchill Livingstone/Elsevier.

Leap, N. and Pairman, S. (2010) 'Working in partnership', in S. Pairman, J. Pincombe, C. Thorogood and S. Tracy (eds), *Midwifery: Preparation for Practice*, 2nd Edition. Sydney: Elsevier.

McCourt, C. and Stevens, T. (2005) 'Continuity of carer: what does it mean and does it matter to midwives and birthing women?' *Canadian Journal of Midwifery Research and Practice*, 4, 3: 10–20.

McCourt, C. and Stevens, T. (2009) 'Relationship and reciprocity in caseload midwifery', in B. Hunter and R. Deery (eds), *Emotions in Midwifery and Reproduction*. London: Palgrave Macmillan.

Page, L. A., Cooke, P. and Percival, P. (2006) 'Providing one-to-one care and enjoying it', in L. A. Page and R. Campbell (eds) *The New Midwifery: Science and Sensitivity in Practice*, 2nd Edition. Edinburgh: Churchill Livingstone.

Sandall, J. (1997) 'Midwives' burnout and continuity of care', *British Journal of Midwifery*, 5, 2: 106–11.

Sandall, J., Bourgeault, I. and Meijer, W. (2001) 'Interprofessional rivalries among maternal-health professions: contemporary perspectives', in R. De Vries, C. Benoit, E. van Teijlingen and S. Wrede (eds), *Birth by Design: Pregnancy, Maternity Care. and Midwifery in North America and Europe*. London: Routledge.

Sandall, J., Page, L.A., Homer, C. S. E. and Leap, N. (2008) 'Midwifery continuity of care: what is the evidence?' in C. Homer, P. Brodie and N. Leap (eds), *Midwifery Continuity of Care: A Practical Guide*. Sydney: Churchill Livingstone/Elsevier.

Saultz, J. (2003) 'Defining and measuring interpersonal continuity of care', *Annals of Family Medicine*, 1, 3: 134–43.

Thorpe, J. (2005) 'A feminist case study of the collegial relationships within a home birth midwifery practice in New Zealand', unpublished Master's degree thesis. Otago Polytechnic, New Zealand.

6 Promoting a sustainable midwifery workforce

Working towards 'ecologies of practice'

Ruth Deery

> ... the nature of the current 'economy of performance' and its corrosive relation with ecologies of practice offer to professionals such an impoverished intellectual and practical diet that professional lives cannot be sustained.
>
> (Stronach *et al.* 2002: 131)

Almost every research project I have undertaken, or been part of, in recent times has produced data from midwives that highlight their dissatisfaction with a work culture of cutting costs, maximizing outputs and meeting targets, and where there is no time to step back and reflect on practice (Deery 2008). Midwives, recently qualified and experienced, have also expressed dissatisfaction with working conditions (Ball *et al.* 2002; Deery and Fisher 2010), clinical support (Kirkham and Stapleton 2000; Deery 2005) and lack of resources (Deery 2009). Some of my recent clinical shifts have been spent with community midwives who said that they did not know how much longer they could keep going. Indeed, one of the midwives told me how she began to get palpitations when she was driving to work. As soon as the Health Centre became visible her anxiety levels rose and she began thinking 'I've so much to do – I don't know how I'll get through the day'. As she was telling me this she was clutching her chest clearly despairing 'of ever catching up or otherwise getting out from under the pressing burden of work' (Lipsky 1980: 37).

My starting point in this chapter is that midwives' sense of well-being is essential for the development of an emotionally,[1] intellectually and economically sustaining work environment. However midwives' sense of well-being is threatened by constant reorganizations in the National Health Service (NHS) in England, where labour and birth are increasingly centralized into larger units and maternity services are often experienced as a production line, run according to an industrial model. Within this model midwives have become interchangeable, harassed workers with 'disparate allegiances' (Stronach *et al.* 2002: 109) who must prioritise keeping the system running (Deery and Kirkham 2006), often with impoverished support and few resources. Like the midwife's situation described above, stress in the workplace and the absence of a safe, supportive environment means that satisfying and meaningful work become difficult to achieve (Deery and Fisher 2010), thus making it almost impossible to contribute to the development of a sustainable workforce.

According to Meadows *et al*. (1992: 209–10) a sustainable society is

> one that can persist over generations, one that is far-seeing enough, flexible enough, and wise enough not to undermine either its physical or its social systems of support . . . would be interested in qualitative development, not physical expansion . . . would use material growth as a considered tool, not as a perpetual mandate . . . would apply its values and its best knowledge . . . choose only those kinds of growth that would actually serve social goals and enhance sustainability.

It would seem sensible then to suggest that a sustainable NHS work environment would meet the needs of the present maternity workforce, at the same time not compromising the ability of our 'up and coming' midwives to meet their own needs. The emergence of small-scale birth centres and midwife-led units has highlighted the effectiveness of increased continuity of care and support for women and midwives (see, for example, McCourt and Stevens 2009; Homer *et al*. 2008). Even though some of these units and schemes were established in the NHS further thought was given by the instigators to the necessity of reciprocity within working relationships.

Reciprocity is an important aspect of the midwife–mother relationship (Hunter 2005; Deery and Kirkham 2006). In several studies where midwives have reported that their relationships with women have been beneficial, rather than a one-way process, a sense of mutual trust has developed (Stevens 2003; Hunter 2005; Deery and Fisher 2010). When relationships are reciprocal midwives feel valued and able to be the midwives they want to be (Curtis *et al*. 2006). Women are also more likely to experience a relationship with a midwife where they feel confident, supported and fully informed (McCourt and Stevens 2009).

McCourt and Stevens (2009) found that peer support within a one-to-one midwifery scheme resulted in reducing stress and burnout. In such schemes midwives are able to choose their work partners and, more importantly, they were able to establish their own group practices. This probably resulted in teams of midwives working together that held similar philosophies of midwifery and views concerning work–life balance (Deery and Kirkham 2006). In a work environment where midwives are supported feelings of safety, trust and reciprocity are likely to become evident. Crucially, support systems and 'best knowledge' are unlikely to develop in environments where midwives work as front-line bureaucrats meeting the needs of the system (Lipsky 1980). When clinical work is overly determined by bureaucratic practices, holistic and authentic forms of care can become stifled, which means that they meet neither the needs of midwives or women. However we are now seeing a number of sustainable work environments being created, like those described above, within public maternity services in a number of countries.

The first part of this chapter introduces a conceptual framework used to draw attention to the 'complicated nexus between policy, ideology and practice' (Stronach *et al.* 2002: 109) that now challenges midwives and managers working in the NHS. The second part of the chapter reports some of the findings from a multi-centered, comparative ethnography[2] undertaken in the north of England. Finally, some suggestions are made to help midwives and managers work towards a more sustainable work environment as they struggle with the realities of clinical practice.

The conceptual framework

I have located my interpretation of some of the findings of the research within Stronach *et al.*'s (2002) conceptualization of professional identity where 'economies of performance' are shaped by bureaucratic structures and imperatives and where potentially, 'practice is poor, too urgent to be planned optimally or too poorly resourced to be effective' (p.131). On the other hand, 'ecologies of practice' develop when midwives draw on a wealth of diverse knowledge, experience and influences that may also include relational and experiential knowledge developed in the private sphere. From an educational perspective, Stronach *et al.* (2002:122) define 'ecologies of practice' as:

> The accumulation of individual and collective . . . experience . . . through which people laid claim to being 'professional' – personal experience in the classroom/clinic/ward, commonly held staff beliefs and institutional policies based on these, commitments to 'child-centred' or 'care-centred' ideologies, convictions about what constituted 'good practice' and so on.

Therefore, I am suggesting that the development of 'ecologies of practice' in midwifery promote the potentially rewarding aspects of commitment to, and sometimes beyond, organizational requirements (for example, caseload midwifery and birth centres), while 'economies of performance' depend on midwives becoming obedient technicians in order to achieve institutionally defined aims and goals. It is not my intention to suggest that midwives work in one clearly defined area or the other. Indeed, and as will be seen later in this chapter, it is interesting to note how some midwives are able to work within an 'economy of performance' and still achieve some degree of job satisfaction. However, some of the data reported suggest that the fulfilling aspects of working within an 'ecology of practice' are succumbing to an increasingly 'risk-focused rhetoric' (Brown and Calnan 2010: 2) approach towards clinical practice; a development that has negative repercussions on the quality of midwifery services, while also contributing to emotional exhaustion and 'burnout' among midwives themselves (see Deery and Fisher 2010 for emotion work and midwifery working practices that are embedded in 'economies of performance' and 'ecologies of practice' respectively. See also Hunter and Deery 2009).

I intend to explore how some midwives can work within the space of creative tension between 'ecologies of practice' and 'economies of performance' that I identified above. For others (including managers), the requirement to meet organizational targets and the pressures of productivity can prevent attempts to develop practice more creatively. Midwives cannot thrive in a system that undercuts 'ecologies of practice' and works against its own intended ethos. However, satisfying and meaningful work where midwives experience clinical practice as nurturing their own growth, facilitating them to 'be midwives to the activities and development of others' (Orbach 2008: 15) can be sustained. Such an approach also promotes 'the best of human nature rather than the worst to be expressed and nurtured' (Meadows *et al*. 1992: 233).

About the study

A comparative ethnographic approach was taken to the study that used the subjective experiences of the researcher and the participants. The intention was to pursue the potential for understanding and challenging the complexity of cultures while attempting to interpret internal and external conditions that affect everyday situations (Carspecken 1996) in clinical practice. Previous research experience has shown that this approach can help to understand the cultural phenomena within a maternity setting and where power, hegemony and institutional working play such an important role (Hughes *et al*. 2002). The social and cultural context of midwifery at the time the study was undertaken subscribed to the values associated with a woman-centered approach. However, these values were often not met in clinical practice because organizational values (for example, meeting performance indicators) were given precedence.

This chapter reports some of the findings from the three maternity units (Sites A, B and C) studied. All were at different stages of developing 'alongside' midwife-led care. During the course of the study radical reconfiguration took place on two of the sites. Site A and C merged leaving a birth centre that was managed by midwives only at Site C and all 'high risk' obstetric care at Site A. The well-established midwife-led unit on Site A was relocated away from the obstetric unit, but still in close proximity, and renamed a birth centre. One of the aims of the research was to identify what cultural and organizational changes would enable NHS maternity care to deliver more effective and efficacious care. Data collection methods comprised focus groups and individual interviews with midwives, midwifery managers, obstetricians and women service users. At the start of the study, non-participant observation was carried out in the midwife-led and obstetric units. Informal shadowing of senior obstetricians also took place.

Some of the findings from preliminary interviews and focus groups with midwives and managers are presented here. Data from the midwifery managers presented an interesting dimension of 'in-between-ness' (Stronach *et al*. 2002: 113) in terms of them feeling like 'piggy in the middle'. The interviews and focus groups were categorized using thematic analysis (Boyatzis 1998); emergent themes were identified and catalogued. As analysis progressed the data were scrutinized for consistency and patterns, and themes were accordingly reassessed and, in some cases, modified. Pseudonyms have been used to protect the identities of all the participants.

Some of the findings

Sarah was an experienced midwife who had worked in a variety of settings. She had found working on the post-natal wards in the hospital too much like an assembly line and had opted to work as a community midwife. She provided a frustrated example of the stressful effects of being on the receiving end of decisions made within an 'economies of performance' model, where she had observed some midwives and managers preferring to conform to the 'dimensions of the work more subject to administrative manipulation' (Lipsky 1980: 188): 'They just get tossed out there and nobody gives a damn, "let's just get them through, get them home and discharge them as quick as possible and so be it".'

When the system takes precedence 'economies of performance' become the preferred way of working, limiting and fragmenting the development of working practices, especially relationship building (Deery and Kirkham 2006). As Sennett (1998: 44) points out, 'what the routine worker lacks is any larger vision of a different future, or knowledge about how to make change'. Sita was an experienced midwife who had worked in all areas in the maternity unit. Her words suggest that she was constantly endeavouring to meet constant demands that were made worse by managers wanting to meet targets:

> There's so much change going on at the moment, in terms of shipping women out quicker and management are on your back to get rid of patients quicker and you just feel constantly harassed that you can't do your job properly, it's awful, it's depressing.
>
> (Deery 2009)

Sandra was an experienced midwife and manager who worked across two sites. Her words reinforce Sita's above, highlighting the tensions that become apparent when 'economies of performance' are collectively experienced as dominating professional practice:

> There's a lot of target driven stuff, they're [senior management] more focused than they ever were, it's not like 18 week waiting lists, it's a different kind of target, risk management, complaints, incident forms and it's all got to be turned round in a certain time.
>
> (Deery 2009)

Therefore, more recognition needs to be given to the fact that people enter midwifery because it offers the opportunity to develop rewarding, sustaining relationships with women within an 'ecology of practice' and where different ways of working can be explored. Julie, a recently appointed midwifery manager, worked on one of the sites where an 'alongside' midwife-led unit operated. She stated that 'midwives should be able to provide one-to-one care for women and provide real support, not in and out, fleeting here, there and everywhere.' Julie's words acknowledged that midwives get caught between 'economies of performance' (e.g. audit, meeting targets) and 'ecologies of practice' (e.g. continuity of care, relationship building). Likewise, as Sandra a more experienced manager stated: 'I feel like the jam in the sandwich, one layer of bread is the staff and the other layer is management and I'm stuck in the middle . . . it's frustrating and for me it's a balancing act, I tend to just absorb it.' Sandra's words appear to suggest that an ability to demonstrate versatility is necessary for a midwifery manager. However such versatility, experienced negatively within an 'economy of performance', is physically, psychologically and professionally detrimental to the well-being of midwives and managers (see Deery and Kirkham 2007) and not compatible with the promotion of long-term sustainability.

Christine had extensive experience of working with disadvantaged and vulnerable women. She thrived on working holistically with women and had been making positive impact with women. Her words below strongly suggest that organizational constraints are inhibiting the development of 'ecologies of practice' in a way that is detrimental to the quality of service provided, while also undermining midwives' engagement with women:

> I was speaking to a community midwife the other day and in the past two weeks she's noticed a big increase in the amount of women that are coming home . . . who haven't established breastfeeding, who are needing extra support and visits which, you know, they just can't provide.
>
> (Deery 2009)

Competing demands on, and of, midwives places them under enormous pressure to control their work situations, where 'ecologies of practice' become inhibited, disabling midwives from working in a way that may be satisfying and rewarding and ultimately contributing to organizational effectiveness. Various (usually unhelpful) coping mechanisms also come into play when midwives and managers have to control their work situations (see Deery and Kirkham 2007).

Diane, with over 30 years' experience as a midwife, suggested that working in an 'alongside' midwife-led unit supported more holistic practice. Despite the fact that Diane was often busy she believed that 'you can still make that effort':

> Even if it's busy you can smile at a woman, you can be nice to her, you can touch her, you can talk to her partner, you can make a bond between yourselves . . . you make your own path and do the absolute utmost that you possibly can for them.
>
> (Deery 2009)

Diane was experienced enough to use the space of creative tension between 'economies of performance' and 'ecologies of practice' to engage with women; this seemed to enable her to achieve a greater sense of job satisfaction than some of her peers. The relational processes of recognition and affirmation that this involves are probably fundamental to human well-being (Fisher 2008), and therefore to empowering practice (Fisher and Owen 2008).

Diane was also keen to point out that:

> Midwifery is not just about babies plopping out, you've got to let the women know you care and that you are there for them . . . some midwives concentrate on the technical bit and not the emotional input that you've got to put in, whether it's easy or difficult.

> (Deery 2009)

The differing approaches to care above highlight workplace tensions and/or the differing strategies adopted by midwives in the face of organizational pressures. Although routinized work can result in a more task-orientated approach to midwifery it can also become a strategy for self-preservation, shielding midwives from some of the toxic effects of a performance culture (see Deery and Kirkham 2007). Therefore, a continued emphasis on the task-orientated 'economies of performance' may lead to a stifling of the potential intellectual challenges that can otherwise characterize the midwife–mother relationship (Kirkham 2000; Deery 2005; Deery and Fisher 2010).

The high value placed on technical competence and efficiency in the NHS leaves little space for the development of 'ecologies of practice' that go beyond managerially defined roles, enabling midwives to draw on a range of clinical and experiential knowledge that cannot be codified. As Sarah's words suggest:

> Midwives need to engage with midwifery in a way that is deeply personal to them, they've got to consciously think about this woman and her situation . . . enter into her world . . . recognize and deal with different situations, acknowledging stress. I think self-development things are essential . . . it's about an inner optimism . . . what is deeply satisfying is having your beliefs and ideals affirmed in some way.

> (Deery 2009)

Working within 'ecologies of practice' also supports the intellectual and creative dimensions of clinical practice, enabling midwives to engage with their role within the dynamics of the midwife–mother relationship in an innovative and problem-solving way (Kirkham 2000; Deery 2005; Deery and Fisher 2010). The midwives who were able to work in this way also appeared to find their relationships with women intellectually stimulating. However, such practices tend to remain unacknowledged and undervalued within the profession. Gerry, who encouraged women to manage their own births and avoid intervention where possible, stated: 'Midwives walk past me, they don't talk to me or I get snide comments, I've actually built up a thicker skin and I think to a certain extent you just have to.'

Gerry's words suggest that the midwives who walk past her prefer to control and manage the birth process, rejecting the opportunity to engage in, and learn, new skills. The consequence of this is that 'ecologies of practice' are not sufficiently role-modelled in a profession that continues to place emphasis on technical competence rather than encouraging the establishment of positive relationships with women and colleagues (Deery and Fisher 2010). One of the midwifery managers expressed a desire to be a more effective role model but found that 'the paperwork was phenomenal . . . I want to be on the shop floor motivating the midwives not always chasing my tail'.

Therefore if commitment is located within 'economies of performance', the work emphasis will be task-based and quantitative, whereas those operating within 'ecologies of practice' will interpret their success in qualitative terms. Diane aspired to work in a way that developed relationships with women but found that in a busy, stressful environment:

> You're not giving your best, you can't give your best. There's always somebody on your back saying, 'can't she [the woman] go home, can't she do this, can't she do that' so you're rushing to do everything all the time and you know the poor woman . . . where is she in all this.
>
> (Deery 2009)

Likewise, Sita found that there were 'good and bad days' but that she also had to

> . . . carry a lot. I think you carry a lot yourself and go home and sound off sometimes. Sometimes it's damned hard and you can go home really frustrated and feel that you've just got through by the skin of your teeth. You are repeatedly handing in incident forms and receiving feedback that we have to work within budgets.
>
> (Deery 2009)

Task-based approaches to care, embedded within 'economies of performance', became the favoured way of working for many of the midwives and managers as this enabled them to distance themselves from the highly demanding work involved in more holistic approaches with women. Such detachment limited and fragmented the development of relationships that become apparent in response to the intellectual and creative commitment that is associated with 'ecologies of practice'.

Fostering 'ecologies of practice' through 'qualitative development'

Referring back to the midwife in the introduction to this chapter – she is hardly likely to be able to sustain her current working pattern given her high anxiety levels within an 'economy of performance' that 'turns around too fast and too unexpectedly for people . . . to retrain, relocate, readjust' (Meadows *et al.* 1992: 211). A more sustainable midwifery environment would be interested in her 'qualitative development' (Meadows *et al.* 1992: 210). Examples of such development can be found in the midwifery literature.

Jones (2000) set up a model of structured reflection, facilitated by a supervisor of midwives, in a newly opened birth centre. The midwives found this experience empowering, providing opportunities to focus on 'casework moments' (Wilkins 1998: 189) and once issues around confidentiality and trust had been agreed the process was valued. Similarly, Derbyshire (2000) facilitated group clinical supervision in a neonatal unit in Exeter. These groups enabled the staff to 'reflect on their professional activity . . . problems in the work area are addressed and solutions found' (Derbyshire 2000: 172). Structured reflection and clinical supervision provide opportunities for midwives to work within an 'ecology of practice' where professional expertise, practice and commitment can be facilitated, developed and encouraged. Crucially, Jones and Derbyshire both worked in small, contained settings (a free-standing birth centre and a small neonatal unit) and where midwives worked to an appropriate, and probably similar, philosophy. As reconfiguration took place during the course of the study reported in this chapter, structured reflection became the 'norm' for the midwives within the newly created free-standing birth centre. Within a safe, trusting space 'ecologies of practice' were fostered and the birth centre is thriving to this day.

However, 'ecologies of practice' are unlikely to develop in large-scale maternity units where the culture can be target driven and overly determined by the rigid and codified practices associated with 'economies of performance'. Community midwives in a different area experienced clinical supervision as time consuming and they did not feel safe enough with each other 'to move from self-protection to self-analysis' (Deery and Kirkham 2007: 81). As a result they resisted the process of clinical supervision, claiming that organizational demands, a lack of support and demanding relationships with women and each other were detrimental to a sustaining work environment (Deery 2005).

Conclusion

The atypical nature of midwifery work means that a 24-hour maternity service almost always has to be offered and often within a resource-contained NHS. Combined with the ever-present threat of being exposed as a 'failing' organization, constant monitoring and a lack of resources can have a highly detrimental effect on staff morale and recruitment and retention (see Ball *et al.* 2002; Hughes *et al.* 2002; Deery 2005). Many health professionals and academics now argue that the proliferation of targets and monitoring systems has become counter-productive, and that many midwives feel increasingly submerged by an ever-present 'audit culture' that involves a plethora of ever-moving targets and performance indicators and a mountain of paperwork, impenetrable bureaucracy and obscure jargon that gets between them and the job (Bryson and Deery 2009). Such an organizational system trains staff to clinically manage and measure aspects of their work, but does not provide time and space to reflect upon and develop their practice (Deery 2005, 2008). Those midwives who found themselves able to work within the tension created when juggling 'economies of performance' and 'ecologies of practice' were usually more experienced, autonomous midwives who did not resent work-related issues encroaching into their home life occasionally (Deery 2008; McCourt and Stevens 2009).

The nature of maternity services and midwives' practice varies between different countries (Page 2008). Also, the problems that undermine 'ecologies of practice' are not exclusive to the NHS in the UK. They will indeed have resonance for many midwives worldwide. When 'economies of performance' are adhered to, the scope for creativity, innovation and commitment may be stifled or eroded. Midwives become deterred from drawing on a wide range of professional and experiential knowledge and the potential for excellent practice is undermined. Unfortunately, midwifery is predominantly based on the need to fulfil managerially defined tasks and where the art of midwifery is fast becoming secondary to performance monitoring and audit. Empowering, creative practice in midwifery depends on enthusiasm and the development of positive working relationships with women and each other. If the potential for these are precluded, midwifery commitment is likely to disappear within an increasingly instrumentalized and non-sustainable working environment.

Notes

1   The benefits of an emotionally sustaining work environment have been discussed elsewhere and will not be addressed in this chapter. See Hunter and Deery (2009) and Deery and Fisher (2010).
2   I am especially grateful to the Health Foundation who funded the research and all who participated in the study. Some of the data presented in this chapter has been presented elsewhere. (See Deery and Fisher, 2010.)

References

Boyatzis, R. E. (1998) *Transforming Qualitative Information, Thematic Analysis and Code Development*. London: Sage Publications.
Bryson, V. and Deery, R. (2009) 'Public policy, "men's time" and power: the work of midwives in the British National Health Service', *Women's Studies International Forum*.
Brown, P. and Calnan, M. (2010) 'The risks of managing uncertainty: the limitations of governance and choice, and the potential for trust', *Social Policy and Society*, 9: 1.
Carspecken, P. F. (1996) *Critical Ethnography in Educational Research: A Theoretical and Practical Guide*. New York: Routledge.
Coffey, A. (1999) *The Ethnographic Self, Fieldwork and the Representation of Identity*. London: Sage Publications.
Curtis, P., Ball, L. and Kirkham, M. (2006) 'Why do midwives leave? (Not) being the midwife you want to be', *British Journal of Midwifery*, 14, 1: 27–31.
Deery, R. (2005) 'An action research study exploring midwives' support needs and the affect of group clinical supervision', *Midwifery*, 21, 2: 161–76.

Deery, R. (2008) 'The tyranny of time: tensions between relational and clock time in community based midwifery', *Social Theory and Health*, 6, 4: 342–63.

Deery, R. (2009) 'A comparative ethnography of obstetric culture and midwife-led care', unpublished research report, University of Huddersfield.

Deery, R. and Fisher, P. (2010) 'Switching and swapping faces: performativity and emotion in midwifery', *International Journal of Work Organization and Emotion*, 3, 3: 270–86.

Deery, R. and Kirkham, M. (2006) 'Supporting midwives to support women', in L. Page and R. McCandlish (eds), *The New Midwifery: Science and Sensitivity in Practice*. 2nd Edition. London: Elsevier.

Deery, R. and Kirkham, M. (2007) 'Drained and dumped on: the generation and accumulation of emotional toxic waste in community midwifery', in M. Kirkham (ed.), *Exploring the Dirty Side of Women's Health*. London: Routledge.

Derbyshire, F. (2000) 'Clinical supervision within midwifery', in M. Kirkham (ed.), *Developments in the Supervision of Midwives*. Manchester: Books for Midwives Press.

Fisher, P. (2008) 'Wellbeing and empowerment: the importance of recognition', *Sociology of Health & Illness*, 30, 4: 583–98.

Fisher, P. and Owen J. (2008) 'Empowering interventions in health and social care: recognition through 'ecologies of practice', *Social Science and Medicine*, 67: 2063–71.

Homer, C., Brodie, P. and Leap, N. (2008) *Midwifery Continuity of Care: A Practical Guide*. Sydney: Churchill Livingstone/Elsevier.

Hughes, D., Deery, R. and Lovatt, A. (2002) 'A critical ethnographic approach to facilitating cultural shift in midwifery', *Midwifery*, 18: 43–52.

Hunter, B. (2006) 'The importance of reciprocity in relationships between community-based midwives', *Midwifery*, 22: 308–22.

Hunter, B. and Deery, R. (eds) (2009) *Emotions in Midwifery and Reproduction*. London: Palgrave Macmillan.

Jones, O. (2000) 'Supervision in a midwife managed birth centre', in M. Kirkham (ed.), *Developments in the Supervision of Midwives*. Manchester: Books for Midwives Press.

Kirkham, M. (ed.) (2000) *The Midwife–Mother Relationship*. London: Macmillan Press.

Kirkham, M. and Stapleton, H. (2000) 'Midwives' support needs as childbirth changes', *Journal of Advanced Nursing*, 32, 2: 465–72.

Lipsky M (1980) *Street-Level Bureaucracy. Dilemmas of the Individual in Public Services*. New York: Russell Sage Foundation.

McCourt, C. and Stevens, T. (2009) 'Relationship and reciprocity in caseload midwifery', in B. Hunter and R. Deery (eds), *Emotions in Midwifery and Reproduction*. London: Palgrave Macmillan.

Meadows, D. H., Meadows, D. L. and Randers, J. (1992) *Beyond the Limits, Confronting Global Collapse, Envisioning a Sustainable Future*. White River Junction, VT: Chelsea Green Publishing Company.

Orbach, S. (2008) 'Work is where we live: emotional literacy and the psychological dimensions of the various relationships there', *Emotion, Space and Society*, 1: 14–17.

Page, L. (2008) 'Being a midwife to midwifery: transforming midwifery services', in K. Fahy, M. Foureur and C. Hastie (eds), *Birth Territory and Midwifery Guardianship: Theory for Practice, Education and Research*. Sydney: Elsevier Books for Midwives, 115–29.

Sennett, R. (1998) *The Corrosion of Character, The Personal Consequences of Work in the New Capitalism*. London: W. W. Norton & Company.

Stevens, T. (2003) 'Midwife to midwife: a study of caseload midwifery', unpublished Ph.D. thesis, Thames Valley University.

Stronach, I., Corbin, B., McNamara, O., Stark, S. and Warne, T. (2002) 'Towards an uncertain politics of professionalism: teacher and nurse identities in flux', *Journal of Education Policy*, 17, 1: 109–38.

Wilkins, P. (1998) 'Clinical supervision and community psychiatric nursing', in T. Butterworth, J. Faugier and P. Burnard (eds), *Clinical Supervision and Mentorship in Nursing*, 2nd Edition. Cheltenham: Nelson Thornes.

7 Sustained by joy

The potential of flow experience for midwives and mothers

Mavis Kirkham

Introduction

When asked to write on midwifery and sustainability, I was struck by the fact that such a request could only be a very modern one. Until recently no one could see such a basic practice as midwifery as anything other than sustainable in itself and contributing fundamentally to sustaining society.

Birth is about relationships. It was, and in many contexts still is, something done by mothers who are supported by midwives and families. Changes over recent years have seen birth move from the home to the hospital and become surrounded by increasingly complex technology and organization. Birth is also the entry to society and how we manage that entry demonstrates our values as a society. We thus have tensions between supportive relationships around birth and our organizations that embody values of hierarchy, efficiency, technology and expert authority. These tensions can create frustration for midwives and mothers; but behind this shines the knowledge of what birth can be.

In this chapter I seek to convey the joyous engagement that birth can be for mothers and midwives and the circumstances that foster such experience, as well as the alienation often reported by both these groups in recent years. The concept of flow, in its several uses, seems an appropriate tool with which to do this.

Organizational flow

I have been worried by the use of the word 'flow' in maternity care for some years now. I was aware of this word being widely used by midwives when we were studying informed choice (Kirkham and Stapleton 2001). The majority of the midwives involved with that large study appeared to 'go with the flow' of obstetric and managerial opinion 'because it made life easier' (Stapleton *et al.* 2002: 607). Since then, the many moves to standardize services through guidelines, policies, procedures and pathways have made the organizational flow more powerful. We found that the pressure to go with the flow of the organization had a divisive effect on relationships, which could be reflected in horizontal violence towards those who did not conform. Midwives certainly ensured that the vast majority of women made what were seen locally as the 'right' choices. A minority of midwives did go against the flow and some excellent care was observed around the facilitation of informed choice. However, this was the work of individuals rather than the strategy in any unit, and these individuals were vulnerable with regard to both the institutional hierarchy and their conforming colleagues (Kirkham and Stapleton 2001).

Management terminology has changed in recent years and this, together with services being centralized, produced concepts such as 'managing patient flow'. Organizational innovations such as triage and its more recent refinements (Cherry *et al*. 2009) followed.

Once one is aware of 'flow' in this sense, it is all around, in the institutional weight carried by authoritative knowledge and the accepted rules of standardized practice, as well as the hospital-wide management concept of 'patient flow'. Controlling this flow enables organizations to run smoothly and is thus a positive outcome of the hierarchical organization of maternity care in and from hospitals. It requires staff and patients to be docile and to give up responsibility, which may be temporarily comforting. Going with the flow necessitates the development of a whole series of coping habits that may be useful in the short term but damaging in the longer run. Such organizational flow and midwives' policing of it may also have a strong undertow for mothers who do not wish to be docile.

For midwives and mothers, going with the organizational flow is a passive experience. It may save time and bring relief in not having to make decisions concerning individuals, but it limits relationships because it ignores individual concerns and it prevents the autonomous activity and skilled judgement that bring high job satisfaction (Marmot 2004).

Flow in positive psychology

The concept of flow is also applied to individuals, where it also implies a strong current, which carries one along, but with very different meaning for the individual. Here the individual is actively and completely engaged with the work in hand.

> ... people in flow exhibit a masterly control of what they are doing, their responses perfectly attuned to the changing demands of the task. And although people perform at their peak while in flow, they are unconcerned with how they are doing, with thoughts of success or failure – the sheer pleasure of the act itself is what motivates them.
>
> (Goleman 1995: 91)

Mihaly Csíkszentmihályi (2008) also identifies flow with concentration, clear and challenging but achievable goals, distorted sense of time, direct feedback on progress and sense of control in activity that is experienced as intrinsically rewarding (not all these attributes have to be present). Ken Robinson calls this state being in ones element or 'being in the zone' (Robinson 2009: 92). Such a state is often linked with demanding physical tasks such as rock climbing (Csíkszentmihályi 2008), or the work of master craftsmen (Sennet 2008). To me this state fits exactly with the descriptions of women who have experienced active and fully engaged labour and birth. It also fits my experience of clinical midwifery at its best, where the midwife enables the woman to feel safe enough to focus on her experience: those times when I know I don't want to do any other job, or to retire.

The positive psychology literature closely associates flow with happiness (Seligman 2002; Robinson 2009). It is also energizing. It 'doesn't take energy away from you; it gives it to you' (Robinson 2009: 93), which is the opposite of feeling 'drained and dumped on' (Deery and Kirkham 2007), as reported by many midwives in the English National Health Service (NHS). The energizing potential of the state of flow fits with my best experience as a midwife and as a mother.

Flow and relationship

Most descriptions of flow concern physical tasks. Such skilled craftsmanship 'tends to focus on relationships; it either deploys relational thinking about objects or . . . attends to cues from other people' (Sennett 2008: 51). Birth, for midwives and mothers, has another person at its centre. Birth is about a network of relationships: the relationship with the baby sustains the mother, even when adult relationships before the birth are experienced as unsupportive. The midwife–mother relationship can build confidence and facilitate the building of other relationships. The midwife can facilitate the pregnant women in building a support network that will sustain her later as a mother (Leap 2010). In labour, the midwife can help the mother to feel 'safe enough to let go' of her other commitments and worries and allow her body to be in control (Anderson 2010).

In the midwife–mother relationship at its best, the midwife is closely engaged with and attentive to the mother. Ideally, this relationship is developed over the course of the pregnancy, so that when the woman labours she and her midwife know each other well. Where such on-going relationships are possible, the midwife builds the relationship to develop mutual trust and respect. When the woman then labours, both can be totally concerned with the labour and the woman's coping with it, all the preliminary work has been done and the focus is entirely upon the tremendous task in hand.

Flow for the mother

Labour and birth can be the ultimate flow experience. I cannot envisage a society where this knowledge is completely lost by women, whatever the other pressures upon them.

Yet 'women birth as they live' (Hastie 2008: 83) and many women experience little autonomy and flow in their lives. This may be because of economic or social deprivation, or it may be because their experience is largely passive and/or stressful, and this experience deeply influences their expectations of birth.

Nevertheless there are groups of women who feel it is important to use their own power in giving birth. They often choose home birth and may be fortunate to be cared for by midwives who share their values. Independent midwives usually serve these women well, offering continuity of care and developing trusting relationships that respect and foster women's confidence in their ability to give birth. Some health services offer similar midwifery services and they are very precious and rare (Davis-Floyd *et al.* 2009).

There are also women who opt for 'freebirthing', choosing not to have professional attendance in their childbearing. This means that they are not constrained by obstetric orthodoxies and generalized policies – they are autonomous. The price of that autonomy is the absence of any medical care.

Sometimes flow is experienced within orthodox maternity services. It tends to manifest most often where trusting relationships between mothers and midwives can develop, which is more likely where services are on a smaller scale, as in birth centres (Kirkham 2003) or small case-holding practices (Davis-Floyd *et al.* 2009). Sometimes flow occurs, unplanned, in the labour wards of large hospitals, often at night, when services are less fragmented and medical and managerial services are less seen. Sometimes flow is seen in highly medicalized situations, where the woman is treated with respect and totally involved with events around the birth. This is difficult to achieve because of the many different relationships and technical issues involved, but for some obstetricians this achievement gives high job satisfaction and greatly improves their clients' experience.

Wherever flow occurs for childbearing mothers it is life enhancing. Mothers look back on this experience as evidence of their own strength at later points when they face challenges as mothers (Edwards 2005). This is important because 'Birth is not only about making babies. Birth is also about making mothers – strong, competent, capable mothers who trust themselves and know their inner strength' (Katz-Rothman 1996: 253).

It is interesting that the experience of labour has been compared with the flow of a strong current: 'If you resist, horror and impediment. If you swim, not pain but sensation!' (Bagnold 1938: 145.) To swim in such circumstances involves total concentration. Where the carer can act as swimming coach antenatally and lifeguard during labour, both parties can find birth to be a flow experience.

Flow for the midwife

Being skilfully engaged in helping women achieve a good birth is really sustaining for midwives. The relationships with women that make this possible are crucial to midwives' job satisfaction (Kirkham *et al.* 2006) and not being able to best use their skills is a key reason why midwives leave midwifery (Ball *et al.* 2002).

All around the world midwives tell stories of facilitating good birth even in difficult circumstances (see, for example, Olafsdottir and Kirkham 2009). Creating and maintaining space where women feel safe to give birth is a real flow activity (Kirkham 2010). The midwife is building trust: the mother's trust in the midwife and most importantly in her own ability to give birth. She usually does this by demonstrating her trust in the mother and her strengths. Thus reciprocal trust and self-confidence is crafted.

In order to achieve such a level of relational skill, the midwife needs the opportunity for on-going care and a degree of autonomy so that she can tailor her care to the individual woman. Where staff have more autonomy, they are more generous in their relationships and can facilitate autonomy in their clients. This has been found in medicine (Kaplan *et al.* 1996) and in midwifery (Hunter 2006; Hunter and Deery 2009). The organization that makes such professional autonomy and continuity of care possible usually means that the midwife is working in a contained setting with a small, known group of colleagues. This may be a small unit or birth centre or a small team within a larger organization (Homer *et al.* 2001 and 2008). Peer support can also then be developed (e.g. Jones 2000; McCourt and Stevens 2009). In such settings midwives relish the responsibility and take great pride in developing their skills (Hunter 2003); on-going skill development is fundamental to the continuing experience of flow at work (Csíkszentmihályi 2008). The mutual support and job satisfaction such midwives experience appears to protect them from high levels of occupational stress and burnout (Sandall 1997; McCourt and Stevens 2009).

Flow and management

It is clearly highly satisfying for midwifery managers to create and maintain a service where midwives and mothers can work together well (Leyshon 2004). Midwifery managers, however, find this very difficult to achieve. They often feel powerless, trapped between two very different value systems: that of midwifery and that of the larger organization (Curtis *et al.* 2003). The values of NHS management are concerned with efficiency, economic use of resources and the processing of women through the maternity care system. Operationalizing these values assumes a high degree of control over the individual's path through the service and the experience of clients and workers. Yet individual midwives and mothers may not feel they are best served by such control. There is thus a real tension between the crafting of systems and the crafting of care for individuals within those systems: 'One reason we may have trouble thinking about the value of craftsmanship is that the very word in fact embodies conflicting values, a conflict that in such institutional setting as medical care is, so far, raw and unresolved' (Sennett 2008: 51).

Organizational values do not include flow, which is concerned with individuals performing at their best. Organizations have more humble and short-term objectives; yet we know that pregnancy and birth have long-term impacts on the health of babies and mothers (Barker 1994; Edwards 2005), as well as the vocation of midwives.

Standardization, fears and dilemmas

In recent years, there have been striking moves to standardize and control clinical practice. This is seen in the rise of micro-management and the growth of rules, whether they are called policies, procedures, protocols or guidelines, which must be followed or careful attention be paid to justifying any other course of action (Griffiths 2009). Such a philosophy of managerial control is often seen as enhancing safety for childbearing women. Yet it invokes a very narrow definition of safety: a live mother and baby at the end of a defined clinical episode. Mothers define safety more widely, in terms of time and in terms of the emotional and physical well-being of their family (Edwards 2005). The English Department of Health has also used much wider definitions:

> Safety is not an absolute concept. It is part of a greater picture encompassing all aspects of health and wellbeing. Each woman should be approached as an individual, and given clear and unbiased information on the options that are available to her, and in this way helped to balance the risks and benefits for herself and her baby.
>
> (Department of Health 1993: 10)

Such a definition fits well with the great potential of childbirth to improve the health and well-being of families, not least by enhancing maternal confidence. Sadly, it is part of a statement of policy for maternity care that was not achieved, although it continues to influence policy rhetoric. The proliferation of rules remains the reality.

'The problem with following external rules is that one's energy must focus outwards on the rules and in doing this one loses sight of one's inner self which is the source of "inner power", wisdom and insight' (Fahy and Hastie 2008: 31). This power is the synthesis of personal values and clinical skills. Focussing outwards on the rules is particularly likely if those rules are changing and become ever more detailed, as many midwives now experience in the workplace. Such attention to rules is just the distraction from or interruption/fragmentation of the task in hand that stops the complete engagement that is flow. 'At both levels, the individual and the collective, what prevents flow from occurring is either the fragmentation of attentional processes . . . or their excessive rigidity' (Csíkszentmihályi 2008: 86). This approach explains why many women see their midwives as 'checking not listening' to them (Kirkham and Stapleton 2001; Edwards 2005), a sad but common indictment of our services.

As rules have proliferated, so have the opportunities to get things wrong and clinical practice has become increasingly fearful. Midwifery practice and education generate fears of doing the wrong thing, and more importantly, of not doing all the small required right things. Such constant anxiety as to the details of practice is destructive in two ways. First, it distracts from the individual woman and our relationship with her. Second, it inhibits the synthesis of clinical knowledge and the development of higher levels of skill: the 'fast and frugal' (Gigerenzer 1999) thinking of the skilled and experienced clinician who has developed manual and relationship skills through practice and engagement in flow. Fear can be useful as skilled awareness that things are not as they should be (Becker 1997). Constant worry as to whether we have done the ever-changing 'right' thing corrodes our ability to pick up small cues as to future problems: the well-honed skills in noticing slight differences, which are often described as intuition. Such worry therefore undermines clinical judgement:

> Flow is a state of self-forgetfulness, the opposite of rumination and worry: instead of being lost in nervous preoccupation, people in flow are so absorbed in the task at hand that they lose all self-consciousness, dropping the small preoccupations . . .
>
> (Goleman 1995: 91)

The proliferation of rules leaves midwives worrying and can have negative effects on mothers. 'If professionalism means "sticking to the rules" midwives are unable to engage with women's decisions that challenge those rules' (Edwards 2005: 183). Yet maternal choice has long been an article of health policy, or at least of its rhetoric (Department of Health 1993 and 2007). We also know that supportive, engaged, continuing relationships between mothers and midwives build reciprocal trust and contribute to good clinical outcomes (Davis-Floyd *et al.* 2009). It is also ironic that where relationships are good clients are highly unlikely to sue clinicians (Gladwell 2005: 40–41), yet fear of litigation is often quoted as the basis of the prevailing fears in maternity services (Kirkham and Stapleton 2001). There is a fundamental tension between standardized practice and individual autonomy (for clients or clinicians) that I have not seen acknowledged in health policy.

This is not to say that midwives do not need continuing education. We clearly do. We also need freedom to learn, from research and from our clients, and to reflect on that learning. Increasing managerial control does not contribute to learning. It creates an ever-growing list of things that midwives can be blamed for, which may be felt to protect the institution but not to enhance the practice of those midwives. It cannot make care sensitive to the needs of individuals, because the check-list of rules must inevitably be generalized to 'fit' all women.

Excellence in maternity care is possible; many women praise their midwives highly. 'Birth models that work' have been studied (Davis-Floyd *et al.* 2009) and we know that these include 'a woman-centred ideology internationally known as the midwifery model of care' (Davis-Floyd *et al.* 2009: 22) and continuing, flexible, mutually respectful relationships between childbearing women and their midwives. This study includes two English examples of such excellent care: the Albany Midwifery Practice that has recently had it's contract with Kings College Hospital terminated because 'we feel that we need to bring all our services in line with the same national clinical and safety guidelines and standards' (Reed 2010: 5) and a free-standing birth centre which, like all similar birth centres has been repeatedly threatened with closure (Walsh 2007).

Where services are centralized and standardized, as they are in England, and run according to market values that valorize cutting costs, staff use of time is more and more strictly controlled. In such circumstances management, far from striving for excellence, tends to fear it (Page 1997). We hear the tragic arguments for closing birth centres or case-holding practices on the grounds of 'equity', meaning the lowest common denominator of service provision. This approach has the sad result of lowering all our expectations of maternity services (Kirkham 2010). The pressures to go with the organizational flow can be overwhelming for midwives, divisive for colleagues and the subsequent routinized care is experienced by mothers as just checking (Edwards 2005) or uncaring (Halldorsdottir and Karlsdottir 1996). Relationships are not part of this model.

Flow and society

Where it is possible for midwives and mothers to engage with the process of birth so as to achieve the experience of flow, there are tremendous social implications. Midwives can support each other and develop 'creative teams' (Robinson 2009: 125) that value diversity and the continuing development of skills (Jones 2000; Hunter 2003). They have sufficient autonomy, role models and motivation to respect, nurture and 'tend and befriend' (Taylor 2002) clients and colleagues.

When we listen to women, rather that just checking their clinical condition, we engage with wider relationships (Kirkham 2010). Continuing reciprocal relationships nurture mother and midwife (McCourt and Stevens 2009). Support networks are established and extended and power moves from the professional towards the mother as she develops knowledge and confidence in her ability to birth and to mother her baby. The development of sustaining relationships around birth, rather than short-term coping strategies (Kirkham 2007), supports and models new dimensions of reciprocal support for mothers and midwives. It also offers ways of living our professional and family lives that are more sustainable because of the web of relationships that supports us.

Where maternity care is local, birth and its attendant networks are part of local life. Where maternity care is offered on a small enough scale to feel human and continuity of care is valued, it is possible to build trusting relationships. For midwives this gives us a secure group of colleagues small enough to know well and the autonomy that makes such a difference to occupational health (Marmot 2004). Mothers too can negotiate personally appropriate care from a known midwife and build a network of support for the future (Leap 2010). Thus anxiety is lessened, social capital is increased and clinical outcomes improved.

The circumstances conducive to flow experiences for mothers and midwives also enable us to learn and develop our skills:

> It is this dynamic feature that explains why flow activities lead to growth and discovery. One cannot enjoy doing the same thing at the same level for long . . . The desire to enjoy ourselves again pushes us to stretch our skills, or to discover new opportunities to use them.
>
> (Csíkszentmihályi 2008: 75)

In midwifery this push to increase skills and knowledge springs from relationships. Midwives are motivated to learn about the particular health conditions and needs of women who they will see again and again and women benefit from the feedback from their midwife's researches. This learning is tailored to need and is mutual. Equity as well as education is thus promoted; both are conducive to good health. Attention span can also be increased where listening is valued and relationships continue throughout a pregnancy; whereas the organizational fragmentation of the industrial model of care tends also to fragment our attention.

Thus the circumstances conducive to flow in midwifery tend to be those where a much broader view of health is taken than is usually measured in clinical outcomes. Such a view includes families' own priorities and the development of community networks and support. This is entirely appropriate for a service that can have such long-term impact upon the health of families. Such a social, rather than a narrowly medical, model of birth facilitates true community development.

The need for change in organizational values

While the circumstances conducive to flow experiences for mothers and midwives are also those linked with good health, the promotion of such experiences is not an aim of health service management. Health services run according to market values, such as the NHS, prioritize efficiency and economy above excellence for staff or clients.

There are other ways or organizing care. 'Birth models that work' can be found in many countries and their characteristics (Davis-Floyd *et al.* 2009: 22–23) are very similar to the circumstances conducive to flow experiences for midwives and mothers. Three main ingredients for positive outcomes are cited again and again in maternity care: 'a close personal and trusting relationship with a midwife in a one-to-one caseload model; a strong belief in childbirth as normal physiology; a familiar environment for birth that enhances and supports the normalcy of childbirth' (Pairman 2006: 85).

The New Zealand model of maternity care is also relevant here (Guilliland and Pairman 1995; Pairman 2010). In New Zealand, midwives can achieve a considerable degree of autonomy and continuity of care as lead maternity carers (LMC) and 'continuity of care and the relationships that are developed with women continue to be the main driving forces for the midwives continuing to practice as LMC midwives' (Wakelin 2006: 3). When midwives there decide to leave midwifery this tends to be because of the sheer pressure of work (Wakelin 2006), whereas English midwives leave because they cannot achieve the autonomy and relationships that sustain their New Zealand colleagues (Ball *et al.* 2002). Thus the New Zealand model is more sustainable, given more midwives, whereas the English model rapidly burns out large numbers of dedicated young midwives.

One model of care that holds out great hope for midwifery in the UK is that put forward by Independent Midwives UK (see van der Kooy 2009 and www.independentmidwives.org.uk). This model would enable independent midwives to provide care for individual women contracted through the NHS. This would mean that any woman could access independent midwifery care without having to pay for it privately, independent midwives would have access to NHS facilities for their clients, and insurance for independent midwives would be available through the NHS. This would enable English women to opt for care similar to that of New Zealand women who choose a midwife as their LMC.

There are wider organizational models, which fit better with a public service and which could be used in health care. Jane Jacobs proposes that there are two moral systems: commercial and guardian. It may well be that the values and practices which suit commercial activity do not fit the 'guardian' activities of public services where loyalty and generosity are traditionally valued (Jacobs 1992) and the same generosity can be applied to the use of time in caring relationships.

Or it may be that the market values underpinning the organization of the modern NHS are out of date in the real marketplace. Some management writers certainly value workers' autonomy, flexibility and trust far more than the NHS. Fairtlough (2005) states that there are 'three ways of getting things done: hierarchy, heterarchy and responsibly autonomy' and health services tend to suffer from 'the hegemony of hierarchy' (Fairtlough 2005: 7). Accountability is a key characteristic of responsible autonomy where central control is replaced by more self-sufficient sub-units. Fairtlough suggests that 'responsible autonomy may be the better alternative to hierarchy in Guardian organizations' (Fairtlough 2005: 60). It is interesting that these alternative ways of organizing foster the relationships and the autonomy that are prerequisites for flow.

Joy

Birth is usually a joyous event and midwifery can be a hugely rewarding job. Yet there is real danger that present systems of maternity care spread anxiety, fear and passivity rather than confidence and joy, without enhancing safety. Such systems cannot be sustainable, since they make mothers unhappy and midwives leave or become 'obedient technicians' (Deery and Hunter 2010).

'The best moments usually occur when a person's body or mind is stretched to its limits in a voluntary effort to accomplish something difficult and worthwhile' (Csikszentmihalyi 2008: 3), rather than being a passive patient or technician. Surely the pursuit of excellence, as flow experience, with its joyous potential should be a major aim of maternity services. Work towards that aim would improve health outcomes, enhance staff retention and increase social capital.

A mother's total engagement with her labour can be seen as the 'most intense initial phase' (Taylor 2010) of the 'primary maternal preoccupation' (Winnincott 1958) so essential to infant well-being and as enabling her later focus on the baby's needs. As such, it is of great social value. Seen in this way, the engagement with the process of birth that can be a flow experience for mother and midwives has profoundly positive social consequences. Yet, in Meg Taylor's view, the fragmentation of care, the low status of midwives and their inadequate numbers

> ... indicates the low status of motherhood generally. I think this low status and social pathology are not coincidental. But if it were to be the case that midwifery could properly fulfil its function by providing holistic care at this uniquely powerful time of transition, a considerable level of social change would be required, requiring a higher status to be accorded to both midwifery and motherhood.
>
> (Taylor 2010: 248)

Yet, 'Birth remakes us and makes us revalue our way of being in the world' (Murphy-Lawless 2006: 444). It is therefore a point at which we should be working for social change. To value flow and joy for mothers and midwives would be a worthwhile aim for real change in maternity services. It would have tremendous consequences

> ... when birth is done differently, it can help us develop an ethical stance that questions this unsustainable, exclusive and inhumane model [of modern maternity care] and starts to revalue connection – connection between mind and body, mother and baby, within families, between woman and midwife, between family and community and between disparate communities sharing similar struggles to make life more humane.
>
> (Edwards 2010: 109–10)

Without such brave aims, I fear that midwifery, as I know and love it, could disappear. Others have changed health systems. A movement for joyous birth could achieve even more than the hospice movement has achieved for peace and dignity in dying. If our service is to continue and be sustainable, systems of organization with underlying values conducive to flow and joy are greatly needed. We know that flow is hard to achieve, but it must be worth consciously working for. When there are precedents and we know how excellence can be achieved and how much it can achieve, can lesser aims be justified?

References

Anderson, T. (2010) 'Feeling safe enough to let go: the relationship between a woman and her midwife in the second stage of labour', in M. Kirkham (ed.), *The Midwife–Mother Relationship*. Basingstoke: Palgrave Macmillan.

Bagnold, E. (1988 originally published 1938) *The Squire*. London: Virago.

Ball, L., Curtis, P. and Kirkham, M. (2002) *Why Do Midwives Leave?* London: Royal College of Midwives.

Barker, D. J. P. (1994) *Mothers, Babies and Disease in Later Life*. London: BMJ Publishing.

Becker, G. de (1997) *The Gift of Fear*. London: Bloomsbury.

Cherry, A., Friel, R., Dowden, B., Ashton, K., Evans, R. *et al.* (2009) 'Managing demand: telephone triage in acute maternity services', *British Journal of Midwifery* 17, 8: 496–500.

Csikszentmihalyi, M. (2008) *Flow*. New York: Harper Perennial Modern Classics.

Curtis, P., Ball, L. and Kirkham, M. (2003) *Why Do Midwives Leave? Talking to Managers*. London: Royal College of Midwives.

Davis-Floyd, R. E., Barclay, L., Daviss, B-A. and Tritten, J. (2009) *Birth Models That Work*. Berkeley, CA: University of California Press.

Deery, R. and Hunter, B. (2010) 'Emotional work and relationships in midwifery', in M. Kirkham (ed.) *The Midwife–Mother Relationship*, 2nd Edition. Basingstoke: Palgrave Macmillan.

Deery, R. and Kirkham, M. (2007) 'Drained and dumped on: the generation and accumulation of emotional toxic waste in community midwifery', in M. Kirkham (ed.), *Exploring the Dirty Side of Women's Health*. London: Routledge.

Department of Health (1993) *Changing Childbirth: Report of the Expert Maternity Group*. London: HMSO.

Department of Health (2007) *Maternity Matters: Choice, Access and Continuity of Care in a Safe Service*. London: Department of Health.

Edwards, N. P. (2005) *Birthing Autonomy: Women's Experiences of Planning Home Birth*. Abingdon: Routledge.

Edwards, N. P. (2010) 'There's so much potential and for whatever reason it's not being realised. Women's relationships with midwives as a negotiation of ideology and power', in M. Kirkham (ed.), *The Midwife–Mother Relationship*, 2nd Edition. Basingstoke: Palgrave Macmillan.

Fahy, K. and Hastie, C. (2008) 'Midwifery guardianship: reclaiming the sacred in birth', in K. Fahy, M. Foureur and C. Hastie (eds), *Birth Territory and Midwifery Guardianship: Theory for Practice, Education and Research*. Sydney: Books for Midwives.

Fairtlough, G. (2005) *The Three Ways of Getting Things Done. Hierarchy, Heterarchy and Responsible Autonomy in Organisations*. Axminster: Triarchy Press.

Gigerenzer, G. (1999) quoted in Gladwell, M. (2005) *Blink*. London: Penguin.

Gladwell, M. (2005) *Blink*. London: Penguin.

Goleman, D. (1995) *Emotional Intelligence*. New York: Bantam Books.

Griffiths, R. (2009) 'Maternity care pathways and the law', *British Journal of Midwifery*, 17, 5: 324–25.

Guilliland, K. and Pairman, S. (1995) *The Midwifery Partnership Model for Practice, Monograph Series, 95/1*. Wellington: Department of Nursing & Midwifery, Victoria University.

Halldorsdottir, S. and Karlsdottir, S. I. (1996) 'Empowerment or discouragement: women's experience of caring and uncaring encounters during childbirth', *Health Care for Women International*, 17: 361–79.

Hastie, C. (2008) 'The spiritual and emotional territory of the unborn and newborn baby', in K. Fahy, M. Foureur, and C. Hastie (eds), *Birth Territory and Midwifery Guardianship: Theory for Practice, Education and Research*. Sydney: Books for Midwives.

Homer, C., Brodie, P. and Leap, N. (2001) *Establishing Models of Continuity of Midwifery Care in Australia. A Resource for Midwives*. Sydney: University of Technology Sydney, Centre for Family Health and Midwifery.

Homer, C., Brodie, P. and Leap, N. (2008) *Midwifery Continuity of Care: A Practical Guide*. Sydney: Churchill Livingstone.

Hunter, B. (2006) 'The importance of reciprocity in relationships between community-based midwives', *Midwifery* 22: 308–22.

Hunter, B. and Deery, R. (eds) (2009) *Emotions in Midwifery and Reproduction*. London: Palgrave Macmillan.

Hunter, M. (2003) 'Autonomy, clinical freedom and responsibility', in M. Kirkham, (ed.), *Birth Centres. A Social Model for Maternity Care*. Oxford: Elsevier.

Jacobs, J. (1992) *Systems of Survival. A Dialogue on the Moral Foundations of Commerce and Politics*. London: Hodder & Stoughton.

Jones, O. (2000) 'Supervision in a midwife managed birth centre', in M. Kirkham (ed.) *Developments in the Supervision of Midwives*. Manchester: Books for Midwives.

Kaplan, S. H., Greenfield, S., Gandek, B., Rogers, W. H. and Ware, J. E. (1996) 'Characteristics of physicians with participatory decision making styles', *Annals of Internal Medicine*, 124: 497–504.

Katz-Rothman, B. (1996) 'Women, providers and control', *Journal of Obstetric, Gynecologic & Neonatal Nursing*, 25, 3: 253–56.

Kirkham, M. (2003) *Birth Centres: A Social Model for Maternity Care*. Oxford: Elsevier.

Kirkham, M. (2007) 'Traumatised midwives', *AIMS Journal*, 19, 1: 12–13.

Kirkham, M. (ed.) (2010) *The Midwife–Mother Relationship*, 2nd Edition. Basingstoke: Palgrave Macmillan.

Kirkham, M. and Stapleton, H. (eds) (2001) *Informed Choice in Maternity Care: An Evaluation of Evidence-based Leaflets*. York: NHS Centre for Reviews and Dissemination.

Kirkham, M., Morgan, R. K. and Davies, C. (2006) *Why Midwives Stay*. London: Department of Health. Online. Available at: www.nhsemployers.org and www.rcm.org (accessed 21 March 2010).

Kooy, B. van der (2009) 'Choice for women and choice for midwives – making it happen', *British Journal of Midwifery*, 17, 9: 524–25.

Leap, N. (2010) 'The less we do the more we give', in M. Kirkham (ed.) *The Midwife–Mother Relationship*. Basingstoke: Palgrave Macmillan.

Leyshon, L. (2004) 'Integrating caseloads across a whole service: the Torbay model', *MIDIRS Midwifery Digest* 14, 1, Supplement 1: S9–S11.

McCourt, C. and Stevens, T. (2009) 'Relationship and reciprocity in caseload midwifery' in B. Hunter and R. Deery (eds), *Emotions in Midwifery and Reproduction*. London: Palgrave Macmillan.

Marmot, M. (2004) *Status Syndrome*. London: Bloomsbury.

Murphy-Lawless, J. (2006) 'Birth and mothering in today's social order: the challenge of new knowledges', *MIDIRS Midwifery Digest*, 16, 4: 439–44.

Olafsdottir, O. A. and Kirkham, M. (2009) 'Narrative time – stories, childbirth and midwifery', in C. McCourt (ed.) *Childbirth, Midwifery and Concepts of Time*. Oxford: Berghahn Books.

Page, L. (1997) 'Misplaced values: in fear of excellence', *British Journal of Midwifery*, 5, 11: 652–54.

Pairman, S. (2006) 'Midwifery partnership: working "with" women', in L. A. Page and R. McCandlish (eds), *The New Midwifery: Science and Sensitivity in Practice*, 2nd Edition. Edinburgh: Churchill Livingstone.

Pairman, S. (2010) 'Midwifery partnership: a professionalising strategy for midwives' in M. Kirkham (ed.) *The Midwife–Mother Relationship*, 2nd Edition. Basingstoke: Palgrave Macmillan.

Reed, B. (2010) 'Choices are not choices if you are not allowed to make them for yourself', *The Practising Midwife* 13, 1: 4–5.

Robinson, K. (2009) *The Element*. London: Penguin.

Sandall, J. (1997) 'Midwives' burnout and continuity of care', *British Journal of Midwifery* 5, 2: 106–11

Seligman, M. E. P. (2002) *Authentic Happiness*. New York: Free Press/Simon and Schuster

Sennett, R. (2008) *The Craftsman*. New York: Yale University Press.

Stapleton, H., Kirkham, M., Thomas, G. and Curtis, P. (2002) 'Midwives in the middle: Balance and vulnerability', *British Journal of Midwifery*, 10, 10: 607–11.

Taylor, M. (2010) 'The midwife as container', in M. Kirkham (ed.), *The Midwife–Mother Relationship*. Basingstoke: Palgrave Macmillan.

Taylor, S. E. (2002) *The Tending Instinct*. New York: Henry Holt.

Wakelin, K. J. (2006) 'Staying or leaving: a study of the sustainability of LMC midwifery practice in an urban region of New Zealand', unpublished Master's degree thesis, University of Victoria.

Walsh, D. (2007) *Improving Maternity Services, Small is Beautiful – Lessons from a Birth Centre*. Abingdon: Radcliffe Publishing.

Winnicott, D. W. (1975) 'Primary maternal preoccupation', in *Through Paediatrics to Psychoanalysis* (a reissue of Winnicott's *Collected Papers*. London, Tavistock 1958) London: Hogarth Press.

8 The birthing environment

A sustainable approach

Carolyn Hastie

Introduction

Birds do it. Bees do it, even bears and humans do it. An instinctive and compelling need to prepare the environment for birth and the care of offspring, known as 'nesting', is common to the females of many living species. The tendency is to seek a safe, out of the way, private place to birth. Depending upon the particular species, preparation for birth can take weeks or merely involve retreating to a secluded, concealed place once labour begins. The birthing process is instinctive, mediated by a genetic programme and deep, ancient brain structures that are common to all mammals. If that birth space is disturbed or the female is threatened in any way, labour will usually slow down. Once the threat has passed, labour will resume. Humans, despite their cognitive brilliance, also require facilitative environments for optimal child-bearing. Disturbances to that environment can have a cumulative effect, rendering a woman unable to birth normally. If the disturbances occur after birth, the exquisitely orchestrated mother/baby interaction patterns that lay the foundation of attachment can be disrupted with lifelong consequences.

The midwife has a time-honoured, powerful and privileged role in creating a facilitative environment for birth. A midwife has the honour of working alongside a woman, being 'with' her, supporting her growth and development as she births new life and becomes a mother. The midwife's capacity-building role extends to supporting each woman to discover who she is and what she is capable of. Midwives have a vital and influential part in ensuring the sustainability of the childbearing process and maternity care. Normal, natural birth is eco-friendly; it doesn't require a great deal in terms of material resources, it does, however, require the loving attention of skilled and caring midwives. Normal birth needs to be protected, promoted and supported because it is the epitome of a human activity with an extremely low carbon footprint.

Following a definition of normal, natural birth and an exploration of why normal, natural birth is important for sustainability, the birth environment and cultural considerations are examined. Finally, suggestions for optimizing a woman's experience and ways that a midwife can support normal, natural, healthy birth for the woman and her baby in a sustainable way are explored.

Why normal birth?

The terms 'normal' and 'natural' birth have created robust discussion among various disciplines and philosophical orientations as attempts have been made to clarify and define what these terms mean. For the purposes of this chapter, 'normal' and/or 'natural' childbirth refers to a healthy psychophysiological process, which occurs at term, resulting in the birth of a healthy baby and placenta and an intact mother. No medical intervention or drugs to relieve pain or aid the birth process are used. Psychophysiology refers to the complex interrelationships between the physiological and psychological aspects of behaviour (Cacioppo *et al*. 2007). A psychophysiological approach to childbirth appropriately acknowledges and integrates the woman's active, mindful agency in her birth process. A psychophysiological approach provides a useful frame-work for conceptualizing normal, natural labour and birth.

Benefits and sustainability of normal birth

There is no doubt that giving birth and being born are critical life events. However, the process is a healthy one which prepares the woman and the fetus for their impending changes. Normal labour and birth rely upon complex, sensitive and intricate psychophysiological and neurobiological interactions which influence and impact the woman's behaviour as a mother and that of her fetus becoming a neonate. The passage of the fetus through the birth canal is accompanied by a sympathoadrenal response that fuels the fetus for the journey and triggers the absorption of the lung fluid in readiness for air-breathing (Olver *et al*. 2004). Inflammatory defence systems are stimulated along with the central nervous system so that the fetus is fully prepared for life outside the mother's womb (Yektaei-Karin *et al*. 2007). On the other hand, babies who are delivered abruptly by Caesarean section are thought to be unprepared neurologically, endocrinologically and physiologically for birth. Caesarean section has been associated with an increased risk of short-term neonatal morbidity (Lee and D'Alton 2008) and longer-term problems such as asthma and allergy (Roduit *et al*. 2009; Tollanes *et al*. 2008); type 1 diabetes mellitus; childhood leukaemia and testicular cancer (Schlinzig *et al*. 2009). Current thinking is that the stress of being born in an abrupt manner causes permanent epigenetic modifica-tions to the fetus/newborn's neuroendocrine pathways that give rise to disease processes. Prenatal stress due to Caesarean delivery is further compounded by hospital practices that separate surgically born babies from their mothers and inhibit mothers' ability to properly engage with their surgically delivered infants.

Healthy normal birth has many benefits for both mother and baby and their relationship. The list of benefits for immediate and long-term health and well-being is growing exponentially as scientists unravel the mysteries of epigenetics, brain architecture and development (Lipton 2005; Rossi 2002). In addition, the period immediately after birth is now recognized as a 'sensitive period' and the way that time is managed and whether mothers and babies have quality, uninterrupted, extended skin-to-skin experience or not has long-term effects on mother–infant interaction and long-term breastfeeding (Bystrova *et al.* 2009). The benefits of breastfeeding are well proven and include protection from childhood abuse and neglect. Reports of maternal neglect are nearly four times more likely for those who do not breastfeed their babies (Strathearn *et al.* 2009). Breastfeeding rates drop when labouring women are given epidurals, intramuscular narcotics and third stage oxytocics (Jordan *et al.* 2009). Given the overwhelming ecological value of breastfeeding to the individual and society, efforts to increase normal birth rates have the added benefit of increasing breastfeeding rates.

Stress in the 'sensitive period' after birth has been found to trigger epigenetic changes that lead to neuroendocrine and behavioural alterations that are frequent features in depression in children and adults (Murgatroyd *et al.* 2009). Newborns have been found to exhibit a distress cry when separated from their mothers (Christensson *et al.* 1995), whereas skin-to-skin experience at birth for babies has been found to reduce the effect of the stress of being born (Bystrova *et al.* 2003). Swaddling the baby at birth was found to both adversely affect the mother's responsiveness to her baby and affect the mother's ability for positive affective involvement with her infant (Bystrova *et al.* 2009). The obvious solution is to reduce newborn stress as much as possible by ensuring the mother and her baby have relaxed, uninterrupted skin-to-skin time. Benefits of skin-to-skin experience are long term. Babies who experienced skin-to-skin time with their mothers smile more and earlier than babies who do not have that experience. Mothers who experienced extra skin-to-skin time with their babies at birth were found to be more responsive to their babies at three months of age; look face to face and kiss their babies more often than the control group who did not have skin-to-skin time. The benefits of extra skin-to-skin time at birth were even more noticeable when the babies were one year old. Mothers who enjoyed skin-to-skin time with their newborns talked more positively to their children; touched and held them more frequently and stayed home longer before returning to professional employment than the mothers who experienced routine care (de Chateau and Wiberg 1984). Healthy, normal births enable women to engage with their newborns more readily, move freely, breastfeed more easily and require little in the way of material and human resources (Tracy and Tracy 2003). Interventions in the birth process on the other hand, increase health care expenditure and resource consumption both in the short and the long term. The midwife's role in protecting, supporting and promoting normal birth can be seen as a core aspect of sustainability for the long-term health and well-being of future generations and the planet.

Birth, brain architecture and the built environment

The built environment is now recognized to either adversely or positively affect the health and well-being of inhabitants (Joseph and Gulwadi 2009). Advances in neuroscience illuminate the role of the brain in the way a person perceives and orientates themselves in unfamiliar places and how the physical environment impacts on cognition, problem solving, pain tolerance and mood (Sternberg and Wilson 2006). Feeling safe and relaxed or unsafe and stressed has associated psychophysiological effects that impact upon health and healing (Leonard and Myint 2009). Aspects of the natural world, such as gardens, pot plants, views, paintings of natural scenes, together with carefully thought-out elements of design such as colour, walkways and signage, are being incorporated in health care buildings because they are known to trigger feelings of familiarity and relaxation in patients and staff. Because people's experiences in health care buildings are enhanced, evidence-based design improves outcomes and contains costs (Ulrich and Zimring 2004).

Hospitals have incorporated birth centres, with baths and en-suite showers, either within or alongside the standard labour ward, seeking to create a familiar, home-like environment in hospitals for women to labour and birth (Design Council 2009). Hospitals have also made changes to the décor of their standard delivery rooms by including less clinical touches such as coloured walls, artworks, pot plants, side tables, quilts and curtains. Other initiatives to help women and their partners feel more at home in hospital include preparation for birth and parenting programmes with a labour ward tour. Couples are encouraged to bring their own pillows, music and other familiar items with them to use in labour.

A survey conducted by the National Childbirth Trust (UK) in 2005 (Newburn and Singh 2005) reported that nine out of ten women thought that the physical environment influenced how easy or difficult it was to give birth. A pilot study (US) conducted in 2009 examined whether minor changes to a standard labour room, creating an 'ambient' birthing environment, affected women's birthing experience (Hodnett *et al.* 2009). Women using the ambient room experienced shorter labours, a reduction in artificial oxytocin augmention and were more mobile than the control group. Changes to the room involved removing the labour ward bed and replacing it with a double-sized mattress and pillows in the corner. Lights were dimmed, the door was kept closed with a sign to knock before entering and birth balls, music players and DVDs were available. There was no difference in the rate of normal birth between the two groups. The researchers reported that resistance to change was evident in staff reactions to the study. Three hospitals refused to participate; 20 per cent of the staff recommended putting the bed back; some disliked the room and others thought it was unsafe. The health care environment involves much more than bricks and mortar. Those who provide the care and the invisible, yet powerful, structures and processes that govern their work life and behaviour have a major influence on both service outcomes and the carbon footprint of maternity care (Lyndon 2008).

Stone age biology in a twenty-first century social world

Every society has culturally-driven rituals, rules, beliefs, rites and behaviours around the birthing process (Dunham *et al.* 1991). The context within which a woman gives birth is similarly variable. In the Western world, societal and cultural change has been rapid over the last few centuries. Changing social circumstances have gained momentum in the last 100 years and accelerated at a dizzying rate in the last 50 years. The evolutionary perspective of the birthing process, as with many of our lived realities, is that our biology has not changed in step with social change (Armelagos *et al*. 2005). The viral-like spread of technology in communication systems and labour-saving devices creates a 'low touch, high tech' social world. Human bodies, however, still require a 'high touch, low tech' approach to care, just as they did in the Stone Age. Expediency and efficiency are the goals of the technological era. The institution of mechanistic assembly-line production systems has revolutionized industry while disrupting the natural world. Expediency and efficiency applied to human biology generates discontinuities between the conditions and environments we evolved under and those we experience today. Evolutionary anthropologists link diseases that plague the Western world to the 'discordance' between genes and culture (Stearns *et al*. 2008).

As cultural and societal changes have gathered momentum, the technological approach has been applied to the birthing process in the same way it has been applied to the food production industry and with a similarly disrupting effect. Fast food has lead to the metabolic syndrome among the general population and fast birth has led to increasing rates of surgical birth and post-traumatic stress disorder among the childbearing population. The assembly line approach to maternity service provision has become expensive (Tracy and Tracy 2003). Maternity service expenditure in terms of dollars and its carbon footprint has spiralled out of control along with the social costs. The spectre of global warming is becoming an omnipresent reality (St Louis and Hess 2008), adding impetus to the need to take an ecological approach to providing maternity services for birthing women.

An ecological approach to the birthing environment

Ecology is the study of the relationships between living systems and their environment (Wilkes and Krebs 1982). The environment, as discussed in this chapter, includes: the people, furniture, artifacts, equipment, design, buildings, geography, rules, beliefs, attitudes, social interactions, behaviours, power dynamics, cultural patterns, rituals and regulations present, involved in or influencing the birth place. The living systems refer to all the people involved in the birthing arena. Birth Territory is a theory that describes how the birth environment functions and how power is used in the birth place. Birth Territory theory puts childbearing women and their need to feel safe and secure in their birthing environment at the centre of consideration (Fahy *et al*. 2008). As sensing and responding to the environment involves both conscious and unconscious processes, women need to feel safe and secure to develop the trust needed to 'let go' of interest in or attention to external cues, so that she is able to focus on her baby and her experience to birth the baby and placenta well. The midwife's role is to keep the environment calm, relaxed and enabling of the woman's process; minimizing any external interruption or distraction of her mindful focus.

The process of labour and birth engages the same genetic switches and hormonal systems that are triggered when making love and having an orgasm. The environmental factors that a particular woman requires to 'let go' and fully engage in satisfying, loving sex are the factors that would be of benefit to that woman when giving birth. Birth and sex, both aspects of the sexual continuum, are mediated by deep, ancient brain structures and genetically programmed primal activities, influenced in either positive or negative ways by environmental factors. An Italian architect, Bianca Lepori, specializes in birth spaces. She writes that the external environment is experienced with at least three bodies: the moving, feeling, dreaming bodies, which are hardwired to respond to cues in the environment (Lepori *et al.* 2008). In his ground-breaking book, *Birth Reborn*, Michel Odent, a French doctor (Odent 1984), brought our attention to the ideal birth environment with his 'salle sauvage' (primitive room). Prenatal care at Pithiviers included singing together around a piano. Birthing care included the constant support of a skilled midwife, warm deep pools and a dimly lit, earth-coloured room with a low-lying double bed. The reputation of the excellent outcomes travelled fast. Women travelled from all over Europe and the US to give birth at Pithiviers. According to Odent, the only obligatory players in the birth environment are the woman and her baby (Odent 2008). There are however, complex social pressures that affect the birthing environment and women's experiences of birth.

A cross-cultural perspective on the birth environment

In the second half of the twentieth century, what has been referred to as the largest uncontrolled and unevaluated experiment in the Western world was introduced for childbearing women (de Jonge *et al.* 2009). Birth was removed from the home and taken to hospital; a place traditionally reserved for the sick and dying. Birthing women were removed from their traditional support system and made to lie on hard hospital beds to labour and birth alone (Leavitt 1986). The birthing position women adopt to give birth indicates how the culture constructs the birth environment; the expectations, attitudes and beliefs of the attendants and how the woman experiences the birth process (Roberts 1989). A fascinating synopsis of the cross-cultural birth environment experienced in traditional societies is given by Niles and Michael Newton (Newton and Newton 2003). In their overview of birth-related practices from traditional pre-literate cultures, the Newton's describe a wide variety of culturally patterned differences that included; pain expression being sanctioned or valued; movement being encouraged or curtailed; women birthing in private or in the middle of normal family activities with children present; birth being viewed as dirty or normal and men being present or excluded. In 18 tribes of 64 cultures, men had their activity restricted and regulated during the birth period, a custom known as 'couvade'. Birthing positions were similarly diverse. A cross-cultural survey found that 68 out of 76 non-European societies used the upright position for birth. The Newtons recorded that 'of these upright positions, the most common was kneeling with 21 cultures represented. The next most common was sitting, with 19 cultures using this method. Fifteen cultures used squatting and five used standing positions'. In some cultures, a variety of birthing positions were adopted by birthing women, because 'the woman makes the choice for herself' (Newton and Newton 2003: 24).

Poles, stakes and ropes were used for pulling, while other devices were used for bracing and pushing by labouring women. The one common thread throughout the different cultures and their patterned practices around labour and birth was the presence and emotional support of another woman or women (Newton and Newton 2003: 22).

The woman–midwife relationship

A survey on what women want in their birth environment by the National Childbirth Trust (NCT) (Newburn and Singh 2005) found women wanted less clinical-looking rooms, access to ensuite toilets and birth pools. However, the key factors 'overwhelmingly' identified as important were the relationship the woman experienced with the midwife and the woman's sense of control. Listening (Declercq *et al.* 2006), being present (Kennedy 2000), providing personalized care and support and providing quality time (Moon *et al.* 1999); confidence in women's ability (Homer *et al.* 2009), along with good communication skills, provision of information, choice, continuity and control, are key attributes of midwifery care that women have repeatedly indicated they want during childbearing (Hodnett 1989). Women's fears about ringing to negotiate when to come into hospital in labour are lessened when midwives are compassionate, understanding and humble on the phone (Eri *et al.* 2009).

These findings have resonances with the field of psychotherapy in which therapeutic outcomes are associated with relationships characterized by empathy, trust, kindness, unconditional positive regard and congruence between the client and the caregiver, who has 'relational presence' (Bohart *et al.* 2002). The midwife with 'relational presence' engages with the woman in a dynamic way to ensure the woman is an active participant in decision making throughout the birth process (Pembroke and Pembroke 2008). When a midwife engages with a birthing woman in this profound manner the woman feels in control. Feeling in control during labour and birth means the woman feels able to trust that her needs will be met and valued and she can get on with the business of having her baby.

As early as 1981, having a sense of control was identified as a key component of maternal satisfaction with the childbirth experience (Humenick 1981). Ellen Hodnett (1989) investigated women's sense of control in the birth environment in a comparison between home and hospital settings.

Hodnett's conclusion was that the optimal birth environment is one which has 'supportive caregivers, few unfamiliar procedures and personnel (and) encourages freedom of expression' (1989: 22). A sense of control is associated with lower levels of circulating glucocorticoids, the product of the body's stress response (Schulkin *et al*. 2005). People's nervous system electromagnetic fields 'tune in' to each other, discerning threat or safety in the social environment with physiological ramifications (Goleman 2006). Perhaps the staff antagonism to the room modifications in the study by Hodnett *et al*. (2009) was physiologically registered by the birthing women, affecting their ability to let go of conscious control and birth in a straightforward manner. Mander and Melenda (2005) examined maternity care systems in the UK and Finland and concluded that the hospital environment may serve to aggravate the woman's perception of the severity of her pain. Their findings could explain why the presence of a doula has been found to be beneficial (Hodnett 2003) and suggest that the presence of the doula may 'ameliorate the hostile environment which the woman encounters in the labour ward'. National Childbirth Trust researchers noted that, although the numbers were too small to be conclusive, women who had Caesarean section births were more likely to have reported that staff had a 'poor attitude', didn't listen to them and were rude and non-communicative (Newburn and Singh 2005).

Staff attitudes have been implicated in rates of transfer from community to tertiary settings (Klein and Westreich 1983). Childbirth Connection in the United States surveyed 1,573 women who gave birth in 2005. The survey report, called Listening to Mothers 2, found huge gaps between the actual experiences of mothers and optimal conditions. Only 2 per cent of women experienced care practices known to support normal birth such as: access to water for pain management; unrestricted movement; upright positions; unrestricted eating and drinking; hand-held recorders for fetal monitoring; giving birth in non-supine positions and pushing according to own urge. The report said that one quarter of the women reported they felt negative feelings during labour such as 'overwhelmed' and 'weak'. One fifth of the women surveyed used words such as 'powerful' and 'unafraid'. The majority experienced medical interventions, despite having said they wished to avoid them. Pressure to be induced, to have an epidural and Caesarean was experienced by many women. Seventy three per cent of women who had an episiotomy were not given a choice in the matter (Declerq *et al*. 2006). In a 1995 UK study, women's feelings that they had been treated kindly and with understanding in labour correlated with their satisfaction with the amount of information they had been given at the time (Fleissig 1995). Women wanted to know how they were progressing; they felt frightened when the midwife was absent or when there was no response to questions such as 'should I push?' The author concluded that poor communication causes unnecessary anxiety for women while noting that both doctors and midwives had difficulty communicating with women who were single or from minority ethnic groups (Fleissig 1995).

What labouring women want from midwives

According to the National Childbirth Trust survey, women value midwifery support, which includes the qualities, in hierarchical order of importance, listed below (Newburn and Singh 2005):

1 being motivated, encouraged and praised for how well they were doing;
2 practical suggestions about position changes and focusing on breathing patterns;
3 trust in the woman's instincts and respecting what the woman wanted to do;
4 reassurance;
5 being friendly, kind and chatty;
6 firm guidance;
7 remaining calm and positive;
8 explaining what was happening;
9 being a constant presence (not leaving the woman on her own or handing over to another midwife);
10 seeming confident and in control of the situation;
11 involving the woman's partner.

Involving and supporting the woman's partner is very important as one group of researchers observed 'having a relaxed partner had a positive effect on women who were then able to focus on their labour without worrying about an anxious partner' (Hauck *et al.* 2008: 467). As we can see from the information in this section, the relationship between the midwife and the woman, together with her partner, is of vital importance to the woman and has been identified as a contributing factor to positive or negative outcomes.

Optimizing the birth environment

Immersion in water is one environmental feature that is associated with feelings of being in a sanctuary for birthing women. A study by Maude and Foureur (2007) found the design and position of the bath/pool was important to women and they appreciated the freedom afforded by being in water and having 'plenty of room to move around'. Most important of all, however, was the sense of a shared philosophy and belief in the normality of birth with their midwives that underpinned the women's opportunity to get into the water. The evidence from the various studies reported in this chapter explains the relationship, the interactions and the care that women want from their midwife. Women want midwives to believe in birth, to believe in them and treat them and their partners kindly. Midwives need to examine their own behaviour and belief systems and ensure their philosophy and beliefs are conducive to normal birth, because the midwife's interaction style and belief system are potent social influences on a woman's childbearing experience.

Midwives need to reflect on every interaction they have with a childbearing woman to ensure that what I have called the 'golden rule' of midwifery – 'every woman should leave your presence feeling better about herself that when she arrived' – is operational. If every midwife lived by the 'golden rule', then her care would be truly woman-centred; she would speak kindly; she would give appropriate, encouraging compliments and comments; she would listen and she would care deeply about the woman's situation and experience.

The following list contains the features considered integral to promoting, protecting and supporting normal birthing psychophysiology (McNabb *et al.* 2006; Romano and Lothian 2008):

- ensure your birth unit has a policy that supports a woman's right of informed refusal as well as informed consent;
- ensure birth rooms are supplied with equipment for normal birth: towels, showers, baths, en-suite toilets, birth balls, birth mats, birth stools, ledges to lean on, space to move, privacy, sign on door 'knock before entering';
- ensure natural elements are present in the birth room: pot plants, pictures of nature, art work, colour.
- avoid medically unnecessary induction of labour;
- ensure evidence-informed decision making;
- prepare the room for the arrival of the woman and her partner; ice, water, dimmed light, running bath;
- greet, introduce self and speak warmly to the woman and her partner on the phone or on arrival in the delivery suite;
- the woman and her partner shown to their own dimly lit room on arrival;
- the features of the room demonstrated to the woman and partner;
- one-to-one continuous labour support;
- privacy;
- warmth;
- quiet;
- elimination of unnecessary questions to minimize cognitive stimulation;
- keep women as upright as possible;
- encourage mobility, support freedom of movement for the labouring woman;
- unrestricted food and fluid; encourage same;
- rest;
- avoid routine interventions and restrictions;
- minimal noise/talking;
- support and suggest breathing and visualization/massage;
- minimal use of CTG; only use if necessary;
- spontaneous second stage;
- encourage non-supine positions in second stage;
- maintenance of quiet, calm environment after birth of the baby;
- immediate skin-to-skin contact with baby.

Conclusion

Birthing normally is optimal, as it has long-term and wide-ranging effects on the individual being born and the mother. Birthing normally has also been shown to have a very powerful role in lowering the carbon footprint of maternity care. This chapter has demonstrated that the environment shapes the way that people behave and function and how women birth. Midwives have been shown to be powerful constructors and influencers of the birth environment. Extensive research has shown that women have clearly articulated what they want from midwives. Each midwife has an ethical and professional responsibility to ensure she has the necessary attitudinal qualities and knowledge base to support childbearing women adequately. Strategies for optimizing the birth environment have been provided and the need for midwives to develop a relational presence has been examined. The evidence is clear; the midwife's role in protecting, supporting and promoting normal birth is a core aspect of sustainability for the long-term health and well-being of future generations and the planet.

References

Armelagos, G., Brown, P. and Turner, B. (2005) 'Evolutionary, historical and political economic perspectives on health and disease', *Social Science and Medicine*, 61: 755–65.

Bohart, A. C., Elliott, R., Greenberg, L. S. and Watson, J. (2002) 'Empathy', in J. C. Norcross (ed.) *Psychotherapy Relationships That Work: Therapist Contributions and Responsiveness to Patients*. New York: Oxford University Press.

Bystrova, K., Ivanova, V., Edhborg, M., Matthiesen, A. S., Ransjö-Arvidson, A. B. *et al.* (2009) 'Early contact versus separation: effects on mother-infant interaction one year later', *Birth*, 36: 110–12.

Bystrova, K., Widstrom, A.-M., Matthiesen, A.-S., Ransjö-Arvidson, A., Welles-Nyström, B. *et al.* (2003) 'Skin-to-skin contact may reduce negative consequences of "the stress of being born": a study on temperature in newborn infants, subjected to different ward routines in St. Petersburg', *Acta Paediatric*, 92: 320–26.

Cacioppo, J. T., Tassinary, L. G. and Berntson, G. G. (eds) (2007) *Handbook of Psychophysiology*. New York: Cambridge University Press.

Chateau, P. de and Wiberg, B. (1984) 'Long-term effect on mother-infant behaviour of extra contact during the first hour postpartum. Follow up at one year', *Scandanavian Journal of Society and Medicine*, 12: 91–103.

Christensson, K., Cabrera, T., Christensson, E., Uvnas-Moberg, K. and Winberg, J. (1995) 'Separation distress call in the human neonate in the absence of maternal body contact', *Acta Paediatric*, 84: 468–73.

Declerq, E. R., Sakala, C., Corry, M. P. and Applebaum, S. (2006) 'Listening to Mothers 11: Report of the Second National US Survey of Women's Childbearing Experiences'. New York: Childbirth Connection.

Design Council (2009) 'Guy's and St Thomas' Hospital: designing a welcome sanctuary for mothers to be'. London: Design Council. Online. Available at: www. designcouncil.org.uk/Case-Studies/All-Case-Studies/Guys–St-Thomas-hospital/ (accessed 24 March 2010).

Dunham, C., Myers, F., Barnden, N., McDougall, A., Kelly, T. *et al.* (1991) *Mamatoto: A Celebration of Birth*. London: Virago.

Eri, T. S., Blystad, A., Gjengedal, E. and Blaaka, G. (2009) 'Negotiating credibility: first-time mothers' experience of contact with the labour ward before hospitalization' *Midwifery*. In press, corrected proof, Available online 18 January 2009. Online. Available at: www.sciencedirect.com/science?_ob=ArticleListURL&_method=list &_ArticleListID=1265057417&view=c&_acct=C000050221&_version=1&_urlVersion =0&_userid=10&md5=42b28fb12171f14394195274f9a236ea (accessed 24 March 2010).

Fahy, K., Foureur, M. and Hastie, C. (eds) (2008) *Birth Territory and Midwifery Guardianship: Theory for Practice, Education and Research*. Edinburgh: Elsevier.

Fleissig, A. (1995) 'Are women given enough information by staff during labour and delivery?' *Midwifery*, 9: 70–75.

Goleman, D. (2006) *Social Intelligence*. London: Hutchinson.

Hauck, Y., Rivers, C. and Doherty, K. (2008) 'Women's experiences of using a Snoezelen room during labour in Western Australia', *Midwifery*, 24: 460–70.

Hodnett, E. D. (1989) 'Personal control and the birth environment: comparisons between home and hospital settings', *Journal of Environmental Psychology*, 9: 207–16.

Hodnett, E. D. (2003) *Continuity of Caregivers for Care During Pregnancy and Childbirth (Cochrane Review)*, in The Cochrane Library, 4, 2003. Chichester, UK: John Wiley & Sons.

Hodnett, E. D., Stremler, R., Weston, J. A. and McKeever, P. (2009) 'Re-conceptualizing the hospital labor room: the PLACE (Pregnant and Laboring in an Ambient Clinical Environment) pilot trial', *Birth*, 36: 159–66.

Homer, C. S. E., Passant, L., Brodie, P. M., Kildea, S., Leap, N. *et al.* (2009) 'The role of the midwife in Australia: views of women and midwives', *Midwifery*, 25: 673–81.

Humenick, S. (1981) 'Mastery: the key to childbirth satisfaction? A review', *Birth and the Family Journal*, 8 79–83.

Jonge, A. de, Geos, B. Y. van der, Ravelli, A. V., Amelink-Verburg, M. P., Mol, B. W. *et al.* (2009) 'Perinatal mortality and morbidity in a nationwide cohort of 529 688 low-risk planned home and hospital births', *British Journal of Obstetrics and Gynaecology*, 116: 1177–84.

Jordan, S., Emery, S., Watkins, A., Evans, J., Storey, M. *et al.* (2009) 'Associations of drugs routinely given in labour with breastfeeding at 48 hours analysis of the Cardiff Births Survey', *British Journal of Obstetrics and Gynaecology*, 116: 1622–32.

Joseph, A. and Gulwadi, G. B. (2009) *Improving the Patient Experience: Best Practices for Safety-Net Clinic Design*. Oakland: California HealthCare Foundation.

Kennedy, H. P. (2000) 'A model of exemplary midwifery practice: results of a Delphi study', *Journal of Midwifery and Women's Health*, 45: 4–19.

Klein, M. and Westreich, R. (1983) 'Birth room transfer and procedure rates – what do they tell about the setting?' *Birth*, 10: 93–98.

Leavitt, J. (1986) *Brought to Bed: Childbearing in America 1750–1950*. New York and Oxford: Oxford University Press.

Lee, Y. and D'Alton, M. (2008) 'Cesarean delivery on maternal request: maternal and neonatal complications', *Current Opinion in Obstetrics and Gynecology*, 20: 591–601.

Leonard, B. and Myint, A. (2009) 'The psychoneuroimmunology of depression', *Human Psychopharmacy*, 24: 165–75.

Lepori, B., Foureur, M. and Hastie, C. (2008) 'Mindbodyspirit architecture: creating birth space', in K. Fahy, M. Foureur and C. Hastie (eds), *Birth Territory and Midwifery Guardianship: Theory for Practice Education and Research*. Edinburgh: Elsevier.

Lipton, B. H. (2005) *The Biology of Belief*. San Rafael, CA: Mountain of Love/Elite Books.

Lyndon, A. (2008) 'Social and environmental conditions creating fluctuating agency for safety in two urban academic birth centres', *Journal of Obstetric, Gynaecologic and Neonatal Nursing*, 37: 13–23.

McNabb, M. T., Kimber, L., Haines, A. and McCourt, C. (2006) 'Does regular massage from late pregnancy to birth decrease maternal pain perception during labour and birth? A feasibility study to investigate a programme of massage, controlled breathing and visualisation, from 36 weeks of pregnancy until birth', *Complementary Therapies in Clinical Practice*, 12: 222–31.

Mander, R. and Melender, H.-L. (2005) 'Birth settings and pain control trends among women in Finland', *British Journal of Midwifery*, 13: 504–09.

Maude, R. M. and Foureur, M. (2007) 'It's beyond water: stories of women's experience of using water for birth', *Women and Birth*, 20: 17–24.

Moon, M., Breitkreuz, L., Ellis, C. and Hanson, C. (1999) *Midwifery Care: Women's Experiences, Hopes and Reflections*. Brandon: Prairie Women's Health Centre of Excellence.

Murgatroyd, C., Patchev, A. P., Wu, Y., Micale, V., Bockmühl, Y. *et al.* (2009) 'Dynamic DNA methylation process persistent effect of early life stress', *Nature Neuroscience*, 12: 1559–66.

Newburn, M. and Singh, D. (2005) *Are Women Getting the Birth Environment They Need: Report of a National Survey of Women's Experiences*. London: National Childbirth Trust.

Newton, N. and Newton, M. (2003) 'Childbirth in cross cultural perspective', in L. Dundes, (ed.) *The Manner Born: Birth Rites in Cross-Cultural Perspective*. Walnut Creek, CA: AltaMira Press.

Odent, M. (1984) *Birth Reborn*. Glasgow: William Collins & Sons.

Odent, M. (2008) 'Birth territory: the besieged territory of the obstetrician', in K. Fahy, M. Foureur and C. Hastie (eds), *Birth Territory and Midwifery Guardianship: Theory for Practice, Education and Research*. Edinburgh: Elsevier.

Olver, R., Walters, D. and Wilson, S. (2004) 'Developmental regulation of lung liquid transport', *Annual Review of Physiology*, 66: 77–101.

Pembroke, N. and Pembroke, J. (2008) 'The spirituality of presence in midwifery care', *Midwifery*, 24: 321–27.

Roberts, J. (1989) 'Maternal position during the first stage of labour', in M. W. Enkin, and M. J. N. Keirse (eds), *Effective Care in Pregnancy and Childbirth*. Oxford: Oxford University Press.

Roduit, C., Scholtens, S., Jongste, J. de, Wijga, A., Gerritsen, J. *et al.* (2009) 'Asthma at 8 years of age in children born by caesarean section', *Thorax*, 64: 107–13.

Romano, A. M. and Lothian, J. A. (2008) 'Promoting, protecting, and supporting normal birth: a look at the evidence', *Journal of Obstetric, Gynaecologic & Neonatal Nursing*, 37: 94–104.

Rossi, E. L. (2002) *The Psychobiology of Gene Expression*. London: W.W. Norton & Company.

Schlinzig, T., Johansson, S., Gunnar, A., Ekström, T. and Norman, M. (2009) 'Epigenetic modulation at birth – altered DNA modulation – methylation in white blood cells after caesarean section', *Acta Paediatrica* 98: 1096–99.

Schulkin, J., Schmidt, L. and Erikson, K. (2005) 'Glucocorticoid facilitation of corticotrophin-releasing hormone in the placenta and the brain: functional impact on birth and behaviour', in J. Schulkin and M. L. Power (eds), *Birth, Distress and Disease*. Cambridge: Cambridge University Press.

St Louis, M. E. and Hess, J. (2008) 'Climate change: impacts on and implications for global health', *American Journal of Preventive Medicine*, 35: 527–38.

Stearns, S., Nesse, R. and Haig, D. (2008) 'Introducing evolutionary thinking for health and medicine', in S. Stearns, and J. Koella (eds), *Evolution in Health and Disease*. Oxford: Oxford University Press.

Sternberg, E. M. and Wilson, M. A. (2006) 'Neuroscience and architecture: seeking common ground', *Cell*, 127: 239–42.

Strathearn, L., Mamun, A. A., Najman, J. M. and O'Callaghan, M. J. (2009) 'Does breastfeeding protect against substantiated child abuse and neglect? A 15-year cohort study', *Pediatrics*, 123: 483–93.

Tollanes, M., Moster, D., Daltveit, A. and Irgens, L. (2008) 'Cesarean section and risk of severe childhood asthma: a population-based cohort study', *The Journal of Pediatrics*, 153: 112–16.

Tracy, S. and Tracy, M. (2003) 'Costing the cascade: estimating the cost of increased obstetric intervention in childbirth using population data', *British Journal of Obstetrics and Gynaecology*, 110: 717–24.

Ulrich, R. and Zimring, C. (2004) *The Role of the Physical Environment in the Hospital of the 21st Century: A Once-in-a-Lifetime Opportunity*. Concord, CA: The Centre for Health Design.

Wilkes, G. and Krebs, W. (1982) *The New Collins Concise English Dictionary*. Sydney: Collins.

Yektaei-Karin, E., Moshfegh, A., Lundahl, J., Berggren, V., Hansson, L. *et al.* (2007) 'The stress of birth enhances in vitro spontaneous and IL-8-induced neutrophil chemotaxis in the human newborn', *Pediatric Allergy Immunology*, 18: 643–51.

9   Sustainable midwifery education

A case study from New Zealand

Sally Pairman

> Education is critical for promoting sustainable development and improving
> the capacity of the people to address environment and development issues
> ... It is critical for achieving environmental and ethical awareness, values and
> attitudes, skills and behaviours consistent with sustainable development and
> for effective public participation in decision making.
>
> (UN Conference on Environment and Development 1992)

The concept of sustainability within education is currently gaining ground
in both formal and non-formal learning in every sector of education around
the world (UNESCO 2009). The key aspects that are said to be integral to
sustainable education are: universal access to education, community participation and collaboration, and 'a curriculum that values creativity, innovation
and critical thinking and which promotes a global perspective applied to
local circumstances' (ATL 2009: 5). The challenges offered to educators and
institutions would seem to be to 'review, rethink and reform' their programme
content and delivery of courses to provide a clearer understanding of an
ecological, participatory worldview (ATL 2009: 1).

These tenets formed the foundation of a new jointly-owned Bachelor of
Midwifery programme commenced in 2009 by Otago Polytechnic and
Christchurch Polytechnic Institute of Technology (CPIT) across the South
Island of New Zealand. Developed collaboratively, the innovative programme
design increased access and flexibility for students that resulted in increased
student numbers. Midwifery teaching staff also gained more flexibility in
their workloads and were able to more effectively manage the demands of
teaching, practice, research and professional activity. Through sharing
resources and with increased student numbers Otago Polytechnic and CPIT
gained economies of scale that enabled cost-effective and efficient programme
delivery while still achieving strong academic standards. The Bachelor of
Midwifery programme at Otago Polytechnic and CPIT is now recognized as
professionally and educationally sustainable and there are positive signs that
once the programme is fully implemented in 2011 both schools will also secure
a sustainable financial position. This chapter provides a brief case study of
the new programme model, how it was developed and how it is being

implemented. It describes a model of sustainable midwifery education that may be useful to other institutions.

A brief overview of midwifery education

New Zealand is a small country with, in 2009, a population of 4.3 million and 62,540 live births (Statistics New Zealand 2010). Midwives are the main providers of the maternity services and in 2004 (the latest figures available) were chosen as Lead Maternity Carers (LMCs) by 75.9 per cent of women (NZHIS 2007). Although New Zealand has had a regulated midwifery work-force since 1904 the scope of practice and educational preparation of midwives has varied over the years in response to the wider context of the maternity and midwifery education systems (Pairman 2005; 2006).

The midwives of 1904 were educated through a direct-entry midwifery programme and practised autonomously in hospitals and the community as the main providers of maternity services (Pairman 2005; 2006). However, over the next 70 years the move to hospitals as the location for childbirth, the increasing involvement of doctors in maternity services and the increased use of technology in maternity care resulted in limitations to the role and scope of practice of midwives. By 1971 midwives mainly worked in hospitals in a more circumscribed scope assisting doctors as the main clinical decision makers in maternity care. Midwifery education had by then become a 'specialty option' for registered nurses undertaking advanced nursing education pro-grammes and direct-entry midwifery education was no longer available (Pairman 2005; 2006).

Through the combined political activity of midwives and women (con-sumers of maternity services) over the decade of the 1980s midwifery autonomy was reinstated in response to women's demands for significant changes to maternity services (Guilliland and Pairman 2010). Women wanted maternity services that were more responsive to their needs, provided choices and that recognized childbirth as a normal family life process rather than a medical event. Women believed that autonomous midwives were essential to bringing about such changes in the maternity services. In 1990 legislation was passed that enabled midwives to once again work within their full scope of practice and provide one-to-one midwifery care for women throughout pregnancy, labour, birth and the post-natal period to six weeks on their own responsibility (Guilliland and Pairman 2010). This legislation also opened the way for direct-entry midwifery education to once again be recognized as a route to midwifery registration. Women were no longer required to first complete a nursing programme and gain registration as a nurse before undertaking education to become a midwife.

In 1992 Otago Polytechnic and Auckland Technical Institute (now Auckland University of Technology, AUT) were the first two tertiary education organizations to be approved to develop and deliver these new three-year direct-entry midwifery programmes. By 1996 direct-entry midwifery programmes had also commenced at Waikato Polytechnic and Wellington Polytechnic (later incorporated into Massey University); Christchurch Polytechnic commenced its programme in 1997. Between them the five institutions prepared approximately 100 graduates each year, through Bachelor's level programmes, who met the standards for registration and commenced work as registered midwives.

Until September 2004 the Nursing Council of New Zealand was the regulatory authority responsible for midwives as well as nurses, and also set the standards for entry to the register of midwives. In 2003 the Health Practitioner's Competence Assurance Act established, among other things, the Midwifery Council of New Zealand (MCNZ), which then took over the regulation of midwives from the Nursing Council. One of the Council's first acts was to conduct a review of the existing five pre-registration midwifery education programmes.

Midwifery Council pre-registration midwifery education review

The Council undertook its review over 17 months from December 2004 to May 2006. It found that although graduates were competent at the point of registration the context of the maternity services had changed significantly over the 10–14 year timeframe during which these programmes had been operating. First, midwives now held a central role as the main caregivers within the maternity services. Second, first-time mothers were older and had more co-existing medical conditions. These changes meant that society had high expectations of midwives to manage the bulk of maternity care. New graduates needed to be both competent and confident in their practice and able to 'hit the ground running' as they entered the workforce. Finally, there was evidence of an existing and worsening midwifery workforce shortage that meant attention had to be paid to attracting midwifery students and improving access to midwifery programmes, ensuring graduates were well prepared for diverse practice, and developing mechanisms to retain registered midwives in the workforce long term (MCNZ 2006).

Following a consultative process with the midwifery community new standards for approval of pre-registration midwifery education programmes and accreditation of education providers were developed (MCNZ 2007a). These were adopted in July 2007 and all five schools of midwifery were notified of the requirement to review their programmes and make curriculum changes that would bring them into line with the new standards, to gain accreditation for the revised programmes from the relevant quality assurance body and to implement the revised programmes in either 2009 or 2010 (MCNZ 2007b).

The new standards sought to increase national consistency by setting more detailed standards; improve access by requiring flexible delivery modes and encouraging collaboration between schools; and increase levels of graduate competence and confidence by increasing midwifery practice hours and expectations, and better preparing midwives for their teaching roles. International consistency was achieved by aligning the new standards where possible with midwifery education standards in the European Union (Nursing & Midwifery Council 2004). This decision meant that the total hours of the programme were increased from 3,600 to 4,800, each academic year was extended from 34 weeks to 45 weeks, minimum midwifery practice hours were increased from 1,500 to 2,400 and minimum theory hours were increased from 1,500 to 1,920. The total credit value of the degree increased from 360 to 480[1] (MCNZ 2007b). Effectively this is the equivalent of a four (academic) year programme delivered over three calendar years, thereby providing significantly increased opportunity for midwifery practice experiences while at the same time producing new graduate midwives within a three-year time frame.

In its new standards the Council recognized the need to increase graduate numbers to help address the workforce shortage and meet the demands of the maternity service. Efforts to increase midwifery student numbers have, in the past, been constrained both by the reluctance of potential students to leave their family/whānau support in provincial and rural areas and by the limited access to midwifery practice experiences that is possible in the main centres where there is also competition from medical and nursing students. By requiring midwifery education to be delivered flexibly and by encouraging collaboration between education providers, the Council aimed to increase access to programmes for women in rural and provincial areas and to increase overall student numbers, which would result in increased graduate numbers. By requiring an extension to the academic year, the Council sought to maximize clinical learning opportunities for midwifery students by enabling access to maternity services and childbirth experiences at all times of the year and not only during the artificially shorter traditional academic year (MCNZ 2009a).

Impetus for change

The Midwifery Council's consultation on its draft education standards provided the impetus for the midwifery staff at Otago Polytechnic and CPIT to consider a collaborative approach to what was clearly going to be a requirement to revise existing midwifery programmes. As the only two midwifery schools in the South Island of New Zealand, the midwifery staff from Otago Polytechnic and CPIT already had well developed and positive relationships.

A key factor driving the need for change was the sustainability of the midwifery workforce and therefore the imperative to increase the number of midwifery graduates. The lecturers realized this provided a unique opportunity to achieve their vision of a transformed educational paradigm within midwifery education that would challenge the traditional style of classroom-based learning and embrace a blended learning approach. The vision included establishing student learning communities in rural and provincial areas of the South Island and building a sense of professional collegiality between midwives in these areas.

Both schools were small, each with approximately 60–70 equivalent full-time students (EFTS) and approximately six–nine full-time equivalent staff (FTE). Although academic outcomes were good, both schools struggled to meet the financial contribution margins expected by their respective organizations. Midwifery education was expensive with its requirement for significant one-to-one midwifery practice experience and individualized clinical supervision and assessment of students. The individualized nature of midwifery practice experience whereby each student had several placements working alongside one or two midwives in the provision of care to individual women and their families also limited overall student numbers such that it was difficult to achieve a cost-effective ratio of staff to students.

As well as financial viability there were other challenges for the midwifery schools. All midwifery teachers experienced multiple demands on their time that were difficult to manage. As lecturers teaching in a degree programme they needed to gain both teaching qualifications and higher degrees as well as demonstrate active engagement in research and ongoing professional development. As members of the midwifery profession lecturers were expected to maintain a practising certificate, which required them to undertake midwifery practice and also meet the Midwifery Council's recertification requirements through ongoing compulsory and elective education and professional activity.

To meet these myriad demands the midwifery staff of both institutions needed to find ways to make their programmes and schools financially sustainable and responsive to employer and professional expectations while at the same time maintaining high academic standards and meeting the needs of students and the wider midwifery profession. The imperative to redesign the existing Bachelor of Midwifery programmes in line with the Midwifery Council's new standards provided Otago Polytechnic and CPIT with an exciting and timely opportunity to develop a new model for midwifery education that would address these wider concerns.

In June 2006 midwifery educators from both institutions participated in a two-day 'retreat' to discuss collaborating on the development of a new programme. There was a longstanding and positive working relationship and philosophically lecturers in both schools shared beliefs about midwifery education. From a practical and resource utilization perspective the benefits of collaboration were obvious. What we did need to work on though was how we would collaborate and how we would ensure equal participation so that neither school would dominate. There were fears on both sides of 'take over' by the other and concern that the schools might lose their unique identities and in turn lose some of what made the schools and programmes successful and attractive to students and to staff. The process of working through these issues has been continuous and we could not have anticipated the level of commitment and goodwill that would be required by us all to make collaboration work.

By November 2006 we had developed a model we believed would address the financial, academic and professional issues we had identified and the heads of each school submitted a joint proposal for collaboration to the chief executives of each organization. The proposal was to jointly develop and implement a common curriculum for the Bachelor of Midwifery programme for the South Island. Expected benefits of collaboration included:

- Shared resources to meet the requirement from Midwifery Council for a revised programme that incorporated new standards for pre-registration midwifery education.
- Growth in student numbers through a new delivery model that enhanced flexibility and increased access for students living at a distance.
- Consistent approach to midwifery education across the South Island and maximisation of midwifery practice opportunities for students.
- Strengthening of existing collegial relationships between schools of midwifery and maximising of scarce resources through collaboration in implementation and delivery of programme.
- Efficiency gains in programme delivery that enable increased time for staff to engage in research and maintain currency in midwifery practice as well as improving financial viability of both schools.

(Pairman *et al.* 2006: 1)

The respective chief executives agreed to support the joint development of a single midwifery programme that would be jointly owned by both institutions and jointly delivered to students across the South Island. This was the first time Otago Polytechnic and CPIT had embarked on such an ambitious collaborative project and the different academic processes of each institution threw up various challenges in the development, approval and implementation phases of the project. To manage these challenges both teaching teams participate in regular meetings to discuss, negotiate and agree on matters of implementation and delivery and to work out together any issues that may arise. The time required for this level of discussion and negotiation should not be underestimated but we believe this effort leads to more robust decisions and a stronger programme in the long run.

Developing the model: a blank sheet of paper . . .

To develop the programme model we took a 'clean sheet of paper' approach to brainstorming our 'ideal' midwifery programme and drafting a curriculum model that captured the notion of a single programme delivered by two providers working in tandem. We sought to retain the strengths and positive and unique aspects of the existing programmes while at the same time developing an innovative educational model that would prepare midwives for the future.

We were influenced by work being undertaken in Scotland and Norway where doctors and nurses were both educated and embedded in rural communities and health services in a bid to keep them working in rural health services (Godden and Aaraas 2005). In Australia medical students were placed in rural medical centres with teaching from rural practitioners for the fifth year of the six-year programme and were able to meet the programme requirements to the same standard as those placed in urban areas (Maley *et al.* 2006). Key factors in the success of the rural placement programmes were adequate resources and infrastructure and supportive teaching and learning processes.

Satellites and student practice facilitators

Increasing access to women outside of the main centres was a key objective to increasing midwifery student numbers and addressing midwifery workforce shortages. Instead of all students accessing midwifery education through programmes delivered on campus in Christchurch (by CPIT) or in Dunedin (by Otago), we designed a model whereby women could remain for large portions of the programme in their local communities where they had existing support mechanisms. Students live in their rural, provincial or urban home base but are grouped together by geographic location to form several linking 'satellites', or student learning groups. Each satellite has an identified midwife known as the Student Practice Facilitator (SPF). The SPF is a local practising midwife who is employed by either Otago Polytechnic or CPIT and is responsible for coordinating local practice activities, running weekly face-to-face tutorials, teaching practical skills and providing pastoral support for students. In the main centres, where the student cohort is larger, students are also divided into small groups and allocated to midwifery lecturers who take on the SPF role for each group. The numbers of students in each satellite group varies from two to ten depending on their geographical location.

We divided the South Island between us with CPIT taking responsibility for all satellites in the upper South Island and on the West Coast and Otago Polytechnic with responsibility for those in the lower South Island and the lower North Island. We commenced the programme in 2009 with satellites in Invercargill, Central Otago, Dunedin/South Otago, Christchurch and Nelson/Marlborough. In 2010 we added satellites in the West Coast, South Canterbury and North Otago. Otago Polytechnic also commenced satellites in the lower North Island in Whanganui, Palmerston North and three groups in Wellington. There is significant communication between the satellites both formally through online tutorials and web-based 'discussion boards' and informally through student-initiated 'Facebook' interaction and email discussion groups.

Teaching and learning: blended delivery

Because midwifery is a relationship between each midwife and each woman (Guilliland and Pairman 1995) it was important that we maintained significant opportunities for face-to-face learning, even though the students were all in small groups that were at a distance from each other and from the main institutional campuses where most of the staff were located. We developed a model whereby teaching and learning takes place through a blend of online learning resources, face-to-face block courses (intensives), online tutorials, weekly face-to-face tutorials with the SPF, face-to-face midwifery practice and self-directed study. All groups, no matter where they are located, access the same electronic learning resources and participate in the same face-to-face 'intensives' where all students attend block courses in the main centres.

While learning in relation to theoretical knowledge, core skills and behaviours is facilitated by midwifery educators within both schools, students also learn alongside experienced midwives practising in the community and in maternity facilities, and through women and families who share their childbirth experiences. The programme draws on an apprenticeship model whereby students gain valuable midwifery practice experience and opportunities to integrate knowledge, skills, practise and professional behaviour through extended placements working one-to-one alongside experienced midwives.

Online learning resources

Online learning resources are provided through the Moodle learning management system. Each course has its own 'shell' on Moodle through which students can access packages of materials that guide their learning activities and reading. Each institution hosts half of the courses on each institution's Moodle platform but all students and staff are able to access all courses. The learning resources are developed mainly through the use of eXe, which offers a number of tools for interactive coursework design. Where large packages of information need to be provided to students such as videos, the material is copied to DVD and posted to students to reduce any problems with Internet connectivity or speed.

The online learning packages are supported with weekly online tutorials that are provided through a web-based virtual classroom, for example Elluminate or Adobe Connect. Students can access the website from computers in any location and join a virtual classroom for discussion in real time. This interactive technology enables students and staff to participate in tutorial discussions while at a distance and these tutorials, along with the face-to-face weekly tutorials with the SPF groups, ensure that students and staff remain connected with each other.

Intensives

Students are also required to attend fortnight-long blocks of face-to-face classes known as 'intensives'. The intensives provide the opportunity for students to build and maintain relationships with each other and with staff and for the delivery of some of the essential face-to-face teaching components of the programme. The intensives are held in Dunedin or Christchurch depending on the institution where each student is enrolled. There are three intensives in year one, three in year two, and two in year three. The focus in the first intensive, on building relationships and a sense of identity as midwifery students, was facilitated by taking students on a two-day overnight camp away from the campus.

Midwifery practice opportunities

Students access much of the required midwifery practice experience in their local community with support and supervision from local midwives. However, all students also require midwifery practice experiences in primary, secondary and tertiary maternity facilities (second and third year), in neonatal intensive-care units (second year), and in rural maternity settings (third year), and are therefore required to move at times to access these placements. For non-facility placements the focus is on students experiencing continuity of care by 'following through' women during pregnancy, labour, birth and the post-natal period. By the second year students are also gaining continuity experiences with midwives by working alongside individual midwives in the care of several women. In year three, students work one-to-one with midwives for long periods of time in a modified apprenticeship model. In most cases the SPFs are able to arrange placements for students in local maternity facilities, with local midwives and with pregnant women who have volunteered in response to newspaper and radio advertising, or at the request of their midwife. In Dunedin and Christchurch these placements are coordinated by one person to prevent duplication.

In developing a programme that can be delivered in the same way to students at a distance and in the main centres we have:

- created a standardized midwifery programme across the South Island;
- attracted more students to the midwifery programme;
- enabled students from diverse geographical areas to access the programme;
- begun to build a sense of professional collegiality and 'ownership' between midwives and midwifery students in satellite areas;
- maximized midwifery practice opportunities for students;
- supported students to undertake the majority of their study in their own area through a blended delivery model;
- enabled flexibility in programme delivery and learning to support students managing home, work and study requirements;
- begun to build learning communities among the student groups;
- enhanced maternity services outside the main centres;
- increased numbers of midwives and retention of midwives in rural and provincial New Zealand.

The programme emphasizes the application and integration of theoretical understandings and knowledge with women-centred midwifery practice across a variety of maternity settings. It recognizes the importance of midwives as practitioners grounded in midwifery's professional frameworks and responsible and accountable in their practice. The programme is designed to assist and guide midwifery students to acquire underpinning knowledge, skills, midwifery practice and professional behaviour essential for effective practice within the Midwifery Scope of Practice and the Competencies for Entry to the Register of Midwives.

Consultation

Consultation with women's organizations, midwives, District Health Boards, Māori, professional organizations, students, External Advisory Committees and others indicated strong support from stakeholders for this new programme model. Māori organizations believed that being able to study largely from home would make midwifery education more accessible to Māori women and would improve retention rates for Māori in the programme. Rural and provincial midwives saw that the opportunity for local women to become midwives would help create a stable long-term midwifery workforce. However, the wider midwifery community also identified potential barriers to successful implementation of the programme. These included existing professional isolation, particularly among rural midwives, lack of competence and confidence with electronic methods of communication including online, and a general lack of access to shared learning, support and professional development opportunities.

To address this concern Otago Polytechnic and CPIT succeeded in obtaining a grant from the Tertiary Education Commission[2] that was used to develop an interactive website to enhance communication and support for midwives, midwifery educators, students and pregnant women. The website, Midwifery Junction[3], provides information about the programme and has specific sections and resources for each user group. For midwives it provides professional development activities and continuing education on topics such as Preceptorship and a private discussion board to facilitate communication between midwives. The website provides a mechanism for information sharing, communication and support for all those involved in the programme.

Sustainability

While midwifery is practised primarily through relationships with women, it also requires midwives to work collaboratively with midwifery colleagues and other health professionals. This programme curriculum is based on the premise that midwifery is a sustainable model of practice, both for midwives and for society. Midwives can model less exploitative and more sustainable health care practices in order to support women and their families.

Sustainability is a key concept integrated throughout the programme encompassing not only environmental sustainability but also social, cultural, economic and emotional sustainability. There are specific sustainability courses in year one and year three and issues of sustainability are integrated into all courses within the programme.

The programme itself is also a model of educational sustainability. While both institutions and both midwifery schools retain their individual identity and utilize separate academic and management processes as required, the programme is jointly owned and delivered collaboratively. There is only one programme document. The online learning resources for each course were developed collaboratively by lecturers from both institutions but the result is a single set of learning resources accessed by all students. The costs of programme development, approval and accreditation processes and online resource development have been shared, making the project affordable for both institutions. The workload involved in this project would not have been possible for a single midwifery school but by combining resources and sharing the work both schools have effectively doubled their staffing numbers for no additional cost. Importantly, the opportunity to share the development and implementation between more midwives has drawn on the skills and knowledge of all staff and strengthened the programme.

The programme model of intensive blocks interspersed with online learning and local tutorials and practice has provided more flexibility for teaching staff to undertake their own midwifery practice or research. Delivery of the programme over 45 weeks of each year has increased the time available for students to undertake the required midwifery practice and it has also maximized access to available childbirth experiences across the year. The number of satellites available has increased access to women outside of the main centres and the blended delivery model has made full-time study flexible, manageable and sustainable for the students. By the active participation of practising midwives in the teaching and supervision of students the programme has become the focus of developing communities of learning and practice, particularly in rural settings. Long term, the programme supports sustainable maternity services in rural and provincial areas by ensuring continuing numbers of midwives for these workforces.

Collaboration between Otago and CPIT in the development and provision of this Bachelor of Midwifery programme has provided economies of scale and cost-effective delivery that will ensure the sustainability of midwifery education at these institutions for many years to come.

Conclusion

As two small separate schools it was almost impossible for the schools of midwifery at Otago Polytechnic and CPIT to be financially viable. Student numbers were too low and the nature of midwifery education meant that staffing numbers needed to be high and were therefore costly. In the small midwifery profession in New Zealand it was not always easy to employ midwives with postgraduate qualifications who wanted to be midwifery teachers. By working together on this jointly-owned and -delivered midwifery programme, these schools of midwifery have gained a more secure financial base that will ensure their survival as entities within their respective organizations.

Through the satellite programme model student numbers have increased as access has improved. Midwifery workforce shortages in rural and provincial areas are beginning to be addressed as women from those areas enter the midwifery programme. Shared resources and shared staffing has made the workloads of all midwifery teachers more manageable. Delivery of the programme is more efficient and there is no indication that the new model is any less effective or that academic standards are lower. On the contrary midwifery students have access to more midwifery practice experience throughout the programme and there are positive indications that the students are developing competence and confidence earlier. While the programme is only in its second year of implementation there are positive signs that this new model is financially, academically and professionally sustainable.

Notes

1   One credit is the equivalent of 10 learning hours. New Zealand Qualifications Authority. Available at: www.kiwiquals.govt.nz/about/credits.html (accessed 4 September 2009).
2   Encouraging and Supporting Innovation (ESI) fund.
3   www.midwiferyjunction.org.nz.

References

Association of Teachers and Lecturers (ATL) (2009) 'Sustainable education: review, rethink and reform', Position Statement, London. Online. Available at: www.atl. org.uk/Images/ATL%20sustainable%20education%20position%20statement.pdf (accessed 20 March 2010).
Godden, D. and Aaraas, I. J. (2005) 'Making it work 2. An articulation of challenges and solutions for health in rural and remote areas'. Conference report. Helse Nord, NHS Grampian, NHS Highland. Online. Available at: www.helse-nord.no/getfile. php/RHF/Prosjekter/Making%20it%20Work/Conference_Report_Making_it_ Work2.pdf (accessed 20 March 2010).
Guilliland, K. and Pairman, S. (1995) *The Midwifery Partnership Model for Practice, Monograph Series, 95/1*. Wellington: Department of Nursing & Midwifery, Victoria University.
Guilliland, K. and Pairman, S. (2010, forthcoming) *Women's Business: The History of the New Zealand College of Midwives from 1986 to 2010*. Christchurch: New Zealand College of Midwives.
Maley, M., Denz-Penhey, H., Lockyer-Stevens, V. and Campbell Murdoch, J. (2006) 'Tuning medical-education for rural-ready practice: designing and resourcing optimally', *Medical Teacher*, 28, 4: 345–50.

Midwifery Council of New Zealand (MCNZ) (2006) *Pre-registration Midwifery Education Review Report*. Wellington: Midwifery Council of New Zealand.

Midwifery Council of New Zealand (MCNZ) (2007a) *Pre-registration Midwifery Education Review – Summary Report*. Wellington: Midwifery Council of New Zealand.

Midwifery Council of New Zealand (MCNZ) (2007b) *Standards for Approval of Pre-registration Midwifery Education Programmes and Accreditation of Tertiary Education Organisations*. Wellington: Midwifery Council of New Zealand.

Midwifery Council of New Zealand (MCNZ) (2009) unpublished letter from MCNZ to Tony Ryall, Minister of Health, 19 August 2009.

New Zealand Health Information System (NZHIS) (2007) *Report on Maternity. Maternal and Newborn Information 2004*. Wellington: Ministry of Health.

Nursing and Midwifery Council (2004) *Standards of Proficiency for Pre-registration Midwifery Education*. London: Nursing & Midwifery Council.

Pairman, S. (2005) 'From autonomy and back again: educating midwives across a century'. Part 1, *New Zealand College of Midwives Journal*, 33: 4–9.

Pairman, S. (2006) 'From autonomy and back again: educating midwives across a century'. Part 2, *New Zealand College of Midwives Journal*, 34: 11–15.

Pairman, S., Baddock, S., Kensington, M. and Anderson, J. (2006) Proposal to CEOs Christchurch Polytechnic Institute of Technology and Otago Polytechnic for collaborative midwifery programme between schools of midwifery at Otago Polytechnic and Christchurch Polytechnic Institute of Technology, 23 November 2006, unpublished paper.

Statistics New Zealand (2010) website: Online. Available at: http://search.stats.govt.nz/nav/ct2/population_births/ct1/population/0 (accessed 3 March 2010).

UNESCO (2009) *Review of Contexts and Structures for Education for Sustainable Development*. Paris: UNESCO.

United Nations Conference on Environment and Development (UNCED) (1992) Promoting Education, Public Awareness and Training, *Agenda 21*, Geneva.

10 Mentoring new graduates

Towards supporting a sustainable profession

Mary Kensington

> We are in the grip of a midwifery crisis with many of us about to retire. In order to have a sustainable workforce we need to train and support our graduates. In the same way we look after mothers – we gently support them, then we step back and let them go – we must do the same with our new midwives. We can assume a side by side role very quickly as they gain confidence and knowledge to operate independently.
>
> (*Midwifery News* 2007: 15)

Midwifery autonomy in 1990 opened up the possibility for a radical change in the way maternity services were delivered in New Zealand (NZ). Today the model of caseloading[1] midwifery in NZ is held up internationally as an ideal model. However, achieving autonomy required an enormous transition and significant changes within the maternity system and midwifery under-graduate education. At times changes have been so great that some midwives have not trusted nor understood the implications of autonomy. For new graduates entering the workforce this has created difficult tensions and times of disillusionment and feeling unsupported. This has seen a recent emphasis placed on how to mentor new graduates for autonomous practice.

The focus of this chapter is mentoring of new graduates as a way of providing professional support for midwives, in an effort to sustain growth and development of the profession by ensuring they make the transition to a confident independent practitioner. The first part of this chapter looks at existing knowledge on mentoring relationships and transition to autonomous practitioners. The concepts of 'mentoring' and 'preceptorship' will be briefly explored as there is much overlap and confusion between these terms and they are often used interchangeably within the literature. The next part of this chapter reports on examples of mentoring within New Zealand where there has been a particular commitment made to mentoring new graduates. Findings from research examining experiences of midwives who were mentored in their first year of self-employed practice (Kensington 2005) will be discussed alongside a follow-up study of midwives who have completed the Bachelor of Midwifery degree from Christchurch Polytechnic Institute of Technology (CPIT) (Daellenbach *et al.* 2006). Since these studies, the commitment of the profession to supporting new graduates has been realized through the first government-funded support for all new graduates called the Midwifery First Year of Practice (MYFP), which was established in 2007 and includes a mentoring component. Further examples of innovative ways to think about sustainable mentoring for midwifery graduates are presented, for example, group mentoring (Lennox 2008, 2009) and e-mentoring (Stewart and Wootton 2005a, 2005b; Stewart 2006).

Literature: what is mentoring?

Athough there is no real consensus on a definition of mentoring, the literature describes the mentoring relationship as a dynamic and complex concept that can be 'naturally or artificially contrived to benefit individuals within a sharing partnership' (Morton-Cooper and Palmer 2000: 39). In classical mentoring the relationship is informal and has as its central focus a partnership based on mutual trust. The relationship is set up naturally and not artificially contrived, whereas formal mentoring, also known as contract or facilitated mentoring, is usually determined by the organization and has a recognized programme of development and support (Morton-Cooper and Palmer 2000). Mentoring involves two people negotiating a relationship in which their personal qualities, philosophies and priorities will interact to influence the nature, direction and duration of the resulting partnership. It is based on mutual respect and common values and, at its core, the process is shared, encouraging and supportive. For the mentored person, having someone who is willing to give them support, encouragement and guidance, enables them to come to terms with their role in the organization or professional setting (Morton-Cooper and Palmer 2000).

Preceptorship

Preceptorship offers a period of support for a defined period of time and endeavours to ease the transition into professional practice or socialization into a new role (Bain 1996). The preceptor role, which is usually assigned, provides orientation and support, and teaching and sharing of clinical skills. It is characterized by a relationship where one person teaches, instructs, supervises or coaches another (Donovan 1990; Bain 1996).

Although mentoring and preceptorship have some similarities, essentially they are discrete and unique. Much of the confusion has arisen in the UK where the term 'mentor' usually relates to a relationship with a student (Watson 2000) whereas 'preceptor' is reserved for the support of a new graduate within an institution. The difficulties and confusion has been compounded by the Nursing and Midwifery Council in the UK adding to the mentor's role 'assessment of competence in a range of appropriate practice skills' when working with the student (Davis 2007: 16; Bray and Nettleton 2007). This creates a moral dilemma for the mentor who on the one hand is providing support and guidance and yet on the other hand is assessing and judging the student's progress (Anforth 1992). This dual role is 'contrary to the values and principles of the traditional models of mentoring' (Nettleton and Bray 2008: 206).

Transition to autonomous practice

The literature confirms that the first months especially, and in some cases the first year, can be a stressful time for newly qualified nurses and midwives as they make the transition from student to a registered practitioner (Gerrish 2000; Jackson 1995; Hobbs and Green 2003; Van der Putten 2008). There is no research, other than the study I undertook, that looks at the transition from student to independent midwife. However, there are a small number of studies that detail the transition from student to a graduate midwife working in a hospital setting. These studies identify similar themes to those studies detailing the transition from student to graduate nurse. These themes are: building confidence; the need to gain clinical experience; adapting to the organizations' needs and culture, and 'fitting in' (Jackson 1995; Hobbs and Green 2003; Van der Putten 2008). Other areas identified in these studies as causing stress are coping with new responsibilities; conflict between one's personal philosophy and the constraints placed by the organization, and balancing conflicting ideologies of woman-centred care within a hospitalized system of maternity care (Brady 2008; Van der Putten 2008).

The studies either identify that clinical support and mentorship or preceptorship was critical during the transition period from student to confident autonomous practitioner (Hobbs and Green 2003; Van der Putten 2008), or recommendations were made for the provision of a formal support structure (Jackson 1995; Brady 2008; du Plessis 2008). Irrespective of where midwives go to work they want support as they transition to a confident practitioner.

Emergence of mentoring in New Zealand

Mentoring appeared in discussions and debates within midwifery literature following the Nurses Amendment Act 1990 (Holland 2001; Kensington 2005). This Act granted midwives professional autonomy, thereby introducing a system of maternity care that enabled midwives to establish themselves as independent practitioners offering their services to women both within the home and hospital (Department of Health 1990). The 1990 Act established midwifery as a separate profession to nursing and approved direct-entry midwifery education. The first six years of independent midwifery[2] within NZ was during a period of much uncertainty and significant changes in the health system (Abel 1997; Barnett and Malcolm 1997; Hornblow 1997). During this time it became increasingly evident that there was a need to develop a system of supporting midwives into independent practice (Kensington 2005).

The move from hospital to independent practice in the community was very new and not trusted. The graduates from the three-year direct-entry programmes were especially affected as there was uncertainty and questions about the suitability of the new midwifery education. There was little faith in their ability to practice outside of the hospital, to the extent that in some parts of the country (for example, Auckland, Lower Hutt and Dunedin) they were only granted a temporary access agreement and needed to be supervised for 20 births, with requirements also made of the supervisor/mentor (Kensington 2005). Effectively these restrictions on new graduates implied that they needed further training.

The push to develop a structured system of supporting midwives appears to have come from two major sources: from the access agreements a midwife required with a maternity facility and from the professional impetus of the New Zealand College of Midwives (NZCOM).

The NZCOM acknowledged that midwives moving into self-employed practice, whether new graduates or experienced hospital midwives, may need support, but emphasized that the nature and existence of such a relationship is the prerogative of the individual midwife. The NZCOM consensus statement on mentoring ratified in 1996 described the nature of the relationship between the two registered midwives as one of partnership where the mentor will listen, challenge, support and guide the mentored midwife. It also clearly stated that the mentored midwife remains responsible for her own practice (NZCOM 1996). This was an important step for the College, because if it had upheld the view that a mentor had control over the mentored midwife's practice, then they would have been agreeing with the restrictive practices of the maternity facilities and would effectively be saying that the new midwifery education was not adequate (Kensington 2005).

Since 1996 there has been continued discussion on mentoring and recognition of the need to develop a mentoring framework (Gray 2006). The discussion raised a number of questions. What kind of support then did midwives graduating from the degree programmes want and what was their experience as they made the transition into professional practice?

Examples of mentoring in New Zealand specific to midwifery

A qualitative study I completed involved in-depth interviews with nine midwives about their experiences of being mentored (Kensington 2005). The participants came from throughout NZ and had all graduated through Bachelor programmes in NZ. Five midwives joined established midwifery practices and had individual mentors within the practice. Three midwives, separately, established practices with other new graduate colleagues and were mentored by midwives outside of their midwifery practice. One midwife joined an established practice and was supported by the entire practice. She chose not to have a named mentor.

In December 2005, midwifery lecturers from the School of Midwifery at CPIT commenced a follow-up study of all the midwives who had graduated through the CPIT Bachelor of Midwifery programme since it began in 1997 (Kensington *et al.* 2006; Daellenbach *et al.* 2006). The follow-up study involved two phases. Initially data was collected through a confidential postal questionnaire and then complemented by focus group interviews. An area of particular interest in this research was to find out what assisted graduates to make the transition from student to midwife. The questionnaire provided an opportunity to collect some quantitative data about the kinds of mentoring relationships midwifery graduates from CPIT arranged and to explore whether these may have implications for workforce retention. The categories for the questions on mentoring emerged from Kensington's research (2005).

Both studies (Kensington 2005; Kensington *et al.* 2006) found that there was considerable variability in what constitutes a mentoring relationship in New Zealand. Some of the participants had mentors from within the practices that they joined, while others arranged mentors from outside the practice. The mentor's role in both groups was overwhelmingly one of providing support and advice, although it is acknowledged that the word 'support' has many meanings. Where the mentor was based within the practice, the participants expected their mentor to be available for either discussion of cases or to attend/assist at labours/births. The majority from both studies had 24-hour access to their mentor. In Kensington's (2005) study mentors had offered to be available 24 hours, seven days a week. These participants stated that the availability and accessibility of their mentor ensured that support and, for some participants, gave them the confidence to extend their practice even further. For the graduates who had a mentor outside of the practice 'support' was different. The support ranged from emotional, business and/or practical support and information, to scheduled meetings to listen, facilitate discussion and assist reflection. Interestingly where graduates did not have a mentor to attend births, many had a practice partner who attended the first births with them.

Other studies (Darling 1984; Spouse 1996) recount similar findings where the mentor's main roles are described as providing support and investing time and energy into the relationship, plus offering advice and strategies to the mentored person. Interestingly, in relation to investing time, none of these studies refer to the mentor being so readily available. The mentor availability in these studies supports the assertion that a positive mentoring relationship enhanced self esteem and increased self confidence in the mentored person (Earnshaw 1995; Morton-Cooper and Palmer 2000). It also supports the proposition that the mentoring relationship is based on an individually negotiated partnership; hence availability will be different for each mentored person.

Factors that were significant for the graduate midwives in Kensington's study (2005) in determining a successful relationship were trust, having a similar philosophy to their mentor, knowing their mentor and choice of mentor. These factors ensured the midwife felt safe, comfortable and secure while they gained further confidence. Feeling safe (50 per cent), knowing their mentor (42 per cent) and having a similar philosophy (46 per cent) were also reported in a postal survey of 684 midwives conducted by Stewart and Wootton (2005a) and supported by NZCOM. Respect of the mentor's midwifery practice (56 per cent) was another important consideration. The literature concurs that successful mentoring relationships are those naturally set up and based on a partnership of trust and mutual respect of each other (Earnshaw 1995; Spouse 1996):

> It was quite difficult really because I wanted someone who I could really trust. That was the big thing for me and feel comfortable with . . . I wanted someone that was very experienced, well not very, it was more trust was a big thing, it was just someone I could trust that I could go to about any queries or concerns . . .
>
> (Anne in Kensington 2005)

> She's got a very strong philosophy as normal and that was really, really important for me . . .
>
> (Robyn in Kensington 2005)

Most of the participants remarked that having an experienced mentor was important, however, what emerged from both studies (Kensington 2005; Stewart and Wootton 2005a) is that a shared philosophy and a positive attitude towards women and midwives were considered equally worthy attributes. This is consistent with Morton-Cooper and Palmer's (2000) description of a mentoring relationship as two people sharing common values and working together to support their philosophies. Similarly, Darling (1984) emphasizes the aspects of mutual attraction and respect between the mentor and the mentored person as key to a successful mentoring relationship. For graduate midwives in New Zealand 'knowing your mentor', 'trust' and 'respect' were clearly identified as significant factors in achieving a successful mentoring relationship.

The graduates understood autonomy and their responsibility and accountability to women and the profession when they were registered as a midwife. However, making the transition to a confident independent practitioner can be challenging and stressful at times. The participants in both studies (Kensington 2005; Kensington *et al.* 2006) identified that they required support to establish confidence in their midwifery practice and to assist at those times they felt uncertain and vulnerable particularly in relation to negative attitudes from some other midwives. Zoe appreciated her mentor because she enhanced her confidence and provided reassurance but also understood that she was accountable for her own practice:

> . . . if anything it gave me more confidence to be independent and do my own bit and they were never threatening or condescending, never made

me feel like I was doing the wrong thing. Or just come and support ...
And then if something wasn't going properly I could say what do you
think and they'd say I think you need to do this now. It wasn't that I
was made to feel that I wasn't knowledgeable or anything. It was just
somebody to reflect the situation back on what was in the room

(Zoe in Kensington 2005)

However, the following excerpt explains why the mentor role could also be
seen at times as a protector (Kensington 2005):

I don't know what the political situation is like elsewhere but I know at
certain shifts at certain times of the day at [the hospital] you might have
a group of midwives that are working, that wouldn't necessarily be very
supportive of somebody that's gone directly out into independent practice
and in a situation like that I needed somebody who would support me,
be around me if I was in a situation where I just needed help and I needed
assistance or I wanted to bounce advice off somebody.

(Sophie in Kensington 2005)

For the graduate, at times there was a real fear of being exposed as incompetent
or doing something wrong, plus an unwillingness of some core midwives to
provide support when asked in secondary/tertiary facilities. The mentor's
presence provided a supportive relationship and gave security. Unsurprisingly
it was during the labour and birth, at a time when midwifery practice can
be unpredictable and demanding, that the midwives felt most vulnerable and
uncertain. The midwives' narratives illustrated how in their first year of
practice they were challenged and tested and often felt as if they were 'on
trial', having to prove themselves and 'do time' (Kensington 2005). They were
not accepted as a 'full' midwife and had to prove their knowledge of practical
skills, use of equipment and that they were competent practitioners. Practical
experience was valued more by their midwifery colleagues than the compre-
hensive theoretical and evidence-based education they receive (Kensington
2005). Surtees' research (2003) also reported a finding of graduates' lack of
practical experience being rated a higher concern than the added value of their
theoretical knowledge. Midwifery was seen as 'essentially a practical profession'
(Surtees 2003: 227).

At times the mentor also took on a protector role when the midwife was with
a client in the secondary/tertiary facility and met an unsupportive environment.
While some core midwives were supportive, graduates also encountered core
staff who were lacking generosity and a willingness to help until they had
proven themselves (Kensington 2005). This was also seen with some of the self-
employed midwives. Lack of support and hostility from other midwives and
health professionals was the most commonly-cited challenge in the graduate
follow-up study (Daellenbach *et al.* 2006). Some of the comments from
respondents included 'hostility (or rather a blatant lack of support) from more

senior experienced midwives'; 'hospital culture of not supporting new graduates'; 'expectation from core staff was that we should know everything as a new grad'; and 'hurtful comments/attitudes' (Daellenbach *et al*. 2006). In these circumstances the mentor's role can be seen as pivotal to the graduate midwife. Of note in this study is that midwives who had a mentor available at any time less frequently reported experiencing hostility/lack of support than respondents who did not have this kind of mentoring. Although not statistically significant, nor generalisable to the wider experiences of new graduates entering into caseloading, it would be worthwhile exploring in further research to see if this form of mentoring relationship is more positive for new graduates.

The research (Kensington 2005; Stewart and Wootton 2005a; Kensington *et al*. 2006) discussed confirms that there are a variety of mentoring arrangements in NZ without suggesting any of these are more beneficial or effective than any other. They also substantiate the viewpoint that graduate midwives want practice support and especially a supportive relationship to assist them in the transition to a confident practitioner (Hobbs and Green 2003; Brady 2008; du Plessis 208; Van der Putten 2008). Mentoring is the word that has been chosen in New Zealand to represent the relationship set up to support a midwife to develop professional confidence (NZCOM, 2000), however practice support is also a valued form of support. Where midwives do not have their mentor attend births they have a practice partner or other midwives to provide support. Practice support sits alongside mentoring in assisting the new graduate to become a confident practitioner.

Midwifery First Year of Practice (MYFP)

In May 2006 the Minister of Health (NZ) announced funding for a two-year pilot to provide professional support for new graduates. The Midwifery First Year of Practice (MYFP) began in 2007 and an evaluation took place in 2008.

The establishment of the MFYP was a culmination of many years' work by the NZCOM to establish a formal mentoring programme for midwives. Research by Kensington (2005) and Stewart and Wootton (2005a) was critical to highlighting the positive aspects when informal mentoring arrangements are successful and also raised some of the more concerning issues new graduates face in the workforce. The research provided the NZCOM with evidence to substantiate its claims when making submissions to the government to make mentoring a priority for workforce concerns.

The vision for the Midwifery First Year of Practice encapsulates the intention of this programme to build a sustainable base for the New Zealand midwives workforce in the future by ensuring graduates are 'well-supported, safe, skilled and confident in their practice' (Clinical Training Agency 2009: 1).

The MFYP offers a structured programme of professional support where graduate midwives have to apply (it is not mandatory) and mentors have to opt in and attend training workshops. Key components of the MFYP programme are mentoring of the graduate midwife; attending compulsory and elective education and development; familiarization with the opposite practice setting (graduate midwives who work as a core midwife in a maternity facility or with a caseload are eligible to apply) and attending a Midwifery Standards Review at the end of the year (Clinical Training Agency 2009). Financial reimbursement is included in this package. Although this programme has formal specifications it does encourage a classical mentoring approach in that new graduates choose their own mentor.

As noted in the previous studies, graduates value the supportive relationship mentoring offers:

> Having Deb as my mentor gave me confidence to ask lots of questions – she never made me feel those questions were very silly – and that gave me so much confidence.
>
> (*Midwifery News* 2007: 15)

For midwives who have previously mentored the MFYP programme has provided official recognition and acknowledgment for a role they have always provided and notes the two-way benefits of a mentoring relationship:

> Mentoring has always been happening but until now we have not had a structured programme in place, and we have never been financially acknowledged.
>
> (*Midwifery News* 2007: 15)

> It has also renewed my enthusiasm by helping remind me why I became a midwife in the first place . . . We learn from them as they are close to the research and all the new knowledge. That keeps us going and also keeps public confidence growing.
>
> (*Midwifery News* 2007: 15)

The two-year pilot was deemed a success and funding has been secured for a further three-year period, 2009–11, with the New Zealand College of Midwives continuing to be the provider (Shaw 2009).

Alternative approaches to mentoring

Group mentoring

Sue Lennox presents a new exciting take on mentoring that challenges the assumptions that one-to-one mentoring should be accepted practice in midwifery. In 2005, Lennox led an action research project where four midwifery clinicians provided mentoring support for one year for four midwifery graduates to facilitate their transition from student to autonomous practitioner working as a caseload midwife (Lennox 2008, 2009). The opportunity had presented itself because four members of a recent graduate group were unable to find a mentor, so they approached Lennox and her colleagues, which resulted with the idea of meeting within a group. For the clinicians, group mentoring provided them with the opportunity to mentor where the one-to-one system had not been possible due to their other work commitments and not having time to commit to a mentoring relationship (Stewart and Wootton 2005a). The group initially attended a peer mentoring workshop and then met weekly. The weekly meeting time was set up as a safe space for sharing experiences where the emphasis was on creating opportunities to share stories, challenge situations and questions but remain non-judgemental and non-critical (Lennox 2009).

The graduates had 24 hours/seven days a week on-call back up available where each of the mentors was available on a rotational weekly basis. Within the first six months 87 calls were received, of which 60 were managed on the phone (Lennox 2009). The peak number of calls came in March, which is not unexpected given that the graduates would have begun practising as midwives in late December/January and often do not begin attending labour/births until March/April. For the rest of the year there were relatively few calls. The new graduates worked in pairs, which was a key to building their professional and clinical confidence. For the first three to six months they would attend labour/births together (Lennox 2009). This finding is similar to that found in other studies (Kensington 2005; Kensington *et al.* 2006) where the new midwives who set up in practice together would support each other at births in the first months. This experience not only provided each midwife with support, but also gave them the opportunity to gain extra experience, which helped to increase their confidence (Kensington 2005; Kensington *et al.* 2006).

The weekly meetings became the linchpin to the success of the group mentoring. They were very structured and all eight members took turns at sharing the facilitation (Lennox 2009). The commitment of all members to attend the meetings, plus the sharing of food and laughter, Lennox (2009) stated was quintessential to the success of this project. The focus of the weekly meetings was on storytelling and sharing experiences. There was much discussion of ethical issues, working collaboratively with others and the complexity of negotiating/managing the working environment – people and systems. There was also opportunity to discuss managing stress and work/life balance (Lennox 2009).

This approach is worthy of serious consideration as an alternative sustainable model of mentoring for midwives who are committed to working within a small group. This model ensures midwifery practitioners/leaders are able to take up the opportunity to mentor and share their knowledge and expertise within a group setting. Group mentoring has the potential to promote diversity of thinking, practice and understanding. For the new graduate it can allay their fear of a mismatch with their mentor and at the same time they are able to share stories/experiences with the practice wisdom of more than one mentor.

E-mentoring

In today's world of technology electronic communication has the ability to offer an alternative creative strategy to providing supportive mentoring relationships to midwives 'disadvantaged by geographical and cultural isolation' (Stewart and Wootton 2005a: 41). E-mentoring includes use of email, online discussion groups, bulletin boards, instant messaging and video conferencing. Although 75 per cent of participants in the NZ survey felt mentoring should be carried out by face-to-face contact and in a formal pre-arranged meeting, it also identified that a number of new graduates were unable to acquire a mentor because of geographical isolation and a shortage of mentors (Stewart and Wootton 2005a, 2005b; Stewart 2006). A pilot study was carried out in 2006 where a NZ midwife mentored two new graduates using a secure email system (Stewart 2006). The mentor and mentored midwives found the experience valuable to the extent that it was continued for the rest of the year. For the mentor the asynchronous nature of email offered flexibility in that it can take place at any time of day or night so readily fits with a midwife's busy life. Interestingly, although the mentored midwives both had face-to-face support they appreciated the opportunity offered through email of time to reflect away from the clinical environment, plus the degree of anonymity offered where the mentor lived in a different place (Stewart 2006). E-mentoring has the potential to provide another sustainable model of mentoring for midwives to consider. As a tool for support and professional development it transcends the barriers of location and culture and provides a greater range of choice for the person being mentored (Stewart 2006).

Conclusion

Mentoring is a viable solution to assist the transition from student to confident and competent practitioner as demonstrated in a number of small studies. Providing support to new graduates working as a self-employed or core midwife has the potential to increase the retention and sustainability of the midwifery profession. Comparable studies (Ehrich *et al.* 2002) in teaching and nursing suggest mentoring does reduce the attrition rate of new professionals/graduates. Supporting new graduates through mentoring programmes will ensure the continued access for women in all settings and enhance consumer and maternity services. To support and nurture new graduates is to protect and invest in the future of midwifery.

Notes

1   Caseloading midwives are those who act as Lead Maternity Carers (LMCs). They may be self-employed or employees of an organization. They provide continuity of care for clients from early pregnancy until six weeks post-natal. A LMC is an authorized practitioner and can be a midwife, general practitioner or an obstetrician who has been selected by the woman to provide her maternity care under Section 88 of the New Zealand Public Health and Disability Act 2000.

2 An independent midwife or self-employed midwife provides continuity of care to individual women and their families and is able to claim from the Ministry of Health for their service fees.

References

Abel, S. (1997) 'Midwifery and maternity services in transition: an examination of change following the Nurses Amendment Act 1990', thesis submitted for a Doctor of Philosophy in Anthropology, University of Auckland.

Anforth, P. (1992) 'Mentors, not assessors', *Nurse Education Today*, 12: 299–302.

Bain, L. (1996) 'Preceptorship: a review of the literature', *Journal of Advanced Nursing*, 24: 104–7.

Barnett, P. and Malcolm, L. (1997) 'Beyond ideology: the emerging roles of New Zealand's crown health enterprises', *International Journal of Health Services*, 27, 1: 89–108.

Brady, V. (June 2008) 'Meaning and perspective – the essence of transition from student to midwife', paper presented at International Confederation of Midwives 28th Triennial Congress, Glasgow.

Bray, L. and Nettleton, P. (2007) 'Assessor or mentor? Role confusion in professional education', *Nurse Education Today*, 27: 848–55.

Clinical Training Agency, (2009) 1/B53: Midwifery first year of practice programme interim specification. Ministry of Health. Online. Available at: www.moh.govt.nz/moh.nsf/pagesmh/8946/$File/consult-interim-myfp.pdf (accessed 3 March 2010).

Daellenbach, R., Kensington, M. and Laurenson, M. (2006) 'Becoming a midwife: a follow-up study of midwives who have graduated from Christchurch Polytechnic Institute of Technology (CPIT)', unpublished report, CPIT.

Darling, L.W. (1984) 'What do nurses want in a mentor?' *The Journal of Nursing Administration*, October: 42–44.

Davis, S. (2007) 'Mentoring: understanding the new standards', *The Practising Midwife*, 10, 6: 16–19.

Department of Health (1990) *Nurses Amendment Act 1990: Information for Health Providers*. Wellington: New Zealand Health Department.

Donovan J. (1990) 'The concept and role of mentor', *Nurse Education Today*, 10: 294–98.

Earnshaw, G. (1995) 'Mentorship: the student's views', *Nurse Education Today*, 15: 274–79.

Ehrich, L., Tennent, L. and Hansford, B. (2002) 'A review of mentoring in education: some lessons for nursing', *Contemporary Nurse*, 12, 3: 253–64.

Gerrish, C. (2000) 'Still fumbling along? A comparative study of the newly qualified nurse's perception of the transition from student to qualified nurse', *Journal of Advanced Nursing*, 32, 2: 473–80.

Gray, E. (2006) 'Midwives as mentors', *New Zealand College of Midwives Journal*, 34: 24–27.

Hobbs, J. and Green, S. (2003) 'Development of a preceptorship programme', *British Journal of Midwifery*, 11, 6: 372–75.

Holland, D. (2001) 'Practice wisdom: mentoring – a personal analysis', *New Zealand College of Midwives Journal*, 23: 15–18.

Hornblow, A. (1997) 'New Zealand's health reforms: a clash of cultures', *British Medical Journal*, 314: 1892–94.

Jackson, S. (1995) 'Do midwives need preceptorship?' *British Journal of Midwifery*, 3, 7: 372–86.

Kensington, M. (2005) 'Mentoring in New Zealand midwifery: the liminal journey the midwife makes in the transition to an independent autonomous practitioner', unpublished Master's degree thesis, University of Otago.

Kensington, M., Daellenbach, R. and Laurenson, M. (October 2006) 'The role of the mentor and practice support for new graduate midwives', paper presented at Women and Midwives, Conscious Guardians, 9th Biennial NZCOM conference, Christchurch.

Lennox, S. (June 2008) 'Group mentorship of bachelor of midwifery graduates into community based midwifery practice', paper presented at International Confederation of Midwives 28th Triennial Congress, Glasgow.

Lennox, S. (September 2009) 'Research evidence challenges accepted wisdom', paper presented at Joan Donley Midwifery Research Collaboration, New Zealand College of Midwives, Nelson.

Midwifery News (2007) 'Mentoring, midwifery first year of practice', *New Zealand College of Midwives Midwifery News*, 47: 15.

Morton-Cooper, A. and Palmer, A. (2000) *Mentoring, Preceptorship and Clinical Supervision: A Guide to Professional Support Roles in Clinical Practice*, 2nd Edition. Oxford: Blackwell Science.

Nettleton, P. and Bray, L. (2008) 'Current mentorship schemes might be doing our students a disservice', *Nurse Education in Practice*, 8: 205–12.

New Zealand College of Midwives. (NZCOM) (1996) Consensus Statement: Mentoring, National Committee meeting, November.

New Zealand College of Midwives. (NZCOM) (2000) Consensus Statement: Mentoring, National Committee meeting, September.

Plessis, D. du (June 2008) 'What is happening to newly qualified midwives?' paper presented at International Confederation of Midwives 28th Triennial Congress, Glasgow.

Shaw, A. (2009) 'The midwifery first year of practice pilot programme', *New Zealand College of Midwives Midwifery News*, 52: 17.

Spouse, J. (1996) 'The effective mentor: a model for student-centred learning', *Nursing Times*, 92, 13: 32–35.

Stewart, S. (2006) 'A pilot study of email in an e-mentoring relationship', *Journal of Telemedicine and Telecare*, 12: 83–85.

Stewart, S. and Wootton, R. (2005a) 'Mentoring and New Zealand midwives: a survey of mentoring practice amongst registered midwives who are members of the New Zealand College of Midwives', *Centre for Online Health*, University of Queensland, Brisbane.

Stewart, S. and Wootton, R. (2005b) 'A survey of e-mentoring among New Zealand midwives', *Journal of Telemedicine and Telecare*, 11: 90–92.

Surtees, R. (2003) 'Midwifery as feminist praxis in Aotearoa/New Zealand', thesis submitted for a Doctor of Philosophy in Education, University of Canterbury.

Van der Putten, D. (2008) 'The lived experience of newly qualified midwives: a qualitative study', *British Journal of Midwifery*, 16, 6: 348–58.

Watson, S. (2000) 'The support that mentors receive in the clinical setting', *Nurse Education Today*, 20: 585–92.

11 Good housekeeping in midwifery practice

Reduce, reuse and recycle

Ruth Martis

> Midwifery is a profession based on promoting normalcy. Essentially it is an art of service, in that the midwife must recognize, respond to and cooperate with natural forces. In this sense the midwife's work is ecologically attuned, involving the wise utilization of resources and respect for the balance of nature.
>
> (Davis 1987: 5)

Midwifery practice interacts with the environment on a daily basis. This chapter intends to encourage midwives to rethink the use of transportation, tele-communications and the consumption of equipment in relation to 'reducing, reusing and recycling' in midwifery practice.

There are no black and white practical sustainable solutions. Any usage of technology, equipment, communication, anything needed to support and sustain life on this planet will have an effect on the environment and on people. It is how the effect is minimized that matters. Professional responsibility and accountability requires midwives to critically reflect what they use in every day midwifery practice and how they interact with the woman and her family.

Midwives must explore their attitude toward the concept of obsolescence; buying for the sake of buying, following the latest market fad, discarding adequate and functional equipment such as a mobile phone, for one with a better look or only slight functional improvement. Good midwifery house-keeping is about maintaining and repairing equipment. This requires a major behavioural change. It also provides an opportunity to share this information with prospective parents.

One effective approach to ascertain what is good housekeeping practice is to assess a product's lifecycle. This includes the materials and energy used, the design and engineering, how it is manufactured and packaged, as well as how it is being transported, sold, used and disposed of at end of its life (Trombetti 2009). Providing manufacturers with clear feedback from a lifecycle perspective will enable reassessment of their product and effective change.

Midwifery by its nature is a low technology and high touch profession (Spencer 2004). Midwives across the world describe themselves as guardians of normal birth (Davis 2004). It has been suggested that midwifery therefore has the potential to stand as a 'carbon footprint model of excellence' for the twenty-first century (Davies 2008). While midwives use a variety of equipment in their practice, being the guardian of normal birth enables the midwife to use appropriate assessment tools and carry out interventions only when they are required.

Elizabeth Davis's (1987) quote at the beginning of this chapter describes midwifery as being attuned ecologically and applying wisdom and respect to nature. In practise this means continually attempting to reduce environmental impact through implementation of sustainable practice. Concerns have been raised about the use of disposable equipment in midwifery practice. Current debate focuses on disposable stainless steel suturing instruments and the accumulation of waste from all disposable equipment (Adler *et al*. 2005).

Reusing or reprocessing disposable stainless steel instruments and other equipment has been documented as positively impacting the environment through reduction in landfill waste and toxic manufacturing by-products. Some critics argue that it is easier for damage and malfunction to occur with equipment produced for one use only, while others highlight the difficulty of removing all potential contaminants such as metal flakes and human tissues from reusable instruments (Sloan 2007). There is no evidence in the literature specifically relating to the benefits of disposable perineal suture packs. Increasingly many midwives use them, supplied through local hospitals influenced by aggressive marketing and consumer-friendly packaging. As routine episiotomies are unnecessary (Carroli and Mignini 2009), episiotomy scissors should be provided in sterilized single packs. These packaging options and commercial practices make it difficult for midwives to make ecologically attuned decisions, especially as reusable stainless steel scissors, forceps and needle holders are far more expensive and seldom used. Davies (2008) argues that there is something special about owning instruments that are precision crafted and feel strong. The less robust substitutes in the pre-packed disposable labour packs, she argues, do not offer the same reassurance.

In addition to pollution and waste, there is the question about what uses more energy; autoclaving reusable equipment or the making and discarding of disposable equipment? While the literature is inconsistent as many variables influence the cost factor, it does appear that the use of disposable equipment is more expensive over time as compared to the initially higher cost of reusable stainless steel equipment, with low cost autoclaving (Yang *et al*. 2000).

Plastic packaging, unsterile and sterile gloves, protective sheets, syringes, containers, cord clamps and cord clamp removers are some of the disposable plastic items used in midwifery practice. Disposable plastic items are marketed as being cheaper and cleaner than sterilizing used equipment without informing the buyer about the environmental factors. Biohazard plastic is usually incinerated, as it reduces waste in landfills and saves health care facilities money. Most plastic is made from polyvinyl chloride (PVC), which is the least recyclable plastic and when manufactured or incinerated emits dioxin into the environment. The accumulation of dioxin has been shown to have carcinogenic effects in humans and animals (Institute of Medicine 2003).

Low-level exposure to dioxin has been associated with decreased birth weight, learning and behavioural problems in children, suppressed immune function and the disruption of hormones (Institute of Medicine 2003).

Another environmental chemical emission, Bisphenol A (BPA), has been recently debated in the literature and media. Bisphenol A is released from polycarbonate plastic during heating, for example, warm liquid being poured into the plastic container. BPA is used frequently to make plastic baby bottles, water bottles and plastic cups, as well as the lining inside food cans. BPA is a synthetic oestrogen similar to diethylstilbestrol (DES) and is linked to an increase in prostate cancer, hormonal changes, decreased sperm production, early onset of puberty (Institute for Agriculture and Trade Policy 2005) and chromosomal changes (Collaboration on Health and the Environment 2009). A study by Schonfelder *et al.* (2002) identifies that BPA accumulates in the placenta, exposing the fetus to BPA before birth. Sugiura-Ogsawara *et al.* (2005) found an association with recurrent miscarriages. This discovery has assisted the emergence of bio-based plastics, which are often vegetable-based using corn, potatoes or rice. While these containers are biodegradable and are addressing the environmental effects of plastic, there needs to be further exploration whether in the long term it produces a carbon neutral effect.

Does this mean that midwifery practice should not include the use of plastic products? Reusing, recycling and reducing the amount of plastics used in midwifery practice would contribute considerably towards a sustainable zero-waste approach.

Jeannine Parvati-Baker (2003) identified the essential tools needed in midwifery practice as the midwife's hands, eyes, ears and heart. If these were the tools midwives applied first in midwifery practice then the principles of sustainable practice would follow naturally (Tritten 2008). For example:

- to touch women with hands for abdominal palpation to ascertain the baby's position and well-being, not with technologies such as ultrasound transducers or disposable tape measures;
- to listen to the baby's heartbeats with the genuine sound detection of a wooden Pinard stethoscope, not with an electronic monitoring tool that uses energy and potentially produces harmful sound waves;
- to use washable, reusable linen rather than disposable plastic/paper sheets;
- to use clean cotton towels and face cloths in labour and birth and for drying the baby, rather than paper towels;
- to use recyclable glass containers for testing and measuring body fluids, not disposable plastic containers;
- to promote upright and mobile labour and birth positions that remove some of the need for expensive technologically advanced delivery beds;
- to use massage and words of encouragement instead of pharmaceutical products for pain relief and the associated plastic equipment requiring incineration.

Observing and assessing labour with 'midwifery eyes', as suggested by Parvati-Baker (2003), would potentially reduce the practice of routine vaginal examination in normal labour and therefore the need for extensive use of sterile gloves and their waste disposal. Plastic cord clamps could be replaced by plaited cotton or silk cord ties, lovingly created by the prospective parents welcoming the baby with a handmade gift. This also encourages their bonding experience with the baby. Lotus birth of the placenta, where the cord remains until natural separation takes place, is another option. Both options reduce the use of plastic. Instead of using the biohazard human waste system for the placenta, it can be buried (Birthtoearth 2010), as a biodegradable option. (See Box 11.1 for further birth kit examples.)

Good housekeeping in midwifery practice also incorporates sustainable recommendations for everyday household items. This includes the use of rechargeable batteries and compact fluorescent light bulbs (CTLs), as well as knowing where and how to recycle. Sharing equipment between midwives, such as a sonic aid, or renting equipment, such as oxygen cylinders, are also ways of acting responsibly. While this appears to be more applicable for midwives working in community settings, with creative thinking this also applies to any maternity setting.

Managing communication is an essential component of good midwifery practice, whether it is writing on paper, using computers, mobile phones or pagers. Midwives have embraced technology to manage their business, keep in contact and cut overheads. Any communication tool needs to be assessed from a lifecycle perspective. This is sometimes difficult to achieve. Contextualization can be one effective approach to developing local sustainable midwifery solutions for communication. The example from the Philippines illustrates this well:

> When I was in the Philippines in an area where there was no access to electricity or to solar powered computers and limited access to paper the practice of women-held notes was the best sustainable option during pregnancy. This meant that all the essential information about the woman and the midwifery care provided was recorded on recycled paper. The woman kept the notes and brought them with her whenever she had midwifery care or needed to leave the island for specialized obstetric care. This worked well, as it reduced the duplication of paper notes and enabled the women to feel empowered. The majority of women were unable to read but they knew about the importance of their notes as a vital communication tool between health professionals. There was rarely an issue about notes being lost.

Where electricity is freely available, digital documentation of care has become the norm. Patient information systems have become more compatible, enabling paperless transfer and networking of health care files between them, including referrals to other health professionals and laboratory and medical

Box 11.1 A birth kit example

Suzie was working as a team midwife for a busy hospital. As a team midwife she was able to attend home births, as well as attending births at a small maternity unit nearby and normal births at the tertiary hospital. Recently, Suzie was challenged by Karen, a pregnant woman, to go 'green'. Suzie critically assessed her birthing equipment and rearranged what she was going to use for Karen's planned homebirth. Here is a sample of what Suzie carried in her birth kit:

- stethoscope and sphygmomanometer;
- wooden pinard;
- latex-free sterile gloves;
- pen and notes for documentation;
- scales for weighing the baby;
- uterotonics;
- tourniquet;
- blood test tubes and vacutainers;
- IV giving set and IV fluids;
- sterile reusable suturing set;
- suturing material;
- local anaesthetics;
- small portable oxygen bottle;
- neonatal bag and mask;
- mucous extractor;
- sterile episiotomy scissors;
- dip sticks for urine testing.

Here is a sample of what Karen provided:

- clean linen and towels;
- clean sanitary pads;
- clean bucket;
- cord ties for the baby;
- biodegradable container for the placenta;
- a mirror;
- hot water bottle;
- torch with rechargeable batteries;
- camera;
- energy drinks;
- snack food.

Suzie used the first five items on her list for the home birth, and everything on Karen's list. It is worth reflecting why this might have been so.

Box 11.2 Requirements for a computer to be identified as eco-friendly

1 Reduced levels of cadmium, lead and mercury;
2 energy efficiency, less than 100 watts usage, led (light-emitting diode) lamps for buttons that need to light up or the use of non-light buttons;
3 recyclable computer casing, e.g. made out of wood or recycled aluminium;
4 smaller size;
5 recyclable packing;
6 ease of up-grade, which means the computer is being used for longer;
7 instructions for use come on a CD, not on printed paper;
8 safe recycling options when the computer is no longer useable;
9 facility to ensure regular back-up of files being stored on the computer;
10 manufacturer's specification state that the computer is carbon neutral.

---

imaging results. Midwives need to consider a number of issues across digital data regarding confidentiality, storage and ethics, which are outside the scope of this chapter.

It has been stated in the media that during the manufacture of desktop and mobile computers, and Personal Digital Assistants (PDAs), more water is wasted, more energy consumed and more toxic waste is created than by the manufacture of automobiles (Paperboy 2007). In response to this, many countries have established Environmental Protection Agencies (EPA) (see for example Environmental Protection Authority of New Zealand (2009), Environment Agency United Kingdom (2010) or United States Environmental Protection Agency (n.d.)) that identify eco-friendly computer standards and encourage computer manufacturers to register their compliance with them (refer to Box 11.2).

Telephones and mobile phones are everyday communication tools within continuity of care midwifery practice. The use of various pager systems, email and online social networking websites such as Facebook has increased. Before considering the impact of these types of communication methods on the environment and climate change, the impact on the woman receiving midwifery care must be considered first. Mobile phones are a quick way to transfer information but can be disruptive during antenatal and post-natal appointments, as well as during labour and birth. It can disturb the trust relationship between the woman and the midwife, as illustrated with Louisa's story:

Louisa, a 26-year-old woman, is expecting her fist baby. She is in strong labor. The light in the room is dimmed and relaxing music is playing quietly in the background. Louisa is coping well. Sarah, the midwife, has been providing continuity of care throughout Louisa's pregnancy. When Sarah's mobile phone rings, she answers the phone. It is one of her other women who thinks she is in labour. The phone call interrupted the atmosphere in the room. Louisa is getting distressed and feels she cannot cope any longer with her contractions. As soon as Sarah is off the phone Louisa asks for an epidural.

While the example above might not be a frequent occurrence it does illustrate how mobile phones are often disruptive during times when providing one-to-one care for women. Sarah Buckley (2005) and Michel Odent (2002) both describe the importance of undisturbed hormones to enable the birth process to unfold in its unique way. Midwives need to be mindful of when and where they answer their mobile phones.

Mobile phone calls, text or SMS messages are often not documented or even deleted. Increasingly midwives record sent or received SMS messages directly into their appointment diary, including time and date of the message. This ensures a documentation trail, which can be transferred at any stage into the woman's notes. Mobile networks do not guarantee immediate delivery (or pick up) of SMS or pager messages. Delivery delays mean that it is sometimes better practice to advise women to make positive contact by phone for urgent issues. Sustainable midwifery practice needs to ensure that all electronic documentation and messages can be easily accessed, are stored securely and are protected against fire; the same principles that apply for preserving paper documentation.

In recent years, health concerns about the use of mobile phones have been raised (Ahlbom *et al.* 2009). Mobile phones are low-power devices that emit and receive radio waves, connecting them to a network. Research has been inconclusive about the effect of radio waves, which have been used for over a century since the radio (wireless) was invented. It has been established that radio waves emitted above a certain level can cause heating effects in the body, but it is unclear if this causes a health concern. There is some evidence that mobile phone use can cause changes in brain activity (Moulder *et al.* 1999) and possibly increase the risk of developing a brain tumour (Myung *et al.* 2009). It is possible to measure the Specific Absorption Rate (SAR) of radio wave energy in humans. International guidelines, adopted by many countries, identify standards for low levels of radio wave exposures. Each mobile phone sold in those countries requires identification of the relative SAR information (Mobile Manufacturers Forum n.d.) (see Box 11.3 for further communication tips).

Mobile phones are owned and discarded at a prodigious rate, contributing to non-biodegradable landfill waste (Sahu and Srinivasan 2008). Many countries now recycle unwanted mobile phone as fundraisers. The Starship Children's

Hospital in New Zealand has frequent mobile phone recycling appeals. Old and unwanted phones are refurbished and sold on by a company, with a percentage of the proceeds donated to the hospital (Starship Children's Health n.d.). Many outlets selling mobile phones and other electronic devices now recycle unwanted electronic equipment. While it is believed that this approach is making some difference with waste disposal, it does not address the concept of obsolescence, as discussed at the beginning of this chapter.

The media has encouraged carbon emission neutrality (Global Platform for Disaster Risk Reduction 2009). It is questionable whether a carbon neutral approach is applicable for good housekeeping in midwifery practice. The New Oxford American Dictionary (2005) defines being carbon neutral as calculating your total climate-damaging carbon emissions, reducing them where possible, and then balancing your remaining emissions, often by purchasing a carbon offset – paying to plant new trees or investing in 'green' technologies such as solar and wind power. The carbon neutral approach is currently debated as being fundamentally flawed as an effective approach to climate change. It does not address attitudinal changes and it may well support 'business as usual' and not lead to any real reduction in energy consumption, and therefore the impact on climate change will be minimal (Smith 2007).

Box 11.3 Sustainable telecommunication tips

1 Do not print out emails unless absolutely necessary.
2 Use unbleached paper.
3 Print on both sides.
4 Hand-held notes for pregnant women.
5 Maintain computer, mobile phones and other technological products regularly and repair. Recycle if beyond repair.
6 Use compatible computer software enabling paperless communication between different patient information systems.
7 Keep mobile phone conversations as short as possible.
8 Hands-free mobile phone kits are available, which will reduce close radio waves, as well as addressing the safety aspect when driving.
9 Clearly document text/SMS messages, including date and time.
10 Mobile phone chargers need to be turned off when they are not charging the phone, otherwise they will continue draining energy.
11 Understand clearly that obsolescence and carbon neutral are two concepts that are ineffective for behaviour change of sustainability.
12 When it is absolutely necessary to purchase a new mobile phone, recyclable options need to be considered. Some companies are now offering mobile phones with biodegradable casing.

Midwives from high-income countries invariably will identify that a car is an absolute necessity for their work, whether this is for use in the community or for travelling to work at a hospital. This expectation seems reasonable at the onset but when explored further, questions of lifestyle and events that created this belief need to be addressed.

Could midwives give consideration to walking or bicycling to work in a hospital setting with set working hours? Car pooling or using public transport could be further options for reducing greenhouse gas emission (Cairns *et al.* 2004). Would it be possible for midwives who work in the community to only provide midwifery care to pregnant women and their families who are living at bicycle distance?

> In my homebirth practice I was able to use the bicycle when clients were not living far from my house. I remember distinctly a mother and baby with breastfeeding challenges, which required me to bicycle to their house every three hours for 72 hours. A good light source, reflective vest and helmet enabled safe night bicycling. I had a sturdy box on the bicycle carrier for my post-natal equipment. Most of the time it worked well although sometimes I required a backpack for additional equipment, e.g. loaning out a breast pump. Bicycling provided me with some physical exercise for which otherwise I had little time with a busy family and home birth practice, while at the same time contributing responsibly to global sustainability.

It is estimated that climate changing greenhouse gases from car driving, oil refining, car manufacture and road and bridge building make the transportation sector responsible for about 45 per cent of energy-related emissions (Baer and Singer 2009). The health impact of climate changes and outdoor air pollution has been discussed and well documented in the literature (Raupach *et al.* 2007; Connie 2007; World Health Organization (WHO) 2009).

There are many considerations that community-based midwives need to make when selecting a vehicle, including economy, load space and reliability. There is also the practical factor for vehicle selection, for example when the midwife has a busy city practice, engaging in many short trips with frequent stopping, or if the midwifery practice includes mainly rural travel and is sometimes over difficult terrain. The purpose of this section is to particularly consider the ecological impact of operating a vehicle (see summary in Box 11.4).

Hybrid cars with both electric and petrol engines are one option and are being marketed as the future answer to reducing greenhouse gas emissions. However, they are still very expensive, and even when used in their best environment of start/stop city driving they still provide only minor savings in the total cost of travel. Development is ongoing in hybrid cars and with many options now appearing, the utility of these may improve significantly in the future (Greenfootsteps 2009). Cost-effective petrol-engine cars, highly efficient diesel cars and fully electric vehicles are other options. Fully electrical cars have a practical daily range of less than 150 km, so therefore are useful only for small city driving. Small diesel cars, though more expensive to service if not regularly maintained, are very economical for longer-distance daily travel (Poudenx and Merida 2007).

The total cost of ownership and environmental impact are not easily compared, but it is still probably safe to comment that the economics, efficiency and emissions of a small diesel car continue to make it the current best choice (Sullivan *et al.* 2004). The use of a manual rather than an automatic car can provide an instant fuel saving of 15 per cent (Troung 2009).

For midwives who have the additional requirements of driving in more difficult rural conditions such as snow, mud, and generally unsealed roads or tracks, there is likely a need to invest in a four-wheel-drive vehicle. This will cost more both in terms of purchase price and running costs. The environmental impact of these vehicles is greater, and 'off-road' oriented vehicles

---

Box 11.4 Tips for any vehicle selection

1 Driving smoothly and anticipating traffic conditions ahead, to minimize the use of braking and accelerating to stay in the flow of traffic, will reduce gas emission.
2 Turning off the air conditioning when it is not needed reduces the load on the engine and therefore will use less fuel.
3 Reducing the drag resistance of the vehicle by:
   • keeping the tyres properly inflated;
   • winding windows up;
   • removing the roof rack if not in use;
   • taking all heavy equipment out of the boot.
4 Using a manual rather than an automatic car can provide an instant 15 per cent fuel saving.
5 Updating driving skills will reduce the risk of out-of-control accidents and help improve driving fuel consumption (note that driver training is frequently tax deductible). If using a four-wheel-drive car regularly, ensure driving skills match the capability of the vehicle.
6 Select a vehicle that is promoted as being mostly recyclable.
7 Ensure that vehicle equipment can be repaired rather than just thrown away.
8 Buy a second-hand vehicle or keep your vehicle longer.
9 Regular maintenance will ensure less greenhouse emission and a longer life for the vehicle.
10 Consider walking, bicycling, car pooling, public transport or clientele base in close proximity.

are considered less safe in terms of stability and crash protection when compared to similar-sized road vehicles. To minimize the ecological impact it is advisable to choose a modern, lighter vehicle, diesel powered, with manual transmission to optimize the two- or four-wheel drive according to the conditions (Sullivan *et al* 2004).

The Australian Government Submission to the UN Framework Convention on Climate Change (2007) published figures that highlight that motorcycles and motor scooters use less fuel compared to other transport methods. Choosing a motorcycle depends on the travel environment (city, country, off-road), but the seat should be low enough to sit on while the rider has both feet flat on the ground and light enough to be picked up if it falls over. Rider protective clothing needs to fit well with substantial body armour and a back protector fitted. This also means a good quality helmet, leather boots and gloves. Appropriate types of lockable carrier fittings need to also be considered to store the birthing equipment safely. In London and Bangkok where traffic often comes to a complete standstill, using a motorbike can be a real option to arrive in time for a birth.

Aviation is an increasing source of climate-changing pollution (Eilperin 2010). In Europe, greenhouse gas emission from aviation increased by 87 per cent between 1990 and 2006 (EU press release 2006). A plane pumps out eight times more CO_2 per passenger mile than a train. Aircraft emissions go directly to the stratosphere and therefore have more than twice the global warming effect than emissions from cars at ground level. A return flight from London, England to Sydney, Australia will release as much CO_2 as all the heating, light and cooking for a house in a year (McCarthy *et al.* 2005).

Air travel is not a common transport in relation to midwifery practice. However, maternal and child health research projects, as well as conferences, require midwives to travel by air. Increasingly conferences are being held online or offered in a virtual environment. The Australian Breastfeeding Association (ABA) has been holding an annual online lactation conference for the past four years, which is well attended and enables access from home to well-known international lactation experts (Global Online Lactation Discussion n.d.). Using teleconferencing means midwives have flexibility to listen and contribute in real time with internationally-recognized speakers, or be part of clinical practice guideline development panel meetings or other opportunities such as mentoring online.

To reduce travel and increase accessibility to midwifery education, a number of education providers have embraced interactive online resources. Some providers are also starting to introduce midwifery students to using virtual life as a platform for practicing real life scenarios. Additionally educators are encouraging students to create online midwifery communities through email lists or other web-based social networks (Stewart 2008).

The issues raised throughout this chapter and the lack of evidence in the literature for sustainable midwifery practice might lead to the encouragement of establishing a 'green midwifery movement'. Midwives need to be able to access unbiased evidence to guide their environmental approach to midwifery practice. They need to be able to discuss ecological issues within a professional forum and share appropriate information with parents. A number of online social networks have already been established by midwives, but they are less known and often found accidently. It would be timely to establish some strong global network fora assisting midwifery to be at the forefront of sustainable best practice.

References

Adler, S., Scherrer, M., Rückauer, K. D. and Daschner, F. D. (2005) 'Comparison of economic and environmental impacts between disposable and reusable instruments used for laparoscopic cholecystectomy', *Surgical Endoscopy*, 19, 2: 268–72.

Ahlbom A., Feychting M., Green A., Kheifets L., Savitz D. A. *et al.* (2009) 'Epidemiologic evidence on mobile phones and tumor risk: a review', *Epidemiology*, 20, 5: 653–55.

Australian Government Submission to the UN Framework Convention on Climate Change (April 2007) National Inventory Report 2005 – Volume 1 (for the Kyoto protocol). 'Ride to work'. Online. Available at: http://ridetowork.org.au/?page_id=20 (accessed 3 March 2010).

Baer, H. and Singer, M. C. (2009) *Global Warming and the Political Ecology of Health: Emerging Crises and Systemic Solutions*. Walnut Creek, CA: Left Coast Press.

Birthtoearth (2010) Online. Available at: www.birthtoearth.com/ (accessed 16 March 2010).

Buckley, S. (2005). *Gentle Birth, Gentle Mothering*. Brisbane: One Moon Press.

Cairns, S., Sloman, L., Newson, C., Anable, J., Kirkbride, A. *et al.* (2004) 'Smart choices – changing the way we travel'. UK Department of Transport. Online. Available at: www.dft.gov.uk/pgr/sustainable/smarterchoices/ctwwt/chapter1intro duction.pdf) (accessed 15 March 2010).

Carroli, G, and Mignini, L. (2009) 'Episiotomy for vaginal birth'. *Cochrane Database of Systematic Reviews*, 2009, Issue 1.

Collaboration on Health and the Environment (2009). 'Girl, Disrupted: Hormone Disruptors and Women's Reproductive Health, A Report on the Women's Reproductive Health and Environment Workshop'. Bolinas: Collaborative on Health and the Environment. Online. Available at: www.healthandenvironment. org/articles/doc/5492 (accessed 13 February 2010).

Connie, A. (2007) 'Climate change and human health', *Geography Compass*, 1, 3: 325–39.

Davies L. (October 2008) 'Carbon footprint model of excellence', Conference proceedings. New Zealand College of Midwives Conference, Auckland, New Zealand.

Davis, E. (1987) *Heart and Hands*. 2nd Edition. Berkeley: Celestial Arts Publishing.

Davis, E. (2004). *Heart and Hands*. 4th Edition. Berkeley: Celestial Arts Publishing.

Eilperin, J. (2010). 'Cutting the global carbon footprint of planes and ships'. *The Washington Post*. 4 January 2010. Online. Available at: http://views.washingtonpost. com/climate-change/post-carbon/2010/01/cutting_the_global_carbon_footprint_ of_planes_and_ships.html (accessed 6 March 2010).

Environment Agency United Kingdom (2010). Online. Available at: www. environment-agency.gov.uk/ (accessed 16 March 2010).

Environmental Protection Authority New Zealand Te Mana Rauhï Taiao (2009) Online. Available at: www.epa.govt.nz/ (accessed 16 March 2010).

EU press release (20 December 2006). 'Climate change: commission proposes bringing air transport into EU Emissions Trading Scheme'. Online. Available at: http://europa.eu/rapid/pressReleasesAction.do?reference=IP/06/1862 (accessed 8 March 2010).

Global Online Lactation Discussion (n.d.) Online. Available at: www.goldconf.com/ (accessed 15 March 2010).

Global Platform for Disaster Risk Reduction (2009). 'The second session of the Global Platform will be carbon neutral!' Press release. Online. Available at: www.prevention web.net/globalplatform/2009/carbon/ (accessed 31 March 2010).

Greenfootsteps (2009). 'Transport options for the present and future'. Online. Available at: www.greenfootsteps.com/transport-and-fuel.html (accessed 6 March 2010).

Institute for Agriculture and Trade Policy (2005). 'Smart plastics guide, healthier food uses of plastic'. Online. Available at: www.iatp.org/foodandhealth/ (accessed 15 February 2010).

Institute of Medicine (2003) *Dioxins and dioxin-like compounds in the food supply: strategies to decrease exposure.* Washington, DC: National Academies Press.

McCarthy, M., Woolf, M. and Harrison, M. (2005) 'Energy bulletin', 27 May, *The Independent*. Online. Available at: www.energybulletin.net/node/6372 (accessed 11 March 2010).

McKean, E. (ed.) (2005) *The New Oxford American Dictionary*. 2nd Edition. New York: University Press.

Mobile Manufacturers Forum (n.d.). 'Specific Absorption Rate (SAR) information'. Online. Available at: www.mmfai.org/public/sar.cfm (accessed on 12 March 2010).

Moulder, J. E., Erdreich, L. S., Malyapa, R. S., Merritt, J., Pickard, W. F. *et al.* (1999) 'Cell phones and cancer: what is the evidence for a connection?', *Radiation Research*, 151: 513–31.

Myung, S. K., Ju, W., McDonnell, D. D., Ji Lee, Y., Kazinets, G. *et al.* (2009) 'Mobile phone use and risk of tumors: a meta-analysis', *Journal of Clinical Oncology*, 27, 33: 5565–72.

Odent, M. (2002) 'The first hour following birth: don't wake the mother', *Midwifery Today*. Spring, 61: 9–11.

Paperboy (19 July 2007) 'Conita technology review. Eco friendly wooden computer'. Online. Available at: www.conita.com/Computers/244.html (accessed 6 March 2010).

Parvati-Baker, J. (2003) 'Instinctive birth: finding the pulse', *Midwifery Today*. Winter, 68.

Poudenx, P. and Merida, W. (2007) 'Energy demand and greenhouse gas emission from urban passenger transportation versus availability or renewable energy: the example of the Canadian Lower Fraser Valley', *Energy*, 32: 1–9.

Raupach, M. R., Marlands, G., Ciais, P., Le Que're, C. Canadell, J. G. *et al.* (2007) 'Global and regional drivers of accelerating CO_2 emissions', *Proceedings of the National Academy of Sciences (PNAS)*. 104, 24: 10288–93.

Sahu, S. and Srinivasan, N. (2008) 'Mobile phone waste. Current initiatives in Asia and the Pacific', *TECH MONITOR*, July–August 2008.

Schonfelder, G., Wittfoht, W., Hopp, H., Talsness, C. E., Paul, M. *et al.* (2002) 'Parent bisphenol A accumulation in human maternal-fetal-placental unit', *Environmental Health Perspective*, 110, 11: A703–A707.

Sloan, T. W. (2007) 'Safety-cost trade-offs in medical device reuse: a Marcov decision process model', *Health Care Manage Science*, 10: 81–93.

Smith, K. (2007) *The Carbon Neutral Myth Offset Indulgences for Your Climate Sins.* Amsterdam, the Netherlands: Transnational Institute.

Spencer, K. M. (2004) 'The primal touch of birth: midwives, mothers and massage', *Midwifery Today*, Summer 70, 11–13: 67.

Starship Children's Health (n.d.). Online. Available at: www.starship.org.nz/index.php/pi_pageid/1659 (accessed 31 March 2010).

Stewart, S. (2008). 'Computer-mediated social networking for mentoring health professionals', in M. Purvis, and B. T. R. Savarimuthu (eds) *Computer-Mediated Social Networking*. Berlin, Germany: Springer-Verlag.

Sugiura-Ogsawara, M., Ozaki, Y., Sonta, S., Makino, T. and Suzumori, K. (2005) 'Exposure to bisphenol A is associated with recurrent miscarriage', *Human Reproduction*, 20, 8: 2325–29.

Sullivan, J. L., Baker, R. E., Hammerle, R. H., Kenney, T. E., Muniz, L. *et al.* (2004). 'CO_2 emission benefit of diesel (versus gasoline) powered vehicles', *Environmental Science and Technology*, 38, 12: 3217–23.

Tritten, J. (2008) 'Technology: stemming the tide'. *Midwifery Today*, Spring, 85: 1–2.

Trombetti, J. (2009) 'DOTmed Industry sector report: disposables'. Online. Available at: www.dotmed.com/news/story/8561/ (accessed 16 March 2010).

Troung, L. (2009) '108 Tips to Raise Your Fuel Economy'. Online. Available at: www.wisebread.com/108-best-fuel-economy-tips (accessed 3 March 2010).

US Environmental Protection Agency (EPA) (n.d.) Online. Available at: www.epa.gov/ (accessed 3 March 2010).

World Health Organization (WHO) (2009) 'Health impact of climate change needs attention'. Online. Available at: www.who.int/mediacentre/news/notes/2009/climate_change_20090311/en/index.html (accessed 9 March 2010).

Yang, R., Ng, S., Nichol, M. and Laine, L. (2000) 'A cost and performance evaluation of disposable and reusable biopsy forceps in GI endoscopy', *Gastrointestinal Endoscopy*, 51, 3: 266–70.

Section three

Supporting an ecological approach to parenting

12 Parents as consumers

Lorna Davies

Despite the claim that we are seeking to leave a better world for our children, we know at another level that we are doing no such thing. We are eating up their future, devouring their resources, recklessly squandering their substance in the pursuit of our here and now; what we may bequeath them is a wilderness, a burnt out and desecrated planet.

(Jeremy Seabrook 1987)

The word 'consumer' is broadly used to describe the users of goods and services generated within an economy. The more we consume, the more rapid the rate of economic growth, which within our current mainstream worldview is held as economic success. Consumer choice has been heralded as holding the potential to improve our lives and drive economies. The word 'consumer' is derived from the Latin word 'consumere', which means to burn up, destroy and devour, but for the last 100 years or so the word has become synonomous with 'pleasure, enjoyment and freedom' (Goldsmith 1996: 118). Consumerism rests on the assumption that the economy will continue to grow. But progressively more economists, as well as ecologists, are beginning to recognize that unharnessed growth is not compatible with finite resources. It has been reported that we have used more goods and services since 1950 than in all the rest of human history (Worldwatch Institute 2008). Increasingly, critics are asking the question 'how much more can the earth take in supporting the drive for more and more?' A question that has been asked by ecopsychologists (a discipline that brings together psychology and ecology) is, does consumerism make us happy? It has been argued that there can be too much choice of consumer products, which can lead to artificially raised expectation, stress and confusion. (Norwood 2006; Irons and Hepburn 2007; Schwartz 2006).

In this chapter it is intended to explore the impact of consumerism on modern parenting with particular reference to concepts such as time poverty and ethical consumerism. The current Western (and increasingly non-Western) generation of reproductive age have been brought up in a consumerist world where, as an established part of that culture, they may find it challenging to stand back and look objectively at the cultural mores. The marketing messages that they have received throughout their lives will almost certainly have influenced their perceptions, their values and their behaviours (Walker 2005: 15). It has been reported, for example, that American children rank Ronald McDonald as second only to Santa Claus in terms of recognition (Boje and Rhodes 2006). Manufacturers, service providers and marketing agents are fully aware of this fact and will use it to their advantage to drive for greater sales of products and services (Baby Products Association 2008).

Expectant and novice parents are wooed with an array of solutions to a range of perceived parenting needs, including feeding, sleeping, monitoring and leisure activities. This specialized group is viewed as a vulnerable and lucrative goal for the many companies who offer goods or services to support the increasingly complex business of becoming a contemporary parent (Falconer 1993).

A significant feature in both Western and increasingly in non-Western societies is that the traditional extended family, who may have provided support, advice and role modeling in previous generations, has in many instances disappeared for many reasons (UNFPA 2009). The number of children within a family group has also diminished over the last half century in Western countries and consequently the acquisition of childrearing skills is not always experiential (UNFPA 2009). Many people will not have even held a baby before giving birth themselves. For that reason many women turn to baby training 'experts' to guide them and periodicals to inform them of what is current in the commercial baby world (Grant 1998). The images that they view in advertising media are usually of contented and confident-looking mothers and healthy happy babies. The message that is conveyed, for some at least, is that it is possible to buy your way to a happy and ful-filling motherhood by purchasing a range of products and services (Thomas 2007).

The marketing potential of expectant parents is without a doubt consider-able, in particular that of first-time parents. Brand loyalty is a key marketing concept and if the consumers are captivated by the product at an important time in their purchasing power history, then they are often hooked for life (Travis 2000). It would seem that the marketing professionals are not only interested in capturing the parents in terms of brand loyalty. Thomas (2007) advises that toy and media corporations, not content with manipulating the insecurities of parents, are accessing and frequently funding research in child development in order to attract the market interest of babies and toddlers.

In the postmodern world, time has become viewed as a precious commodity of which we never seem to have enough (Perlow 1999). In order to free up more time, we employ the use of labour-saving devices and services at an unprecedented level, and yet our lives still seem to be conspicuously 'time poor'. Time poverty is an expression used to describe people who, while having a good level of disposable income through employment, have relatively little 'downtime' for rest and relaxation (De Graf 2003: 1). Consequently, we spend a lot of capital and effort seeking ways of easing our demanding schedules.

This has spawned a host of products and services designed to create more time, such as mobile phones, microwave meals and fast-food outlets. Anything that frees up our time is usually viewed as a valued commodity. This trend extends into childcare practices, where time-saving gadgets abound.

If babies were to be considered commodities, they would probably rate as one of the most expensive investments that we could make in our lifetimes. There are varying estimates around what a new baby will cost and these vary from country to country. The 'Cost of a Child' survey from Liverpool Victoria Friendly Society (2010) estimates that on average a child in the UK will cost £194,000 to raise until the age of 21. Of course this is only an estimate and it may be possible to bring up a child within a much tighter budget. Nonetheless, it would be easy to subscribe to the 'work more to earn more to buy more' ethic, which may ironically mean spending less time with the children for whom we are working excessively hard in order to 'fund'.

As one mother in a newspaper article related to the Liverpool Victoria report stated:

> When finding out we were expecting a little girl, we had many trips to the shops to buy cot mattress, clothes, nappies . . . we didn't think about the future with how many things you have to buy. The list is endless. We are spending most of our money on items of clothing and toys, because you want your child to have the best.
> (Liverpool Victoria Friendly Society 2010)

A recent Australian study identified that people are working longer hours, with many staff not taking leave entitlements. This corresponds with reports of children who are overscheduled with extra-curricula activities and disturbingly high numbers of people and children, and sometimes very young children, suffering from depression and anxiety (Shepanski and Diamond 2007). Paradoxically, what children and particularly babies need is time, space and relationships that provide a wealth of relaxed and stimulating time as the basis for healthy growth and development (Walker 2005).

The concept of risk has become an inevitable part of life and the childbearing period is no exception, with risk assessment forming one of the first encounters between a woman and her care provider in pregnancy. Risk assessment can be perceived as being driven by fear avoidance tactics. We fear a less than positive outcome and believe that we can manage it by identifying it (Symon 2006). Women who are expecting a baby or who have recently given birth may have many fears. Fear is believed by some theorists of human motivation to be a necessary part of the human condition designed to encourage parents to protect their young (Maslow 1943).

However, it would seem that some manufacturers have identified a potential susceptibility during this period and have used it as an opportunity to advertise items that promise to buy peace of mind. The sales of fetal heart monitors directly to women are one such example, as the following quote demonstrates: '. . . can give you the peace of mind that your baby is safe and well at all times throughout your pregnancy, no matter where you are' (Bumps to Kids 2009).

What the marketing blurb fails to address, is the fact that electronic fetal heart monitors are an invasive form of monitoring. The ultrasound waves created by the machine cross through maternal tissue to locate the fetus and subsequently create a sound, which is transmitted as an echo. We do not really know if there are safe levels to such exposure, even on low frequency and for short periods of exposure. Additionally, midwives and doctors are educated to interpret the heart sounds. Would a woman without this underpinning knowledge be able to detect any subtle changes that may lead a health professional to act upon?

In November 2009 the *British Journal of Medicine* (Chakladar and Adams 2009) published a case study outlining the tragic case where a woman presented with a stillbirth after attempting to auscultate her baby's heart sounds at home with an electronic fetal heart monitor. A recent Cochrane review by (Mangesi and Hofmeyr 2007) states that we should be more aware of women's perceptions of reduced fetal movements, which are associated with stillbirth and intrauterine death. This is reiterated in the current NICE guidelines for antenatal care (2003), which recommends that women who suspect a reduction in their baby's movements should contact their care provider. The most worrying aspect of this sad scenario is that it fostered a reliance on technology that underplayed other significant signs that all may not have been well with the baby, such as reduced fetal movements.

Davis-Floyd (2001) refers to a reliance on technology as the *super-valuation* of the scientific and technocratic: the supremacy of the rational, medical model. Many midwives recognize the limitations of this technocratic model and stress the need to 'rehumanize' birth (Anderson and Davies 2004). It cannot be denied that technology does have a place in maternity care, but it must be used appropriately and with due care and attention. The ethics of a company who sell such equipment to women, under the auspices of ensuring the well-being of their babies, are surely questionable.

Health services have been drawn into the commercial world of sales before birth, offering a conduit between parents and products by allowing companies to market free samples to health service staff and 'patients'. This may be the response of a cash-strapped health service, or may be intended as an act of altruism, but whatever the reason the message could be interpreted as condoning the products. The public on the whole trust health professionals and therefore would expect them to give unbiased and evidence-based advice about the use of products and equipment. Giving advice about not using baby products for at least a month after birth (Trotter 2008: 244) may sound a little hollow when the woman finds a complimentary sachet of baby bath and shampoo in her room on the post-natal ward.

Some enterprising companies have freed the manufacturers from the need to establish a direct link with parents-to-be, by creating a one-stop shop in the form of complimentary packs that can be obtained via the health service or even from local retailers. They contain a range of 'try before you buy' samples as well as coupons for products and magazine samples. The fact that the production of disposable nappies may be causing environmental damage (Women's Environmental Network 2003) or that follow-on formulas could be viewed as a way of circumventing the International Code of Marketing of Breast-milk Substitutes on the part of the baby formula company are not alluded to by the companies or presumably the health services.

There would appear to be a device designed for every conceivable situation within the world of the twenty-first century infant. Long gone are the days when a layette listed baby gowns and mittens as the must-have items. From jogging strollers to a digital wireless video monitor with night-light lullaby cameras, the act of shopping for a baby has taken on a new turn, which may be a reflection of our ever-increasing reliance on and need for technology. A quick glance at the iPhone website reveals a feast of uses for the must-have applications relating to parenting, including a labour contractions monitor that emails the information to your care provider and a baby monitor that phones you automatically if the baby cries.

It could be argued that this 'school of software' approach to childcare is undermining an ancient and instinctive response on the part of parents (Wickham 2004). Do we have so little faith left in our primal senses that we need a machine to tell us what to do and when with our bodies and our babies? This is the antithesis of what Jean Liedloff describes in her classic text, *The Continuum Concept* (1985), where she argues that we are designed to occupy a specific ecological niche and in order to achieve a state of equilibrium and well-being, we need to inhabit the conditions that evolution has led us to expect. Liedloff suggests that if the pre-programmed needs of babies are not met, they are hindered from fully developing and maturing. She also stresses that the conditions that babies are pre-programmed to meet means being with their mothers at all times (which she described as 'in arms'), sleeping with them and being fed by them in response to their cues. Meeting these needs actually costs very little in terms of material outlay, but does cost in time provision.

There are many parents who have adopted attachment parenting, which fulfills the conditions outlined by Liedloff (1986) and feel that it works for them in terms of their ethos and lifestyle. There is research to suggest that children who experience the principles do appear to have advantages in life in terms of self-esteem and autonomy (Bosmans *et al.* 2006; Karavasilis *et al.* 2003). However, when we consider the cultural context that we inhabit in Western society, where separation has been the modus operandi for parenting for the last century at least and where women usually return to the workplace within a few months after birth, the notion of attachment parenting is something that may need to be approached with sensitivity. Perhaps more attention should be paid to improve the quality of parent–child interactions and means of forming attachment within our own cultural context as a starting point. Ensuring unlimited skin-to-skin contact following birth would be a good starting point. Parents could be encouraged to indulge in a 'babymoon' (a play on the idea of a honeymoon) where they are advised to take the phone off the hook, lock the front door and concentrate on becoming a family for the first few days at home after having their baby. We could take a leaf from the example of Scandinavian countries where a humanistic approach to social policy includes guaranteed rights to childcare, shared access to parental leave and cash payments for home-based care (Leira 2002).

It may be useful at this juncture to explore some of the driving forces behind the products on the market. The Baby Products Association (BPA) is a UK-based organization that was set up with the objective of promoting the baby and nursery products sector in both the UK and Europe. The BPA has led a long-term campaign for over 10 years that aims to discourage parents from using second-hand nursery goods. In a leaflet endorsed by a leading parenting magazine, parents are advised that buying second-hand equipment such as prams, stair gates and high chairs is 'gambling with your child's safety'. We should acknowledge that not all second-hand equipment is free from fault and danger and that care should be taken when purchasing a previously-owned object. Clearly in light of the knowledge that we now have about the association between used mattresses and Sudden Unexpected Death of Infants (SUDI) (Fleming *et al.* 2002), it would be remiss of any midwife not to advise a mother to buy a new cot mattress. However, why couldn't a family cut their costs by buying a new mattress and using a second hand cot frame?

The campaign raises a number of other concerns. First, this cannot be considered good housekeeping. If single use of a product leaves it faulty and danger prone, then perhaps we need to be looking seriously at the quality of the products that the organization is supporting and be asking why they are not made to a more robust standard that would enable multi-use. The campaign does not take into consideration the fact that much recycling of nursery equipment may take place within families, where items are handed down for subsequent babies within the same family and the history of the product is well known. This is an ageless practice, which has probably served families well since time immemorial.

The target group for the manufacturers and advertisers could be perceived to be a 'market of vulnerability', where families understandably want to provide the best that they can for their children. The tone of the campaign could lead one to suspect that the mark of a good parent is to provide a baby with the most contemporary and stylish equipment available. Where does this leave families on low incomes who are having to work within a very tight budget? What they require is practical advice on what baby products they actually need; what safety checks may be needed for pre-used equipment and where such checks could be carried out.

Last, but by no means least, is the environmental argument. The product in question, be it a hardwood cot, a plastic mobile or baby shampoo, has cost a considerable amount of ecological currency during its production, marketing and transportation. Its disposal will equally leave its mark on the environment. The legitimate single use of any product should therefore be held up for scrutiny and items reused wherever possible.

Having explored a range of facets relating to consumerism and parenting it may be useful to return to the earlier question of 'does consumerism make us happy?' Empirical studies have consistently shown that there is only a tenuous link between wealth and happiness and that once beyond poverty, further economic growth does not appreciably improve human happiness (Inglehart 1990). Myers (1993) suggests that happiness diminishes when we compare what we have with what we want; what we have with what we expected to have by now and what we have when compared to others.

Could it be that this is precisely the status quo that manufacturers are fighting hard to preserve in the marketing area of new parenting? By preying on a range of motivational factors such as egotism, guilt and fear, are they aiming to perpetuate a constant demand for their products. If new parents are consciously or unconsciously comparing themselves to the happy, smiling, successful-looking model parents in sales catalogues and advertisements how must that leave them feeling as parents if they cannot achieve that measure for whatever reason?

Pregnancy and early parenthood are times of great change in people's lives. It is a time when some begin to question their existing values and beliefs and look beyond the sphere of their own needs, as for the first time they find themselves responsible for the needs of another individual (Davies 1994). They might also reflect on how their present lifestyle will influence the lives of their children. This may lead them to question the quality of the food they eat, the water they drink and the quality of their local environment, as well as broader global issues such as sweatshop child labour. These parents may feel encouraged to buy more organic foodstuffs, fair-trade products and locally-produced goods.

This growing trend is termed as ethical consumerism and is characterized by those who choose to purchase goods and services that cause minimal harm to or exploitation of humans, animals and/or the natural environment (Harrison *et al.* 2005). It can be argued that ethical consumers have had a significant effect on retail and service industries over the last few decades by demanding goods and services that do not lead to environmental degradation or global injustice (Harrison *et al.* 2005). However, ethical consumerism has also been criticized as an oxymoron that does little more than to create niche markets for products that result in a value-added price premium (Purvis 2006). The growth of 'eco- friendly-baby' stores that market BPA-free bottles and amber teething necklaces could possibly be held up for scrutiny on this count. No one could argue against the fact that that we should be making an effort to change our lifestyles as much as possible, and considering what we buy is significant, but it would be short-sighted to believe that 'greening' our shopping trolleys is primarily what we have to do. Ethical purchasing decisions are unlikely to bring about the level of change that is almost certainly required to effect a pardigm shift on the scale of the Brundtland Report call to meet 'the needs of the present without compromising the ability of future generations to meet their own needs' (Brundtland 1987).

However, a more compelling case emerges from the debate around what makes us happy that may help to faciliatate a more profound change. It has been said that personal happiness and well-being are equated with autonomy, achievement and the development of deep interpersonal relationships, and less with the acquisition of material wealth and goods (Kahneman and Sugden 2005).

The relationship that a midwife has with a woman in pregnancy is a unique one. This is particularly so when both the woman and the midwife are privileged enough to work within a continuity of carer model, and get to know each other over a number of months, during a period where personal growth figures significantly for the woman. If relationships are a significant factor in achieving happiness, then could the midwife serve an important role, which stretches far beyond addressing the physical needs of the woman? If sustainability is about relationships and communities then it may be that the midwife could play a key role in helping to facilitate the relationship between mother and baby, which has been acclaimed as the prototype of all relationships (Odent 1999). This could be introduced during pregnancy by encouraging the woman to connect with her baby, and continued by holding space for the woman during labour and birth and by promoting the development of the relationship following birth as identified in Chapter 8 by Carolyn Hastie.

Midwives could use the antenatal period to help the woman to connect with others in her community by offering childbirth and parenting education that promotes relationships, helping the women to establish their own new network of friends and support (see Chapter 15 by Mary Nolan). By encouraging the active involvement of the woman's partner or her family members, again she has the potential to help to strengthen existing relationships.

To revisit the concept of the super-valuation of the scientific and technological (Davis-Floyd 2001), midwives as fundamentally 'low-tech, high touch' (DeVries and Barroso 1997: 253) practitioners could place greater value in their art to support their scientific knowledge. This may result in a decreased reliance on technology and a greater faith in tacit skills and understanding as discussed by Ruth Martis in Chapter 11. This may have the secondary effects of encouraging women to have greater faith in their bodies and fostering self esteem. If people are happy with who they are then they are less likely to need to augment their lives with consumerism (Hamilton 1998). We need to become much more eco-aware in our lives generally. What could be a better place to start than with our newest arrivals and their families?

Our current consumer patterns are not sustainable in the long run in either the shopping mall or within the milieu of contemporary health care. It would be easy to convince ourselves that attempts to address issues of such magnitude are overwhelming and that any actions that we may undertake, insignificant.

It has to be recognized that the current delivery of health care provision does little to embrace the principles of sustainability, as is discussed elsewhere in this book. However, we should not underestimate the might of the individual and should embrace the fact that in raising consciousness by what we say and do, we are in a position to facilitate change in attitudes and behaviour. As companions on the birthing journey of women, midwives should be able to role model, educate and assist in decision making around environmental concerns and ecological well-being as much as we currently do around birth preferences.

References

Anderson, T. and Davies, L. (2004) 'Celebrating the "art" of midwifery', *The Practising Midwife*, 7, 6: 22–25.

Baby Products Association (2008) 'Market Assessment Executive Report'. Mumbai: Bharat Book Bureau.

Boje, D. M. and Rhodes, C. (2006) 'The leadership of Ronald McDonald: double narration and stylistic lines of transformation', *The Leadership Quarterly*, 17, 1: 94–103.

Bosmans, G., Braet, C., Van Leeuwen, K. and Beyers, W. (2006) 'Do parenting behaviors predict externalizing behavior in adolescence, or is attachment the neglected 3rd factor?' *Journal of Youth and Adolescence*, 35, 3:354–64.

Bumps to Kids (2009) Online. Available at: www.b2k.co.nz/shop/product.aspx?id=c6bb4354-48f4-42a9-8227-8d3ed3e7a6b6 (accessed 21 December 2009).

Brundtland, G. H. (1987) 'Our common future – call for action', *Environmental Conservation*, 14: 291–94.

Chaklader, A. and Adams, H. (2009) 'Dangers of listening to the fetal heart at home', *British Medical Journal*, 339, 4: 308.

Davis-Floyd, R. (2001) 'The technocratic, humanistic, and holistic paradigms of childbirth', *International Journal of Gynecology and Obstetrics*, 75, S1: 5–23.

Davies, L. (1994) 'Ecological midwifery', *Midwifery Matters*, 61: 8–10.

De Graf, J. (ed.) (2003) *Take Back Your Time: Fighting Overwork and Time Poverty in America*. San Francisco: Berrett-Koehler Publishers.

DeVries, R. and Barroso, R. (1997) 'Midwives among the machines. Re-creating midwifery in the late twentieth century', in H. Marland and A. Rafferty (eds), *Midwives, Society and Childbirth: Debates and Controversies in the Modern Period*. New York: Routledge.

Falconer, K. (1993) 'Bumping up the profits', *The Guardian*, 23 February 1993.

Fleming, P. J., Blair, P. S. and Mitchell, E. A. (2002) 'Mattresses, microenvironments, and multivariate analyses', *British Medical Journal*, 325 (7371): 981–82.

Goldsmith, E. (1996) *Resource Management for Individuals and Families*. New York: West.

Grant, J. (1998) *Raising Baby by the Book: The Education of American Mothers*. New Haven, CT: Yale University Press.

Hamilton, C. (1998) 'Measuring changes in economic welfare: the genuine progress indicator for Australia', in R. Eckersley (ed.) *Measuring Progress*. Melbourne: CSIRO Publishing.

Harrison, R., Newholm, T. and Shaw, D. (2005) *Ethical Consumer*. London: Sage.

Inglehart, R. (1990) *Culture Shift in Advanced Industrial Society.* Princeton, NJ: Princeton University Press.

Irons, B. and Hepburn, C. (2007) 'Regret theory and the tyranny of choice', *The Economic Record,* 83, 261: 191–203.

Kahneman, D. and Sugden, R. (2005) 'Experienced utility as a standard of policy evaluation', *Environmental & Resource Economics,* 32: 585–87.

Karavasilis, I., Doyle, A. B. and Markiewicz, D. (2003) 'Associations between parenting style and attachment to mother in middle childhood and adolescence', *International Journal of Behavioral Development,* 27, 2: 153–64.

Leira, A. (2002) *Working Parents and the Welfare State: Family Change and Policy Reform in Scandinavia.* Cambridge: Cambridge University Press.

Liedloff, J. (1986) *The Continuum Concept: In Search of Happiness Lost.* Cambridge, MA: Da Capo Press.

Liverpool Victoria Friendly Society (2010) 'Cost of a child survey'. Online. Available at: www.lv.com/media_centre/press_releases/lv=%20cost%20of%20a%20child (accessed 9 January 2010).

Mangesi, L. and Hofmeyr, G. J. (2007) 'Fetal movement counting for assessment of fetal wellbeing'. *Cochrane Database Systematic Review.* Online. Available at: http://mrw.interscience.wiley.com/cochrane/clsysrev/articles/CD004909/frame.html (accessed 13 January 2010).

Maslow, A. H. (1943) 'A theory of human motivation', *Psychological Review,* 50, 4: 370–96.

Murphy-Lawless, J. (2006) 'Birth and mothering in today's social order: the challenge of new knowledges', *MIDIRS Midwifery Digest,* 16, 4: 439–44.

Myers, D. (1993) *The Pursuit of Happiness: Discovering the Pathway to Fulfillment, Well-being, and Enduring Personal Joy.* NY: Harper Collins.

National Institute for Health and Clinical Excellence (2003). 'Antenatal care: routine care for the healthy pregnant woman'. Online. Available at: www.nice.org.uk/guidance/CG62 (accessed 12 January 2010).

Norwood, Franklin B. (2006) 'Less choice is better, sometimes', *Journal of Agricultural & Food Industrial Organization,* 4, 1, Article 3. Online. Available at: www.bepress.com/jafio/vol4/iss1/art3 (accessed 14 January 2010).

Odent, M. (1999) *The Scientification of Love.* London: Free Association Books.

Perlow, L. A. (1999) 'The time famine: toward a sociology of work time'. *Administrative Science Quarterly,* 44, 1: 57–81.

Purvis, A. (2006) 'Choice: The curse of the green consumer?' *The Green Magazine.* Online. Available at: www.greenfutures.org.uk (accessed 6 January 2010).

Schwartz, B. (2006) *The Paradox of Choice. Why More is Less.* New York: Harper Perennial.

Seabrook, J. (1987) 'Agenda: bringing up baby to enjoy the wealth of the nation – uses and abuses of children', *Guardian,* 24 August 1987.

Shepanski, P. and Diamond, M. (2007) *An Unexpected Tragedy: Evidence for the Connection Between Working Patterns and Family Breakdown in Australia.* Sydney: The Relationships Forum.

Symon, A. (2006) *Risk and Choice in Maternity Care: An International Perspective.* Edinburgh: Elsevier.

Thomas, S. G. (2007) *Buy, Buy Baby: How Consumer Culture Manipulates Parents and Harms Young Mind.* Orlando, FL: Houghton Mifflin Harcourt.

Travis, D. (2000) *Emotional Branding: How Successful Brands Gain the Irrational Edge.* New York: Crown Business.

Trotter, S. (2008) 'Neonatal skincare and cordcare: implications for practice', in L. Davies and S. McDonald (eds), *Examination of the Newborn: A Multi Dimensional Approach.* Edinburgh: Churchill Livingstone.

United Nations Population Fund (UNFPA) (2009) 'State of the world population'. Online. Available at: www.unfpa.org/swp/2009/en/ (accessed 13 December 2009).

Walker K (2005) *What's the Hurry?: Reclaiming Childhood in an Over Scheduled World.* Oakleigh, VA: Australian Scholarship Group.

Wickham, S. (2004) 'A crying shame', *The Practising Midwife*, 7, 2: 27.

Women's Environmental Network (2003) *Disposable Nappies: A Case Study in Waste Prevention.* London: WEN.

Worldwatch Institute (2008) *State of the World 2008: Innovations for a Sustainable Economy*, NY: W. W. Norton & Company.

13 Breastfeeding and sustainability

Loss, cost, 'choice', damage, disaster, adaptation and evolutionary logic

Carol Bartle

In the beginning there was breastfeeding

Breastfeeding is as old as human life itself. Infants are born into the same environment as always – their mothers. It is the context, milieu and the cultures affecting their mothers that have altered. This does not change infant needs and instinctive newborn behaviours. The growth and survival of humans has been dependent on breastfeeding women, wet-nursing,[1] breastmilk, close women-kin, allomothers[2] and extended family support structures. Hrdy writes: 'For thirty-five million years primate infants stayed safe by remaining close to their mothers day and night. To lose touch was death' (1999: 97).

Staying close not only provided warmth and protection from the environment, but food and protection from illness and death, in the form of immunologic transfer, maternal milk production and delivery. Hrdy observes that modern babies are 'under pressure' to adapt and 'learn to cope with the unnatural expectations of modern parents' (1999: 97).

The loss of the more than ample embrace of breastfeeding for infant health and development is significant. Apart from the necessity for the newborn infant of the colostrum immunization, described as an 'aperitif with consequences', continued lactation has been a 'key player in the evolution of animals who were both social and intelligent' (Hrdy 1999: 145). Mary Wollstonecraft describes a breastfeeding role in the health and well-being of women:

> Nature has so wisely ordered things that did women suckle their children, they would preserve their own health, and there would be such an interval between the birth of each child that we should seldom see a houseful of babes.
>
> (1978: 315)

Maternal survival, breastfeeding and a degree of mother-wellness are necessary for optimal support of infant development in the majority of the world's countries and imperative for natural fertility control in many countries. It has been reported that within the World Health Organization's global dataset of 65 per cent of the world's infant population aged one year or less, only

35 per cent are exclusively breastfed between birth and four months of age.[3] In the Philippines, on average, less than half the infants born are exclusively breastfed by three months of age and by six months less than 25 per cent are exclusively breastfed.[4] Lauer *et al.* (2006) report that as many as 1.45 million lives are lost due to suboptimal breastfeeding in 'developing countries'.

Loss and cost: breastfeeding is more than 'just' nutrition

If breastfeeding was 'just' about nutrition it would be a loss, as even a brief look at the research evidence about the composition of breastmilk nutrients, and the superiority of this fluid gold, demonstrates clearly that artificial reproduction of this almost magical elixir will never be possible. This is even without contemplation of the positive immunological effects of breastmilk and the wonder of breastfeeding. Nutrition is but one of the significant components of breastfeeding lost with the decline of global breastfeeding cultures. Maternal long-term health and increased survival is another in regard to risk reduction for various diseases such as breast cancer,[5,6,7,8] ovarian cancer,[9,10] osteoporosis[11,12] and heart disease.[13,14]

A New Zealand magazine article[15] noted that the London School of Economics and the Optimum Population Trust stated in 2009 that condoms were the cheapest way to reduce carbon emissions. Costs quoted were about US$7 a tonne, as opposed to other low-carbon technologies, which start at about US$24 a tonne. Lactational amenorrhoea – natural fertility and breastfeeding, which fosters optimal health in mothers, child-spacing and a reduction of unwanted pregnancies – did not rate a mention, despite the article discussion about the lifetime carbon footprints[16] of new humans and the associated pressure on resources such as water, food and space.

Lactational amenorrhoea (LAM) is linked to optimal breastfeeding, mother–baby contact and reduction in conception and pregnancy due to ovulation suppression. Exclusive breastfeeding for six months, and continuation of breastfeeding for up to two years and beyond, with the addition of appropriate foods from six months, is optimal. Hrdy (1999) describes breastfeeding as the foundation of family planning in primates, including people. Lactational amenorrhoea for 18 months is described as requiring, on average, about 80 minutes of a baby suckling at the breast per day, which occurs over a minimum of six breastfeeding episodes (Hrdy 1999). Other factors described as important by Hrdy were maternal nutritional status, workload and environmental conditions.

It has been suggested that lactational amenorrhoea is responsible for the prevention of more pregnancies in 'developing' countries than all the other methods of contraception available (Madani *et al.* 1994). Radwan *et al.* (2009) found a 98 per cent protection rate against pregnancy after childbirth for six months in a cohort of 593 women in the United Arab Emirates. Duration of LAM was significantly related to the age of the infant when formula and solid foods were introduced. Most women in Western countries can access cheap contraception so an argument may be that LAM is not so important in the Western context. However, even in relatively affluent countries, when sustainability is added into the argument, with manufacturing and transport costs of condoms and other contraceptive devices, the picture changes. Breastfeeding contributes to carbon-neutral family planning with associated sustainable fringe benefits.

Not-breastfeeding costs related to maternal, infant and young child health are factors in the multifaceted non-sustainability of the current global dominance of artificial feeding. Labbok (1994) discussed the potential cost savings in the US health-care system that could be achieved by supporting mothers to breastfeed for as little as 12 weeks. Cost savings were estimated at US$2.4 billion annually. Drane (1997) used data on relative risk and population-attributable risk per cent from epidemiological studies to estimate cases of illness in breastfed and formula-fed infants, pre-term and full term, for varying prevalence of exclusive breastfeeding. It was estimated that a minimum of Aus$11.5 million could be saved each year in Australia if the prevalence of exclusive breastfeeding at three months was increased from 60 per cent to 80 per cent. Drane based this cost estimate on four illnesses, and educational costs associated with neuro-developmental impairment only, so costs were considered to be underestimated. Smith *et al.* (2002) estimated costs for the Australian Capital Territory of treating selected infant and childhood illnesses associated with early weaning from human milk, and found significant costs related to early weaning in the estimated range of Aus$1–2 million annually. When the study findings were extrapolated nationally, estimated savings were Aus$60–120 million annually.

Frick (2009), an American health economist, examined the use of economics to analyse policies promoting breastfeeding. Frick states that the infant formula market does not represent 'perfect' competition as a market but rather 'monopolistic' competition. Frick describes perfect competition as a market producing a uniformly nutritious infant formula product at minimum cost, sold to consumers at a similar cost regardless of the manufacturer of the goods. This is obviously not the reality of the modern infant formula market. Frick describes the monopolistic competitive market as one where manufacturers use substantial resources to differentiate themselves from each other and compete on 'quality' rather than price. Frick states that the result of this is a market not operating efficiently to produce goods at a minimum cost, with the benefit to infants and families of a broad range of products being unclear. When determining costs in the area of infant and young child nutrition 'the cost of the goods used to produce nutrition, time used to produce nutrition and costs or risks associated with various ways of providing nutrition' (2009: 184) require evaluation. Frick suggests an economic evaluation tool critical for analysing breastfeeding and infant nutrition. A 'cost-consequence' analysis provides the tool for describing costs and benefits and when utilized alongside a 'cost of illness' study this assists with understanding lifetime costs associated with ill-health conditions.

Stuebe and Schwarz (2009) confirmed that infant feeding decisions significantly affect mother–child health outcomes globally, even in settings with clean water and good sanitation. Not-breastfed infants are exposed to increased risk of infections and non-infectious morbidity and mortality. Stuebe and Schwarz argue for a change to the commonly used 'breast is best' rhetoric to a statement identifying the real issue – the risks associated with infant formula feeding.

McNiel *et al.* (2010) re-analysed and reviewed the risks associated with formula feeding to work towards a repositioning of breastfeeding as a natural normative behaviour in the minds of women's and children's health care providers. Reconfiguring reported statistics to reflect risks of formula use rather than benefits of breastfeeding was the aim. A limitation of any such analysis, and this was identified and discussed by McNiel *et al.*, is that few studies use infants exclusively breastfed for six months as the comparison group and the definitions of 'breastfeeding' or 'exclusivity' of breastfeeding are not standardized by any means. Despite this limitation McNiel *et al.* found some statistically significant associations between formula usage and health risk and recommended that infants exclusively breastfed for six months are the standard against which other forms of feeding are compared. The researchers noted that if more studies had included six months of exclusive breastfeeding they would expect 'more findings to achieve significance' (2010: 56).

Akre examines the costs of not breastfeeding and suggests an elevation of the 'global economic implications of child feeding mode' (2009). Consequences of decisions to either observe or disregard the 'hominid blueprint for the natural age of weaning' is portrayed as having 'complex and lifelong economic implications for individuals and society as a whole' (2009: 22). Akre's concluding paragraph includes this statement: '200 million years or so of mammalian evolution should be worth something in terms of our default position being intrinsically weighted in favour of breastfeeding' (2009: 23).

The amount of expenditure on health costs, which could be significantly reduced, represents another aspect of the sustainability argument related to decisions about infant feeding and weaning.

Choice: breastmilk substitutes, cost and waste

The dominance and spread of breastmilk substitutes and infant formula feeding could be described as a global disaster. It may not be as obvious as a war, a tsunami, a hurricane or an earthquake, and for the majority of people who have become accustomed to living embedded within bottle-feeding, infant-formula cultures even a shadow of such a suggestion is likely to be considered outrageous, radical and extreme.

Infant formula feeding represented as a simplistic, easy and equal choice, 'competing' against breastfeeding, which is often portrayed as more difficult, unachievable for many women, painful, embarrassing, body-wrecking, sleep-depriving, time-consuming and a drain on the modern mother who needs to undertake paid work, play, get away from her baby, and wear clothing without wet patches and breastmilk stains. It is a carefully manufactured marketing message, a reflection of cultures where women, mothering, breastfeeding, parenting and children are unsupported and undervalued, a deep sadness, and a tragic loss. As the visionary economist E. F. Schumacher (1974) suggests, in his study of economics, 'as if people mattered', 'nothing makes economic sense unless its continuance for a long time can be projected without running into absurdities' (p. 20). Costs of widespread infant formula use and intensive dairying are running into absurdities in multiple ways.

The cost, to the purchasing consumer, of the artificial milk product on the shelf represents a miniscule part of the total negative cost to the planet and human health. Increasing numbers of dairy herds, unnatural intensive farming methods potentially involving bovine growth hormones, the resulting need for expensive antibiotic use for chronic mastitis-sick cows, the associated damage to land and infrastructures, pollution, significant water contamination and water wastage and consumption, increase in greenhouse gases, manufacture of powdered milk, production of novel ingredients to add to the product, packaging, transport internally on roads and overseas by air and sea, waste products created by both the manufacturing process and the packaging designed to entice product usage, add up to a giant carbon footprint and contribute to an unsustainable future. As Gabrielle Palmer states, 'a woman can produce hundreds of litres of the super-fluid breastmilk for a zero carbon footprint' (2009: 346).

Projected sales of baby food were reported at US$20.2 billion annually by Palmer, with infant formula sales accounting for two thirds of this. Palmer provides a comprehensive list of the waste associated with infant formula feeding. For example, tins for packaging infant formula to supply 1 million babies use 23,706 tonnes of metal and the paper resources amount to 341 tonnes, plus the added costs of all the paper promotional material supplied to not only parents but paediatricians, nurses, midwives and other health workers. Palmer reports that just one of the many baby bottle and teat manufacturers reported distribution of 20 million bottles a year, and to add to this is the problem of non-biodegradable/non-recyclable tetra-pak cartons used for liquid ready-to-feed products.

Frick (2009) points out that all resources are scarce and as the world has a finite amount of land available for cultivation, there is a finite amount of food to meet the nutritional needs for all societies. Reasons for destroying the natural resource of forests and destroying the natural resource of breastfeeding are described by Gabrielle Palmer as being the same – 'for immediate profit' (2009: 4), with disregard for the future and sustainability. Soy is an important part of the diet of many dairy herds and this may now contribute up to 10 per cent of the bovine diet. Soy trade expansion is responsible for vast areas of deforestation in Brazil, Paraguay and Argentina (Friends of the Earth 2008). The 2008 Friends of the Earth report estimated that the livestock sector is responsible for 18 per cent of global greenhouse gas emissions and that deforestation is also a significant source. Schumacher discusses what is economic and what is uneconomic. He points out that economic growth may be, 'pathological, unhealthy, disruptive or destructive' (Schumacher 1974: 40). Broad-scale activities that are non-sustainable and ignore the costs to the environment, and human and animal health cannot be economic as ultimately they will not exist.

Damage: dairy and water

> ... and so you don't even know whose fields this food came from? That sounds terrible. It could be poisoned.
>
> (Kingsolver 1999: 320)

Breastfeeding leaves no footprints and we know where it comes from. It usually travels directly, and safely, with warmth and love to the littlest, most vulnerable of consumers via their mothers' breasts – the shortest 'food-mile' surely? No other animals, equipment, farmers, workers, manufacturers, transporters or retailers are involved in these intimate events, which therefore removes potential for product sabotage due to greed,[17] accidental product contamination or miscalculation.[18] When infants require the gift of donor milk from another lactating woman the breastmilk still travels with warmth and love from another woman, who either cares enough about an infant and mother she knows, or cares enough about anonymous unwell infants that she donates her breastmilk.

In a polluted world where human and animal bodies are exposed to chemicals and breastmilk contains contaminants that ideally should not be there, it is still recognized that breastfeeding and breastmilk remain optimal over all substitute milks. Penny Van Esterik points out that:

> Breastfeeding as risky behaviour and artificial feeding as a way of saving children from their mothers' contaminated milk is a travesty brought about by industrial processes, advances in technical surveillance, and new ways of thinking about woman's bodies.
>
> (2002: vi)

When the natural capital of breastmilk and breastfeeding are unrecognized and support for breastfeeding women under-resourced, this presents an opportunity for the outsourcing of infant feeding, using modified dairy products, leading to substantial financial gains for a few.

As long ago as 1988, ex-National Party MP in New Zealand, Marilyn Waring, wrote about the failure to include reproductive functions and breastfeeding in terms of their economic value, a failure to count women's work as being of value in fact. Smith and Ingham (2001) have also contributed to this important body of work by highlighting how economic production is underestimated when GDP measurements exclude the value of unpaid work. Waring, in her work, was attempting also to draw attention to the degradation of natural assets arising from the additional production of animal milk supplies and the costs to the land arising from this accelerated production and depletion of natural assets.

As New Zealand is a country heavily investing in the dairy industry with increasing numbers of dairy herds and a big export market for milk powder, examination of the environmental costs of such intensive dairy development, which contributes to a significant portion of the global infant formula market, is of interest. A New Zealand Parliamentary Commission for the Environment report (2005), which examined intensive farming, sustainability and the environment, stated that between 1994 and 2002 the dairy cow numbers in New Zealand increased by 34 per cent. In the same period the production of milk solids on a per hectare basis increased by 34 per cent and milk solid production per cow increased. The report noted that use of synthetic fertilizers based on fossil fuels was also increasing on dairy farms and that the total energy input into the average NZ dairy farm had doubled over the preceding 20 years, mainly due to the increase in nitrogen fertilizer. The report also commented on irrigation and the amount of water used for intensive dairy farming. Significant levels of irrigation are required for dry regions of NZ, such as the Canterbury and Otago regions in the South Island, and irrigated dairy farms use nearly double the electricity of non-irrigated dairy farms plus their use of nitrogen fertilizers is much greater – 135 kg of nitrogen fertilizer per hectare for an irrigated farm compared to 68 kg on a non-irrigated farm. Water quality was discussed in this report and it was stated that many rivers draining farmland were unsuitable for swimming because of animal faecal contamination with poor water clarity and nuisance algae growth caused by excess nutrients in the water. Nitrate contamination of water was identified as a concern, as groundwater quality in aquifers that exist under pastoral farming areas, particularly dairying areas, tended to have elevated nitrate concentrations that sometimes exceeded the acceptable levels for drinking water standards.

It is not uncommon in the United States to see public health alerts when nitrate contamination of water in some areas exceeds safe levels. At such times warnings are broadcast to advise parents not to use the water for reconstituting powdered infant formula. Excess nitrates may cause a condition called 'blue baby syndrome' where the oxygen-carrying capacity of red blood cells is dangerously compromised causing methemoglobinemia (Fawell and Nieuwenhuijsen 2003). Methoglobulin is a form of haemoglobin that does not bind oxygen and illness can occur when high concentrations are reached. It has also been suggested that animal faeces contamination in water causing high concentrations of bacteria is linked to methemoglobinemia alongside elevated nitrate levels (Powlson *et al.* 2008).

The New Zealand Parliamentary Commission for the Environment report (2005) stated that intensive dairying areas are typified by rivers in poor condition. Since 2005 the dairy industry and milk production have escalated further within New Zealand with bids to develop even more intensive dairy farms. The MacKenzie Guardians organization[19] represents people in the South Island of New Zealand concerned about water quality, increased dairy farming and environmental degradation. Their website (2009) reports deteriorating water quality in lowland streams and increasing contamination of water in rural communities. They also report 110 applications to take, use and discharge up to 90 million cubic metres of water a year from high country rivers, streams and lakes in the MacKenzie Basin, which is in the South Canterbury region of the South Island of New Zealand. Applications to develop intensive dairy farms with 18,000 cows housed in battery-cow farms consisting of cubicles, where cows will live for eight months of the year, 24 hours a day, seven days a week, were also reported. Plans to irrigate more than 27,000 hectares of the MacKenzie Basin, which is a naturally dry landscape described as 'a natural desert which is surprisingly biologically rich', is currently meeting resistance from the MacKenzie Guardians and others concerned about sustainability. The drive to produce more milk to turn into milk powder for export appears to ignore costs to the environment, water issues, pollution or cruelty to dairy cows.

This is, of course not an issue exclusive to New Zealand. *The Ecologist* online publication from 2 March 2010[20] reported plans to build a new super-dairy farm housing 8,100 cows in Lincolnshire, which would produce an estimated 250,000 litres of milk per day. *The Ecologist* also suggested that the furore over this proposed development masked the fact that most milk produced in the UK already comes from industrial-scale dairy farms. The picture in the US is much the same with reports of the emergence of large dairy farms housing over 15,000 dairy cows[21] and a reported large number of herds being injected with the controversial artificial bovine growth hormone (rBGH) to increase milk yield. Dairy cows do suffer adverse health effects from rBGH exposure, and even though the evidence for harm to humans is as yet inconclusive, there are concerns. For example, the increased use of antibiotics to treat rBGH-induced mastitis in cows promotes the development of antibiotic resistant bacteria.[22] Dairy farms with more than 500 cows have been reported as injecting more rBGH into cows than medium- and small-herd farmers with 54 per cent usage in large herds, 32 per cent in medium and 8 per cent for small-herd farmers. Cows injected with rBGH are more susceptible to infections and also use more feed to produce milk at demanding levels. All this leads to more pollution, pesticide use for the feed crops and an estimated 10 billion pounds of nitrogen fertilizer introduced into fields and waterways each day.[23]

David Merritt (2010), a New Zealand writer and poet, created a poem in 2010 entitled 'I am inorganic 2'. Here are a few sections from this work:

> I am inorganic and of course I am a monoculturalist, I grow grass by the tragic overuse of nitrates and phosphates onto six inches of fragile topsoil. You can watch my land wash away every shower, rainstorm and flood.

I am inorganic so all my milk produce now ends up encased in leeching plastics, both here and abroad. I am mechanised to the max

I am the inorganic dairy farmer.

My cows belch and fart methane.

I don't care because I am part of the backbone of the nation, above reproach and most environmental laws, represented by lobbyists, spinners, analysts, soothsayers, thinktank experts, industry sector groups and conservative, corrupt, rightwing politicians.

There is no end in sight for this poem [either].

Disaster: testing sustainability – infant survival and disaster

Rebecca Solnit's (2009) words about disaster being never terribly far away, ring very true to those who have suffered in a disaster, or because of a disaster, and for those who have watched so many disasters unfold in global media reports recently. Naomi Klein also discusses the 'steady stream' of global disasters, 'military, ecological and financial' (2007: 426). Torjesen and Olness (2009) report at least one large crisis every week that requires external assistance and in 2008 there were 321 disasters, which killed 236,000 people and affected 211 million people, of whom half were children.

Complex humanitarian emergencies are defined as humanitarian crises with political instability, armed conflict, massive population displacement, severe food shortages, social disruption, and collapse of public health infrastructures (Brennan and Nandy 2001). The negative impact of these emergencies on women and children is extreme. Callaghan and Rasmussen *et al.* (2007) estimated that Hurricane Katrina affected 56,100 pregnant women and 74,900 infants. In such situations the circumstances that may have made formula-feeding 'acceptable, feasible, affordable, sustainable and safe' *(AFASS)* (Lhotska *et al.* 2009) no longer exist; chaotic and unsafe conditions have replaced them. Therefore, the only safe option for an young infant is to be breastfed, or wet-nursed, preferably by an HIV-negative woman. Poor sanitation, lack of water, contaminated water, shortage of fuel and supplies and no electricity are among the major issues.

Interrupted breastfeeding and inappropriate complementary feeding heighten the risk of malnutrition, illness and mortality, and uncontrolled distribution of breastmilk substitutes, for example in refugee settings, can lead to early and unnecessary cessation of breastfeeding (WHO/UNICEF 2003). Support for pregnant women, breastfeeding mothers, continued breastfeeding, relactation and wet-nursing saves infant lives and prevents further morbidity.

Some mothers in Haiti, after the massive earthquake in January 2010, were reported in the media as refusing to breastfeed for fear of passing on their depression.[24] One 22-year-old mother interviewed in an emergency maternity tent was asked if she was going to breastfeed her day-old baby. This mother's answer was that she was sad she could not breastfeed and she would not give the baby her milk for six months. This mother was also unsure what she was going to feed her baby.

A widely reported story on the internet after Hurricane Katrina told the story of a young mother and new baby stranded on a rooftop with family members for five days with no access to food or clean water. After being rescued and hospitalized the baby sadly died, and when health workers asked the mother about her own health she apparently asked for assistance with drying up the milk in her lactating breasts. It appears that no family members on that rooftop considered that the baby could have been saved by breastfeeding; some reports suggested that it was as if the 'memory of breastfeeding' had been lost.[25]

As well as a possible 'loss of memory' of breastfeeding, misconceptions about lactation and breastfeeding are common in complex emergency situations, including the suggestion that shock and trauma cause mothers to lose their breastmilk. A temporary inhibition of oxytocin and the milk ejection reflex is not uncommon when breastfeeding mothers are acutely stressed, but given the right information and remedial, mutually comforting mother–baby contact this can be remedied and life-saving milk will flow once more.

In sub-Sahara Africa, breastmilk is known as 'siindjii' in the Djoula language. This expression is made up of two words, sii means life and djii means water – the water that supports and preserves life (Hoffman *et al.* 2009). Breastfeeding provides the 'water' that supports and preserves life and it is the only safe, sustainable infant feeding method in all complex emergency situations.

Evolutionary logic and the limits of adaptation

Human beings are destroying habitats on earth so that there are no longer safe havens for animals, mammals and birds to live, shelter and sustain themselves, displacing other humans, destroying land to create monocultures of single genetically-engineered crops, intensively farming herds of animals, and contributing to global climate change, which in turn contributes to a rise in natural disasters with subsequent tragic loss of life and land. Human beings are also in danger of slowly and tragically demolishing the habitat necessary for breastfeeding to survive – the mother – by the creation of cultures where women are unsupported and breastfeeding becomes endangered, untenable, undesirable, unmanageable and in itself an unsustainable maternal activity. Human being and planet Earth adaptation can only go so far. Natural resources are not infinite. When they are gone, they are gone forever. Infants are adaptable but at what cost? Globally only 34.6 per cent of infants less than six months are exclusively breastfed (WHO, 2009). At what point does the continued escalation of ill-health and associated costs of not-breastfeeding become more noticeable to more people and generate significant action on behalf of governments.

Rebecca Solnit (2009) suggests that the human activity of home improvement, rather than work towards world improvement, seems to have triumphed, with private well-being holding supremacy over public good. Breastfeeding is quite unique as it represents a form of home-improvement that really will lead to world improvement in terms of sustainability, environmental benefit and health. Considering the argument presented by Solnit (2009), where she suggests that human-beings reset themselves to their inbuilt altruistic behaviours and help each other in disaster communities, just like machines resetting themselves to their original settings following a power outage, then perhaps increasing health disasters will lead to the 'resetting' of breastfeeding cultures.

Freidman suggested that only a crisis, real or perceived, produces real change. He also suggested that what actions are taken during these crisis times '. . . depends on the ideas that are lying around' (in Klein 2007: 6). Currently, the global breastfeeding culture remains non-robust and infant formula feeding is often the dominant 'lying-around' discourse in the majority of countries. However, breastfeeding remains the only sustainable, safe way to feed and protect infants in non-disaster times, as well as during times of disaster and emergency.

The human rights of an infant to be breastfed have been debated. Outside of the human rights argument is another highlighted by James Lovelock (1995). Lovelock suggests that humans were not considering the consequences of their actions and that for the species to survive human rights are not enough. Humans also need to take care of the earth. As the main protagonist in Marilynne Robinson's novel *Gilead* says: 'This is an interesting planet. It deserves all the attention you can give it' (2004: 32). Lactation and breastfeeding are maternal endeavors of compelling evolutionary significance. They deserve recognition as strong links to the wellness, sustainability and survival of planet Earth and as much more than the optimal means to feed an infant and young child. Breastfeeding women deserve all the support, protection and attention we all can give them.

Notes

1 Wet nursing – when a lactating woman breastfeeds an infant other than her own. See Fildes, V. (1988). *Wet Nursing: A History From Antiquity to the Present.* Oxford: Basil Blackwell.
2 Allomother refers to an individual, other than the infant's mother, who takes care of the infant.
3 WHO Nutrition Data Bank, which covered 94 countries at this time, https://apps.who.int/nut/db_bfd.htm.
4 http://www.worldbreastfeedingtrends.org/report/WBTi-Philippine-2008.pdf.
5 Stuebe, A. M., Willett, W. C. and Michels, B. (2009) 'Lactation and incidence of premenopausal breast cancer: a longitudinal study', *International Medicine*, 169: 1364–71
6 Collaborative group on hormonal factors in breast cancer (2002) 'Collaborative reanalysis of individual data from 47 epidemiological studies in 30 countries,

including 50,302 women with breast cancer and 96,973 women without the disease', *The Lancet*, 360: 187–95.

7 Freudenheim, J. L., Marshall, J. R., Graham, S., Laughlin, R., Vena, J. E. *et al.* (1994) 'Exposure to breastmilk in infancy and the risk of breast cancer', *Epidemiology*, 5, 3: 324–31

8 Zheng, T., Holford, T. R., Mayne, S. T., Owens, P. H., Zhang, Y. *et al.* (2001) 'Lactation and breast cancer risk: a case-control study in Connecticut', *British Journal of Cancer*, 84, 11: 1472–76.

9 Jordan, S., Siskind, V., Green, A.C., Whiteman, D. C. and Webb, P. M. (2010) 'Breastfeeding and the risk of epithelial ovarian cancer', *Cancer Causes and Control*, 21, 1: 109–16.

10 Titus-Ernstoff, L., Rees, J. R., Terry, K. L. and Cramer, D. W. (2010) 'Breastfeeding in the last born child and risk of ovarian cancer', *Cancer Causes and Control*, 21, 2: 201–07.

11 Blaauw, R., Albertse, E. C., Beneke, T., Lombard, C. J., Laubscher, R. and Hough, F. S. (1994) 'Risk factors for the development of osteoporosis in a South African population: a prospective analysis', *South African Medical Journal*, 84, 6: 328–32.

12 Melton, L. J., Bryant, S. C., Wahner, H. W., O'Fallon, W. M., Malkasian, G. D. *et al.* (1993) 'Influence of breastfeeding and other reproductive factors on bone mass in later life', *Osteoporosis International*, 3, 2: 76–83.

13 Stuebe, A. M., Michels, K. B., Willett, W. C., Manson, J. E., Rexrode, K. and Rich-Edwards, J. W. (2009) 'Duration of lactation and incidence of myocardial infarction in middle to late adulthood', *American Journal of Obstetrics & Gynecology*, 299, 2: 138.e1–138.e8.

14 Schwartz, E. B., Ray, R.M., Stuebe, A. M., Allison, M. A., Ness, R. B., Freiberg, M. S. and Cauley, J. A. (2009) 'Duration of lactation and risk factors for maternal cardiovascular disease', *Obstetrics and Gynecology*, 113, 5: 972–73.

15 Barnett, S. (2009) 'Baby blues: Your reproductive choices are affecting the global environment', *New Zealand Listener*, October 3: 55.

16 The measure of an individual's contribution to global warming (Lynas, 2007).

17 The melamine tragedy, China 2008. Six infants were reported to have died and almost 30,000 children became ill after drinking infant formula intentionally laced with melamine to 'boost' protein levels in milk that had been watered down. Melamine is a plastics component and when combined with a related compound, cyanuric acid, can cause kidney stones and kidney failure.

18 The International Baby Food Action Network compiles lists of infant formula recalls due to processing and manufacturing errors and contamination. See http://www.ibfan.org.

19 'The aims of the Mackenzie Guardians are to promote the protection of the natural/ naturalistic wildlife, water, vegetation, heritage and landscape values of the Mackenzie Country. Mackenzie Guardians believe that the values of this unique area need to be conserved for the enjoyment and well-being of present and future generations.' From http://mackenzieguardians.co.nz/about.

20 http://www.theecologist.org/News/news_round_up/431805/most_uk_milk_ already_from_industrialsized_dairy_farms.html.

21 'Profits, costs and the changing structure of dairy farms'. Economic Research Service USDA. http://www.efs.usda.gov/publications/err47/err47b.pdf.

22 The American Cancer Society at http://www.cancer.org/docroot/PED/content/ PED_1_3x_Recombinant_Bovine_Growth_Hormone.asp.

23 See www.sustainable.org/issues/rBGH.

24 See http//www.google.ca/reader/shared/chase/jodinechase (accessed 29 January 2010).

25 Hurricane Katrina reports at:
    www.medindia.net/news/healthinfocus/World-Breastfeeding-Week-2009-55543-
    1.htm
    www.co.durham.nc.us/departments/publ/News_Releases/News_Release.cfm?ID
    =1111.

References

Akre, J. (2009) 'From grand design to change on the ground: going to scale with a global feeding strategy', in F. Dykes and V. H. Moran (eds), *Infant and Young Child Feeding: Challenges to Implementing a Global Strategy*. Oxford: Wiley-Blackwell Publishing.

Brennan, N. J. and Nandy, R. (2001) 'Complex humanitarian emergencies: a major global health challenge', *Emergency Medicine*, 13: 147–56.

Callaghan, W. M., Rasmussen, S. A., Jamieson, D. J., Ventura, S. J., Farr, S. L. *et al.* (2007) 'Concerns of women and infants during natural disasters such as Katrina: the population at risk', *Maternal and Child Health Journal*, 11, 4: 307–11.

Drane, D. D. (1997) 'Breastfeeding and formula feeding: a preliminary economic analysis', *Breastfeeding Review*, 5, 1: 7–15.

Fawell, J., and Nieuwenhuijsen, M. J. (2003) 'Contaminants in drinking water: environmental pollution and health', *British Medical Bulletin*, 68:199–208.

Frick, K. D. (2009) 'Use of economics to analyse policies to promote breastfeeding', in F. Dykes and V. H. Moran (eds), *Infant and Young Child Feeding: Challenges to Implementing a Global Strategy*. Oxford: Wiley-Blackwell Publishing.

Friends of the Earth (2008) 'What's feeding our food? The environmental and social impacts of the livestock sector', Online. Available at: www.foe.co.uk/resource/briefings/livestock_impacts.pdf (accessed 21 February 2010).

Hoffman, J., De Allegri, M., Sarker, M., Sanon, M. and Böhler, T. (2009) 'Breast milk as the "water that supports and preserves life" – socio-cultural constructions of breastfeeding and their implications for the prevention of mother to child transmission of HIV in sub-Sahara Africa', *Health Policy*, 89: 322–28.

Hrdy, S. B. (1999) *Mother Nature: Natural Selection and the Female of the Species*. London: Chatto & Windus.

Kingsolver Barbara. (1999) *The Poisonwood Bible*. London: Faber & Faber.

Klein, N. (2007) *The Shock Doctrine: The Rise of Disaster Capitalism*. New York: Metropolitan Books.

Labbok, M. H. (1994) 'Breastfeeding as a cost effective preventative health measure', *International Journal of Gynecology and Obstetrics*, 47, Suppl: 555–61.

Lauer, J. A., Betran, A. P., Barros, A. J. D. and Onis, M. de (2006) 'Deaths and years of life lost due to suboptimal breast-feeding amongst children in the developing world: a global ecological risk assessment', *Public Health Nutrition*, 9, 6: 673–85.

Lhotska, L., Norton, R. and McGrath, M. (2009) *Guidance on infant feeding and HIV in the context of refugees and displaced populations, Version 1.1*. United Nations High Commission for Refugees (UNHCR): Geneva.

Lovelock, J. (1995) *The Ages of Gaia: A Biography of Our Living Earth*. Oxford: Oxford University Press.

Lynas, M. (2007) *Collins Gem Carbon Counter*. London: Harper Collins.

MacKenzie Guardians (2009) Online Available at: http://mackenzieguardians.co.nz/ (accessed 14 March 2010).

McNiel, M. E., Labbok, M. H. and Abrahams, S. W. (2010) 'What are the risks associated with formula feeding? A reanalysis and review', *Birth*, 37, 1: 50–58.

Madani, K. A., Khashoggi, R. H., al-Nowaisser, A. A., Nasrat, H. A. and Khalil, M. H. (1994) 'Lactation amenorrhea in Saudi women', *Journal of Epidemiology and Community Health*, 48: 286–89.

Merritt, D. (2010) 'I am inorganic 2'. *Inorganic*. Whanganui: Landroverfarm Press.

Palmer, G. (2009) *The Politics of Breastfeeding: When Breasts are Bad for Business*. London: Printer & Martin.

Parliamentary Commissioner for the Environment, New Zealand (2005). *Growing for Good: Intensive Farming, Sustainability and New Zealand's Environment*. Wellington: Parliamentary Commissioner for the Environment.

Powlson, D. S., Addiscott, T. M., Benjamin, N., Cassman, K. G., De Kok, T. M. et al. (2008) 'When does nitrate become a risk for humans?' *Journal of Environmental Quality*, 37, March/April.

Radwan, H., Mussaiger, A. O. and Hachem, F. (2009) 'Breastfeeding and lactational amenorrhoea in the United Arab Emirates', *Journal of Pediatric Nursing*, 24 1: 62–68.

Robinson, Marilynne (2004) *Gilead*. London: Virago.

Schumacher, E. F. (1974) *Small is Beautiful: A Study of Economics as if People Mattered*. London: Abacus.

Smith, J. P. and Ingham, L. H. (2001) 'Breastfeeding and the measurement of economic progress', *Journal of Australian Political Economy*, 48:51–72.

Smith, J. P., Thompson, J. F. and Ellwood, D. A. (2002) 'Hospital system costs of artificial infant feeding: estimates for the Australian Capital Territory', *Australian and New Zealand Journal of Public Health*, 26, 6: 543–51.

Solnit, R. (2009) *A Paradise Built in Hell: The Extraordinary Communities That Arise in Disaster*. New York: Penguin.

Stuebe, A. M. and Schwarz, E. B. (2009) 'The risks and benefits of infant feeding practices for women and their children', *Journal of Perinatology*, 1: 1–8.

Torjesen, K. and Olness, K. (2009) 'International child health: state of the art', *Current Problems in Pediatric and Adolescent Health Care*, 39: 192–213.

Van Esterik, P. (2002) *Risks, Rights and Regulation: Communicating About Risks and Infant Feeding*. Penang: World Alliance for Breastfeeding Action (WABA).

Waring, M. (1988) *Counting For Nothing*. Wellington: Allen & Unwin.

Wollstonecraft, M. (1978) *Vindication of the Rights of Women*. Middlesex: Penguin (originally published in 1792).

World Health Organisation/UNICEF (2003) *Global Strategy for Infant and Young Child Feeding*. Geneva: WHO.

World Health Organization (2009) WHO Executive Board 126th session provisional agenda item 4.6, 19 November 2009. 'Infant and young child nutrition quadrennial progress report', Online. Available at: http://apps.who.int/gb/ebwha/pdf_files/EB126/B126_9-en.pdf (accessed 29 January 2010).

14 The pregnant environment

Megan Gibbons and Jean Patterson

> I look at my watch. Five minutes! I look down at the stick. Two lavender
> lines . . . Unmistakable. Now there are two of us.
>
> (Steingraber 2003: 10)[1]

Introduction

Pregnancy is an incredibly complex state of being and each unique episode
brings its own character and challenges according to the conditions present
in the life of the woman at the time. In most cases, the pregnancy will
flourish and a healthy, well baby and mother will result. However, there are
a multitude of factors that may influence the pregnancy and subsequent
outcomes. Midwives need to be able to provide holistic care in order to
facilitate appropriate responses to each woman's and baby's needs.

In this chapter we explore some of the common environmental and lifestyle
factors that pose identified or potential risks to women and their babies during
pregnancy. These include the environmental hazards of radiation, some heavy
metals, synthetic compounds and drugs, all of which have the potential to
cause harm to a growing baby during pregnancy.

The classic environmental text by Rachel Carson, *Silent Spring* published
in 1962, identified some of the devastating effects of environmental toxins
and warned that their 'presence casts a shadow that is not less ominous
because it is formless and obscure' (Carson 1962: 188). Almost half a century
later, it is estimated that there are more than 70,000 synthetic chemicals
utlilized commercially and approximately 1,000 new chemicals are introduced
each year. (US FDA 2007). For most of these, the potential effects on embryos
and fetuses are unknown.

There are numerous examples of different forms of environmental toxins
that have led to devastating outcomes. In the early 1960s, at around the time
Carson was writing, women around the world were prescribed Thalidomide
for morning sickness, a synthetic oestrogen, which had not been subjected to
any rigorous clinical testing. As a result, thousands of babies were born with
limb defects. Many studies have found a correlation between cases of low birth
weight, neural-tube defects, choanal atresia, cardiac defects and drinking-water

contamination (Infante-Rivard 2004). Studies on the level of endocrine disruptors created in the production of pesticides and plasticizers indicate that these may affect the function of sex and thyroid hormones and suggest that exposure to these *in utero* may compromise fertility in adult life (Barrett *et al*. 2009). This leads us to consider the fact that the effects on babies exposed to the toxins *in utero* may have a much longer-lasting impact, including on future generations. Angier, reflecting on being pregnant with her daughter, refers to her as her 'matryoshka', her Russian doll. She explains 'At twenty weeks' gestation, the peak of a female's oogonial load, the fetus holds 6 to 7 million eggs' (1999: 2).

Some of the potential teratogenic agents of pregnancy are listed in the remainder of the chapter. It should be acknowledged that this is an enormous subject area and there are many more agents than we could consider for inclusion. The intention of the discussion of agents in this chapter is to raise awareness so that women may take the initiative wherever possible, to avoid or minimize their exposure to these toxins.

> Organogenesis begins with three flat layers and one week later produces a coiled, segmented object that looks like an architectural detail on the end of a stair banister.
>
> (Steingraber 2003: 15)

Radiation exposure

Radiation is the process of the release of energy from one body, which travels in a straight line though space (Pergament *et al*. 1993). It is everywhere in our environment and we are exposed to low levels every day. This background radiation emanates from space, soil, air, building materials, power lines, microwaves, and even from the food we eat. Radiation is classified as non-ionizing or ionizing. Non-ionizing radiation comes from the lower end of the electromagnetic spectrum, which includes visible light, microwaves and radio waves, and does not have the energy needed to remove an electron from an atom or molecule, whereas ionizing radiation does. Its source comes from unstable, often decaying atoms, which shed energy to regain stability (Pergament *et al*. 1993).

Prenatal radiation exposure can occur when a woman inhales or ingests radioactive particles in air or food (Health Physics Society n.d.). The most sensitive period for effects on the fetus is between 2 and 15 weeks of pregnancy. Radiation exposure *in utero* can affect growth and development, cause anomalies, predispose the individual to cancer and adversely affect brain function and IQ in later life. Where exposure to radiation is low, less than the equivalent of 500 chest X-rays, the risk to the baby is very low for developing abnormalities, however the risk of cancer in later life remains (Health Physics Society n.d.). After the sixteenth week of pregnancy the risk to the unborn baby decreases unless the exposure is large; more than the equivalent of 5,000 chest X-rays (a level of exposure that would cause radiation sickness in the mother) (Health Physics Society n.d.).

Radiation is measured in RADs (radiated absorbed dose), but when estimating health risk the measurement is usually recorded in roentgens (rem) (Pergament *et al.* 1993). Everyone is exposed to daily background radiation amounting to around 300 millirem each year (Health Physics Society n.d.). Most standard medical tests have dose rates below the 5,000 millirem though some speciality tests are above this dose, which increases the risks at particular gestation stages. While pregnant women would rarely experience such large doses of X-rays it is always best to avoid unnecessary exposure. Therefore women requiring an X-ray should inform the technician if they are pregnant and discuss with their doctor whether an alternative procedure would be more appropriate (Centre for Disease Control and Prevention 2006).

> The discs three layers are the original tribes of Israel. All body parts originate from one of them.
>
> (Steingraber 2003: 15)

Pregnant women exposed to ionizing radiation in their work environment, such as those performing or assisting with lengthy fluoroscopic investigations, are at increased risk (Damilakis *et al.* 2005). Women in these roles need to consider how they might limit their exposure during pregnancy.

The heavy metals

> The internal anatomy of a human placenta closely resembles a maple grove: the long columns sent out by the embryo into the uterine branch lining during the first few weeks of pregnancy quickly branch and branch again until, by the end of the third month of pregnancy, the treetops of an entire forest press up against the deepest layers of the womb.
>
> (Steingraber 2003: 30)

In common with the inevitable exposure to radiation in the environment women are unable to avoid some inhalation or ingestion of toxic metal traces. The degree of risk is largely related to area of residence and lifestyle or work activities. Heavy metals such as lead, cadmium and mercury are not required by our bodies for cell growth. Rather, absorption of these metals in significant quantities has been demonstrated to affect human growth and development, particularly that of the developing fetus.

Lead (Pb)

Lead is used in production and smelting processes and in paints and finishes, batteries and potteries. It is also used in activities such as stained-glass or jewellery making (Ministry of Health 2008). During flooding lead is washed into storm water drains and waterways (Organization of Teratology Information Specialists (OTIS 2010). Most people have low levels of lead in their bodies absorbed through their lungs or ingested with food and water. Only small amounts are absorbed through the skin, but this can be transferred to food when working with lead (Gundacker *et al.* 2002).

Lead stored in the body usually gravitates to the bones from where it is only slowly released (Gomaa *et al.* 2002). Where blood levels exceed 10µg/dl it can affect the shape and motility of sperm (OTIS 2010). In pregnancy, lead stores from the mother cross to the placenta and high blood lead levels are associated with an increased risk of miscarriage or premature birth (Gundacker *et al.* 2002; OTIS 2010). Cognitive brain development is also affected as is memory and it is thought that this may contribute to the later onset of adult psychiatric disorders (Opler *et al.* 2008). High lead levels are also found in the hair samples of children with Attention Deficit, Hyperactivity Disorder (ADHD) and autism in some, but not all, studies (Curtis and Patel 2008). Breastfeeding, however, confers some protection for cognitive development (Williams and Ross 2007). So while lead is found in breastmilk, it is usually at lower levels than in infant formula. This contamination in formula can be compounded when contaminated water is used to mix the formula (Gundacker *et al.* 2002; Ministry of Health 2008).

> At one end of the line, a bump rises up like a miniature volcano with a tiny crater at its summit. This line is called the primitive streak, the bump is called the primitive node and its crater the primitive pit.
>
> (Steingraber 2003: 15)

To reduce the risk of further lead accumulation during pregnancy, women are advised to avoid using lead-based paints or engaging in renovation projects on older houses. Home drinking-water sources should also be checked for lead levels, particularly if well water is used or water is reticulated through lead pipes. Hand washing is particularly important after handling soil when gardening or, engaging in hobbies that involve working with lead or lead-based products Women are advised to eat a diet rich in the trace elements of calcium, iron and zinc, which are associated with less lead absorption. (OTIS 2010).

> From its perch in the cells near the primitive node, sonic hedgehog directs the development of body parts such as the brain, intestines and limbs.
>
> (Steingraber 2003: 16)

Cadmium (Cd)

Cadmium is a soft blue-white metal found in relation to zinc. It is used in the manufacture of bearings, and alloys with low melting points to reduce friction and metal fatigue. It is also used in atomic fission reactors. Because of its special properties cadmium was used widely in the 1950s and 1960s but when its toxic effects were realized industrial limits were instituted in most industrialized countries (Kippler *et al.* 2009).

Toxins including cadmium are released into the air from factories, incineration plants and smelting processes, with the risks of exposure greater for those who work in, or live near, these installations. Soil and water are contaminated from these sources though significant contamination in some areas is the result of the widespread use of phosphate fertilizers in agriculture (Williams and David 1977). People who smoke tobacco are particularly at risk of inhaling cadmium as the lungs are very efficient at absorbing it (Williams 1998). This was confirmed by Richter *et al.* (2009), who found older smokers in their study had toxic levels of cadmium.

Cadmium accumulates in bone and kidney tissues with high levels of exposure leading to kidney failure (Williams 1998). It also accumulates in the human placenta where it interacts with the transport of micronutrients to the fetus (Kippler *et al.* 2009) affecting birth weight and later IQ development (Tian *et al.* 2009). A potential association between autism and exposure to heavy metals, including cadmium, was found by (Windham *et al.* 2006). However, it is acknowledged that these complex conditions need also to be understood in terms of the social and home circumstances (Williams and Ross 2007).

Women can reduce their exposure to cadmium by avoiding exposure from contaminated sites or workplaces, not smoking and maintaining good hand hygiene. If working with solders that contain cadmium, it is important to do so under a fume hood to filter and ventilate the workspace. A well-balanced diet rich in sources of zinc, magnesium and iron is recommended, as it confers a protective effect for most heavy metal toxicity (Kippler *et al.* 2009; Messaoudi *et al.* 2009).

> At week eleven of pregnancy, no further assembly is required: the embryo is knighted a fetus and simply grows bigger until it is ready for birth.
>
> (Steingraber 2003: 14)

Mercury (Hg)

Mercury is a valuable metal in industry. It is liquid at room temperature and not readily oxidized due to its density. It also alloys well with other metals, with the exception of iron, and vaporizes easily when a current is applied. This makes mercury ideal for use in fluorescent lights (US EPA/Wisconsin Department of Natural Resources 1997).

Like lead and cadmium, mercury finds its way into the air, soils and waterways (Ministry of Health 2008). It is a by-product in petroleum refining, lime and cement manufacture, smelting and refining of non-ferrous metals, including copper and aluminium. It is also present in fossil fuels of wood and coal. Vapour from these sources travels large distances and can cause respiratory problems followed by neurological disturbances and other organ effects (Hujoel *et al.* 2005). Inhaled mercury vapour readily crosses the placenta and accumulates in the fetus due to mercury's high lipid solubility. In children, exposure can lead to brain and nervous system damage and developmental delay (Axelrad *et al.* 2007; Ministry of Health 2008). Thus, where possible, mercury has been replaced by other products. However, its stable qualities mean that it is still used in switches, fluorescent lighting and to calibrate sensitive measuring apparatus (US EPA/Wisconsin Department of Natural Resources 1997).

When mercury leaches into the waterways, bacteria and algae convert it to its organic form of methyl-mercury (MeHg). This moves up the food chain, becoming concentrated in the larger fish species such as tuna and shark (Huffling 2006). Inland fish such as trout may also have higher levels of mercury if caught in lakes or rivers in geothermal areas (Ministry of Health 2008). Methyl-mercury can cross both the placental and blood brain barriers and affect fetal brain development and function. In later life children exposed *in utero* may experience difficulties with language development, memory and some motor functions.

Studies of hair samples of populations who consume diets rich in seafood have produced conflicting results in regard to mercury levels (Gerhardsson and Lundh 2010). Even in populations where whale meat is consumed the beneficial long-chain-free fatty acids in the meat appear to confer a moderating effect on mercury toxicity (Williams and Ross 2007). Fish is a good source of protein and the oily varieties such as mackerel, sardines, herring, salmon and green-lipped mussels are rich sources of valuable long-chain omega-3 fatty acids recommended in pregnancy. So while it is safest to choose fish from the lower end of the food chain (McDiarmid and Gehle 2006) it is considered safe to eat fresh or canned tuna up to three times a week as the fish used for canning are generally smaller fish, which have not accumulated large stores of mercury in their systems (Bowden 2010).

> Organogenesis is . . . fantastical. Sometimes it seems like a magic show. At other times its like origami, the formation of elegant structures from the folding of flat sheets.
>
> (Steingraber 2003: 14)

Concerns about the mercury content of dental amalgam may deter women from seeking dental care during pregnancy. However, a population case-controlled study found that women who had at least one amalgam filling during pregnancy were not at risk of having a baby of low birth weight (Hujoel *et al.* 2005). Alternative resin-based amalgams may be considered, but these have been found to leach oestrogen-like molecules associated with adverse pregnancy outcomes in animal studies (Hujoel *et al.* 2005).

Toxic chemicals in our environment

... [watching] the embryological anatomy of the vertebrate brain ... is like watching a rose bloom in speeded up time. Or like spelunking in an unchartered cave.

(Steingraber 2003: 109)

The widespread use of chemicals to control weeds and pests means that it is virtually impossible to avoid coming into contact with these residues; even when not actively involved in using them. Herbicides and pesticides are sprayed not just in agricultural settings but also to control weeds on roadsides around public buildings and parks (Quackenbush *et al.* 2006). In addition many homeowners use these products to control garden weeds and pests.

Herbicides

There are a variety of herbicides designed to target particular weed species. One common component of household and general-purpose herbicides is glyphosate (Richard *et al.* 2005). Glyphosate residues find their way into the water and soil and into the food chain. They are also absorbed through the skin during the manufacturing process or when mixing or spraying weeds.

Glyphosate was tested on human placental cells. Even at dilutions 100 times lower that those recommended for use, the cytochrome P450 aromatase activity, critical for cell reproduction, was affected in placental cells (Richard *et al.* 2005). Studies on rats exposed to high doses of glyphosate resulted in the death of some of the female rats and discovery of bone defects in their fetuses (Dallegrave *et al.* 2003).

Phenoxy-herbicides

These are used for the control of broad-leaved plants and exposure has been associated with several cancers in humans, and exposure during pregnancy has been associated with early pregnancy loss (Arbuckle *et al.* 1999). Studies in rats showed changes to their liver cells (Sulik *et al.* 1998).

Dioxin

The name dioxin is frequently used to identity a wide range of compounds, including the halogenated aromatic compounds, which have as their basis a dioxin core skeleton. These enduring and unwelcome molecules are a man-made by-product of incineration processes, the manufacture of plastics, pesticides and paper bleaching. Since the late 1980s advances in chemical and environmental management practices have resulted in a reduction in dioxin emissions in New Zealand (Ministry of Health 2009).

Exposure to dioxins is largely through the food chain as the compounds deposited on soil and plant surfaces are consumed by grazing stock (Ministry of Health 2009). Where water run-off is contaminated, dioxin accumulates in the larger fish and mammal species in a similar way to that of methylmercury. Dioxins are believed to cause a variety of neuro-development, immunological and carcinogenic effects (Ministry of Health 2009). Though in exposed populations where large emissions of dioxins are experienced, other social and environmental factors can compound and confound the studies (Huffling 2006).

Small amounts of dioxin can also be absorbed through the skin when inhaling cigarette smoke (Huffling 2006). The accumulated dioxin burden persists for many years in body fat and in the liver and has a half life of 7–11 years; this is dependent to some extent on the amount of body fat present. Elimination occurs slowly over time in faeces with small amounts lost in urine. Elimination also occurs in the breastmilk, from which the infant absorbs 95 per cent with the level in the infant reaching the equivalent level in the mother after six months of breastfeeding. However, by around 10 years of age dioxin levels are equivalent with those of formula-fed children (Ministry of Health 2009).

Advice to pregnant and breastfeeding women is about healthy lifestyle choices. These include avoiding unnecessary exposure to emission sites, eating a well-balanced diet and managing weight gain, as well as eliminating surface contamination with careful hand hygiene and washing fruit and vegetables well before cooking or eating (Ministry of Health 2009).

Pesticides and PCBs

> The language of human brain development borrows its vocabulary from botany, architecture and geography. There are lumens, islands, aqueducts and isthmuses.
>
> (Steingraber 2003: 109)

Organochlorines are organic compounds, which contain at least one covalently-bonded chlorine atom. They are highly lipophyllic and designed to target the nerve cells in insects, creating hyper-excitability and/or depression and convulsions (Coats 1990). In addition to the production of insecticides and fungicides, these compounds are used in electrical and other industrial processes. Organochorine is carried in vapour form, contaminating soil and water. Contamination moves up the food chain as grazing animals, birds and fish species are exposed to the residues, which become concentrated in the fatty tissues (Williams and Ross 2007).

These chemicals persist in the environment and present risks to women and their babies. Organochorines readily cross the placenta and are associated with neurodevelopment effects (Sagiv *et al.* 2010). A potential association was also found between Attention Deficit, Hyperactivity Disorder (ADHD) and low levels of organochlorines measured in the umbilical cord serum of children whose mothers lived near a Polychorinated Biphenols (PCB) waste dump

(Sagiv *et al.* 2010). Further exposure to these chemicals can occur through breastfeeding. However, the properties of breastmilk protect neurological development and appear to compensate for any additional exposure from this source (Williams and Ross 2007).

Recreational drugs

> The twelve cranial nerves go forth like apostles to make contact with the far-flung, newly developing eyes, ears, tongue, nose etc.
>
> (Steingraber 2003: 110)

Smoking

Smoking during pregnancy is known to have increased risk of complications (Rogers 2009), the baby being born prematurely and too small (small for gestational age) (Yakoob *et al* 2009). Low birthweight as a result of small for gestational age or prematurity is known to be associated with coronary heart disease, type 2 diabetes and being overweight in adulthood, in addition to complications in childhood. Smoking during pregnancy is strongly associated with poverty, lower levels of education, poor social support, depression and psychological illness, which can make it more difficult to provide effective intervention. In New Zealand the smoking rates during pregnancy reduced from 22.9 per cent in 2004 to 19.2 per cent in 2007 (NZCOM 2009).

In a Cochrane review of smoking cessation programmes (Lumley *et al*. 2010), there were 52 trials identified – all were in high-income countries and the effectiveness was about 6 per cent. All effective interventions demonstrated reductions in low birthweight babies and preterm births.

Alcohol

Alcohol readily crosses the placenta, therefore fetal blood alcohol levels will be similar to maternal levels, and it may affect fetal neurological and behavioural development (Strandberg-Larsen *et al*. 2009). Alcohol may interfere with metabolic processes and the supply of nutrients from the woman to her baby, and hence its growth and development. Fetal alcohol syndrome (FAS) is the most widely recognized outcome of maternal alcohol intake during pregnancy. It is characterized by intrauterine and post-natal growth restriction, characteristic facial features, and adverse effects on brain function, which may lead to neuro-developmental symptoms (Ministry of Health 2008). It has been recognized that there are, however, a range of effects from exposure to lower amounts of alcohol *in utero* that are more difficult to diagnose. This has been termed fetal alcohol spectrum disorder (FASD). The effects may include some or all of the following: attention deficit, hyperactivity disorder; immature behaviour; lack of organization; learning difficulties; poor abstract thinking; poor adaptability; poor impulse control; poor judgement; and speech, language and other communication problems (Elgen *et al.* 2007). The lower limit of alcohol intake at which no adverse effect will occur for any developing fetus has not as yet been determined and may not exist. In light of this knowledge it would be prudent for women to seriously consider avoiding alcohol during pregnancy.

Illicit drugs

We can generally categorise illicit drugs as opioids, stimulants, hallucinogens and cannabis. While they all have different effects, they all cross the placenta and enter the fetal circulation. They also affect the mothers' health and interfere with her ability to support the pregnancy; there is an increased risk of miscarriage, premature labour and placental abruption. There are a number of consequences that have been found for the infant these include: pre-term birth; low birthweight; birth defects; growth restriction and small head size; impaired neuro-development; poor motor skills; learning disabilities; behavioural problems; and increased risk of infection (Schempf and Strobino 2008). In addition, if the drugs are taken in late pregnancy the newborn infant may be drug dependent and suffer withdrawal symptoms (Oei and Lui 2007). Users of illicit drugs may also have other health and social issues and so the health provider may need to approach the issue sensitively and use appropriate referral services. The best advice is to eliminate use if the woman is a social user and reduce use in the case of addiction with support from suitable agencies.

Summary

> I realize that I am beginning to perceive her as sentient being – as a child- and myself more and more as her mother.
>
> (Steingraber 2003: 112)

In the light of our increasing knowledge of the potentially harmful effects of many environmental toxins, one may imagine that industries and government would be taking on greater responsibility to ensure the environment is safe for pregnant women and their babies. However, ironically, the spotlight in the last few decades seems to be increasingly focussing on the pregnant woman. Many women who are pregnant find themselves under close scrutiny in relation to what they eat or ingest. As Daniels (1997) notes in relation to fetal hazards, mothers are held to blame, while the hazards associated with toxins in food, water and the air that have been caused by pollution from private corporations or governments are virtually ignored.

Midwives and other health professionals need to support women and provide information that enables them to make informed choices around matters relating to exposure to work- or lifestyle-based hazards that may threaten the health and well-being of both her and her unborn baby. Some exposure in our daily lives to radiation, heavy metals, herbicides and pesticides is inevitable, even in countries where the most dangerous chemicals are banned and there are controls on the disposal of toxic wastes. Nonetheless, women seeking the best start for their baby and the ongoing safety of themselves and their families may be able to modify some aspects of their lifestyle to avoid unnecessary exposure to environmental toxins. Changes such as eating well, not smoking, avoiding alcohol or psychoactive substances, and maintaining a healthy weight are all advised. In addition women are best to avoid direct contact with herbicides and pesticides, and practice good hand hygiene after gardening or caring for pets.

As part of pre-conceptual counselling, or care during pregnancy, an assessment of a woman's lifestyle and environment may be helpful (McDiarmid and Gehle 2006). Such an evaluation could cover household tasks, work roles and hobbies, plus any potential for high levels of exposure to the environmental toxins discussed in this chapter. Information could then be shared about activities and lifestyle, which offer the optimal circumstances for the health and well-being of the woman, her new baby and her family.

> And then something is rushing through me like a waterfall of snowmelt down a mountain and suddenly there is space inside me and a tremendous sense of relief . . . Spiky feathers of wild, luxuriant black hair. Dusky skin, greased with vernix that is smooth as the first lotion. Lips I recognize from a school photo of myself in the first grade. Oh. Who are you? Two eyes open, black as mystery. They ask, 'And who are you?'
>
> (Steingraber 2003: 200)

Note

1   Sandra Steingraber is an acclaimed ecologist and author, who uses personal and professional insights to explore ecological issues and offers suggestions on how we can help to protect our environment and ourselves. In her book *Having Faith – An Ecologist's Journey to Motherhood*, she invites us to share the intimate ecology of motherhood. Her wonderful imagery and inimitable lyrical style, are offered in this chapter to remind us of the remarkable transformation that is taking place during pregnancy.

References

Angier, N. (1999) *Woman, An Intimate Geography*. Boston, MA: Houghton Mifflin Company.

Arbuckle, T. E., Savitz, D. A., Mery, L. S. and Curtis, K. M. (1999) 'Exposure to phenoxy herbicides and the risk of spontaneous abortion', *Epidemiology*, 10, 6: 752–60. Online. Available at: www.ncbi.nlm.nih.gov/pubmed/10535791 (accessed 6 February 2010).

Axelrad, D. A., Bellinger, D. C., Ryan, L. M. and Woodruff, T. J. (2007) 'Dose-response relationship of prenatal mercury exposure and IQ: an integrative analysis of epidemiologic data', *Environmental Health Perspectives*, 115, 4: 609–15.

Barrett, J. Gonzalez, S., Sarantis, H. and Varshavsky, J. (2009) 'Girl, Disrupted: Hormone Disruptors and Women's Reproductive Health, A Report on the Women's Reproductive Health and Environment Workshop'. Bolinas: Collaborative on Health and the Environment. Online. Available at: www.healthandenvironment. org/articles/doc/5492 (accessed 23 March 2010).

Bowden, J. (13 February 2010) 'Know-how, can do. Is canned fish a healthy addition to a regular diet?' *Listener*, 48.

Carson, R. (1962) *Silent Spring*. Boston: Houghton Mifflin Company.

Centre for Disease Control and Prevention (2006) 'Possible health effects of radiation exposure on unborn babies.' Online. Available at: www.bt.cdc.gov/radiation/ prenatal.asp (accessed 2 February 2010).

Coats, J. R. (1990) 'Mechanisms of toxic action and structure-activity relationships for organochlorine and synthetic pyrethroid insecticides', *Environmental Health Perspectives*, 87: 255–62.

Curtis, L. T. and Patel, K. (2008) 'Nutritional and environmental approaches to preventing and treating autism and attention deficit hyperactivity disorder (ADHD): a review', *Journal of Alternative and Complementary Medicine*, 14, 1: 79–85.

Dallegrave, E., Mantese, F., Coelho, R. S., Pereira, J. D., Dalsenter, P. R. *et al.* (2003) 'The teratogenic potential of the herbicide glyphosate-Roundup in Wister rats', *Toxicology Letters*, 142, 1–2: 45–52. Online. Available at: www.sciencedirect.com/ science (accessed 12 February 2010).

Damilakis, J., Perisinakis, K., Theocharopoulos, N., Tzedakis, A., Manios, E. *et al.* (2005) 'Anticipation of radiation dose to the conceptus from occupational exposure of pregnant staff during fluoroscopically guided electrophysiological procedures', *Journal of Cardiovascular Electrophysiology*, 16, 7: 773–79.

Daniels, C. (1997) 'Between fathers and fetuses: the social construction of male reproduction and the politics of fetal harm', *Signs*, 22, 3: 579–615.

Elgen, I., Bruaroy, S. and Laegreid, L. M. (2007) 'Complexity of foetal alcohol or drug neuroimpairments', *Acta Paediatrica*, 96, 12: 1730–33.

Gerhardsson, L. and Lundh, T. (2010) 'Metal concentrations in blood and hair in pregnant females in Southern Sweden', *Journal of Environmental Health*, 72, 6: 37–41.

Gomaa, A., Howard, H., Bellinger, D., Schwartz, J., Tsaih, S. *et al.* (2002) 'Maternal bone lead as an independent risk factor for fetal neurotoxicity: a prospective study', *Pediatrics*, 110, 1: 110–18.

Gundacker, C., Pietschnig, B., Wittmann, K. J., Lischka, A., Salzer, H. *et al.* (2002) 'Lead and mercury in breast milk'. *Pediatrics*, 110, 5: 873–78.

Health Physics Society (n.d.) Radiation Exposure and Pregnancy, Online. Available at: www.hps.org/documents/pregnancyfactsheet.pdf (accessed 15 February 2010).

Huffling, K. (2006) 'The effects of environmental contaminants in food on women's health', *Journal of Midwifery & Women's Health*, 51, 1: 19–25.

Hujoel, P. P., Lydon-Rochelle, M., Bollen, A. M., Woods, J. S., Geurtsen, W. *et al.* (2005) 'Mercury exposure from dental filling placement during pregnancy and low birth weight risk', *American Journal of Epidemiology*, 161: 734–40.

Kippler, M., Goessler, W., Nermell, B., Ekström, E. C., Lönnerdal, B. *et al.* (2009) 'Factors influencing intestinal cadmium uptake in pregnant Bangladeshi women- a prospective cohort study', *Environmental Research*, 109, 7: 914–21.

Lumley, J., Chamberlain, C., Dowswell, T., Oliver, S., Oakley, L. *et al.* (2010) 'Interventions for promoting smoking cessation during pregnancy'. *The Cochrane*

Database of Systematic Reviews, Issue 3. Online. Available at: www.cochrane.org/reviews/en/ab001055.html (accessed 4 March 2010).

McDiarmid, M. A. and Gehle, K. (2006) 'Preconception brief: occupational/environmental exposures'. *Maternal and Child Health Journal*, 10: S123–S128.

Messaoudi, E., El Heni, J., Hammouda, F., Said, K. and Kerkeni, A. (2009) 'Protective effects of selenium, zinc, or their combination on cadmium-induced oxidative stress in rat kidney', *Biological Trace Element Research*, 130, 2: 152–61. Online. Available at: www.springerlink.com/content/566617v711v37672/ (accessed 13 February 2010).

Ministry of Health (2008) *Food and Nutrition Guidelines for Healthy Pregnant and Breastfeeding Women: A Background Paper*. Wellington: Ministry of Health.

Ministry of Health (2009) 'Dioxins fact sheet'. Online. Available at: www.moh.govt.nz/moh.nsf/pagesmh/8078/$File/dioxins-practitioners-serumtesting.pdf (accessed 2 February 2010).

New Zealand College of Midwives (NZCOM) (2009) 'Smoke free outcomes with midwife lead maternity carers'. A report prepared for the Ministry of Health. New Zealand College of Midwives.

Oei, J. and Lui, K. (2007) 'Management of the newborn infant affected by maternal opiates and other drugs of dependency', *Journal of Paediatrics and Child Health*, 43: 9–18.

Opler, M. G., Buka, S. L., Groeger, J., McKeague, I., Wei, C. *et al.* (2008) 'Prenatal exposure to lead, σ-aminolevulinic acid, and schizophrenia: further evidence', *Environmental Health Perspectives*, 116, 11: 1586–90.

Organization of Teratology Information Specialists (OTIS) (2010) 'Lead in pregnancy'. Online. Available at: www.otispregnancy.org/otis-fact-sheets-s13037#5 (accessed 12 February 2010).

Pergament, E., Stein, A. K. and Miller, J. L. (1993) 'Radiation and pregnancy'. *Illinois Teratogen Information Service*. Online. Available at: www.fetal-exposure.org/resources/index.php/1993/12/01 (accessed 3 February 2010).

Quackenbush, R., Hackley, B. and Dixon, J. (2006) 'Screening for pesticide exposure: A case study', *Journal of Midwifery & Women's Health*, 51, 1: 3–11.

Richard, S., Moslemik, S., Sipahutar, H., Benachour, N. and Seralini, G. E. (2005) 'Differential effects of glyphosate and Roundup on human placental cells and aromatase', *Environmental Health Perspectives*, 113, 6: 716–20.

Richter, P. A., Bishop, E. E., Wang, J. and Swahn, M. H. (2009) 'Tobacco smoke exposure and levels of urinary metals in the US youth and adult population: the national health and nutrition examination survey, 1999–2004', (NHANES) *International Journal of Environmental Research, Public Health*, 6: 1930–46.

Rogers, J. M. (2009) 'Tobacco and pregnancy', *Reproductive Toxicology*, 28, 2: 152–60.

Sagiv, S. K., Thurston, S. W., Bellinger, D. C., Tolbert, P. E., Altshul, L. M. *et al.* (2010) 'Prenatal organochlorine exposure and behaviours associated with attention deficit hyperactivity disorder in school-aged children', *American Journal of Epidemiology*, 171, 5: 593–601. Online. Available at: www.ncbi.nlm.nih.gov/sites/entrez (accessed 2 February 2010).

Schempf, A. H. and Strobino, D. M. (2008) 'Illicit drug use and adverse birth outcomes: is it drugs or context?' *Journal of Urban Health*, 85, 6: 858–73.

Steingraber, S. (2003) *Having Faith – An Ecologist's Journey to Motherhood*. New York: Berkley Books.

Strandberg-Larsen, K., Grønboek, M., Andersen, A.M., Andersen, P.K. and Olsen, J. (2009) 'Alcohol drinking pattern during pregnancy and risk of infant mortality', *Epidemiology*, 20, 6: 884–91.

Sulik, M., Pilat-Marcinkiewicz, B., Sulik, A., Barwijuk-Machala, M., Sulkowska, M. *et al.* (1998) 'Fetotoxic effect of 2,4-dichlorophenoxyacetic acid (2,4-D) in rats', *Roczniki Akademii Medycznej w Bialymstoku*, 43: 298–308. Online. Available at: www.ncbi.nlm.nih.gov/sites/entrez (accessed 2 February 2010).

Tian, L. L., Zhao, Y. C.,Wang, X. C., Gu, J. L., Sun, Z. J. *et al.* (2009) Effects of gestational cadmium exposure on pregnancy outcome and development in the offspring at age 4.5 years. *Biological Trace Element Research*, 132: 51–59, 48.

US Food and Drugs Administration (USFDA) (2007) 'US Department of Health and Human Services'. Online. Available at: www.fda.gov/ (accessed 21 March 2010).

US EPA/Wisconsin Department of Natural Resources (1997) *Wisconsin Mercury Sourcebook*. United States Environmental Protection Agency. Online. Available at: www.epa.gov/glnpo/bnsdocs/hgsbook/ (accessed 15 February 2010).

Williams, C. H. and David, D. J. (1977) 'Some effects of the distribution of cadmium and phosphate in the root zone on the cadmium content of plants', *Australian Journal of Soil Research*, 15, 1: 59–68. Online. Available at: www.publish.csiro.au/paper/SR9770059.htm (accessed 1 February 2010).

Williams, J. H. and Ross, L. (2007) 'Consequences of prenatal toxin exposure for mental health in children and adolescents. A systematic review', *European Child & Adolescent Psychiatry*, 16, 243–53.

Williams, P. (1998) 'Food toxicity and safety', in J. Mann, and A. S. Truswell (eds) *Essentials of Human Nutrition*. Oxford: University Press.

Windham, G. C., Zhang, L., Gunier, R., Croen, L. A. and Grether, J. K. (2006) 'Autism spectrum disorders in relation to distribution of hazardous air pollutants in the San Francisco Bay area', *Environmental Health Perspectives*, 114, 9: 1438–44.

Yakoob, M. Y., Menezes, E. V., Soomro, T., Haws, R. A., Darmstadt, G. L. *et al.* (2009) 'Reducing stillbirths behavioural and nutritional interventions before and during pregnancy', *BMC Pregnancy Childbirth*, 9 (Suppl 1): S3.

15 An ecology of antenatal education

Mary Nolan

In the United Kingdom, the Royal College of Midwives has defined its vision for the future of childbearing and the maternity services as follows:

> The College believes that a policy of maximizing normal birth in the context of maternal choice is safe, and, further, that it offers short and long-term health and social benefits to mothers, children, families, and communities. Such a policy is more likely to succeed if childbirth is placed within a social and family context.
>
> (Sue Macdonald, Education and Research Manager,
> launching *The RCM 10 Top Tips for a Normal Birth
> for Midwives and Mothers*, 2 June 2008)

The resources needed for normal birth are those that women already possess; their internal resources consist of their instinctive understanding of how to give birth to their babies, and their external resources are the support provided by the people who love them and who will be with them during labour. All of these resources operate more powerfully when birth takes place in a 'social and family context', which is within the woman's home or in a home-like birth centre where she is surrounded by professionals with knowledge of and trust in the normal process of birth. Under such circumstances, birth can be ecological – that is, it makes few or no demands on non-renewable sources; it becomes a sustainable process.

Antonovsky's theory of salutogenesis (1987) supplies a highly appropriate model for the delivery of ecological maternity services and of education for birth and parenting. Within this model, people facing health problems in their lives need to understand the sources of those problems in order to tackle them. A heavy smoker suffering from chronic bronchitis needs to understand that his problem is linked to his smoking habit, and then to have information about the consequences of continuing to smoke, or of quitting. Once people understand the root cause of their health issue, they need to locate resources to help them move towards recovery. Internal resources include their own motivation to get better and desire for an improved quality of life, while outside resources might comprise medication, treatments, support from family and friends, voluntary groups and social networks.

Pregnancy is not an illness. Nonetheless, the model of salutogenesis is applicable because pregnancy *is* a health challenge for women the world over. It is a time of emotional lability, of psychological transition and of staggering physical changes in the woman's body. All of these constitute a challenge, even if one of maintaining health rather than combating illness. In order to meet this challenge, women need to understand what is happening to their bodies, become aware of and reflect on the changes that pregnancy is making in their lives, anticipate the demands of labour and birth, and plan how to care for and nurture their new baby within the individual contexts of their lives.

Salutogenesis presumes that the resources a person can draw on to cope with health challenges come from within herself as well as from outside. If pregnancy and birth are seen by the woman, her family and her health carers as illness processes, the resources she will turn to are those provided by the medical profession. She will draw on her internal resources only to enable her to conform to the illness-orientated advice she is being given. If she sees pregnancy and birth as normal, though *extra-ordinary*, processes, which are integral to a woman's life, the resources she draws on will be different. She will apply the familiar strategies for coping with discomfort and pain, which she has developed through childhood and into adulthood to the discomforts of pregnancy and the pain of childbirth; and she will seek support from the people to whom she normally turns for help in challenging situations, namely her family and friends.

The illness model of pregnancy and birth is resource-intensive in that it requires a range of health care personnel and equipment for undertaking investigations during pregnancy and surveillance of the unborn baby during labour, while underplaying, if not ignoring, the resources the woman herself has to cope with pregnancy, birth and parenthood. The independence that should characterize her adult status is taken away from her as she is encouraged to rely on others to control her pregnant and labouring body and to interpret what is happening to her using a vocabulary drawn from pathology as opposed to the vocabulary of intuition and innate understanding, which is used by women themselves.

Adult education is, according to Malcolm Knowles (1990), an enterprise in which adult learners are given the opportunity to achieve greater adulthood, to become more independent and better able to deal with their world. It is a vital part of the maturation of adults as they move from being a dependent personality toward being a self-directed human being. Its aims are perverted when it undermines learners' ability to seek out information, to enter into partnership with knowledgeable others, and ultimately to make the decisions they feel are right for them.

Antenatal education is provided at a time that has been described as '*the* teachable moment' in adults' lives because it is provided during that visionary nine months when women and men are inspired to reflect on their lives and to make changes in line with their aspirations for themselves and their children. The label 'teachable moment' (TM) has been used to describe naturally occurring health events that can motivate individuals to consider their health behaviours (McBride *et al.* 2003). Such education has also been charged with the responsibility for developing a 'critical mass' of health care users (Enkin *et al.* 2000: 26), a mass of people who can critically evaluate whether health services are truly responding to their individual needs, and challenge when they find the impact of health care on their lives to be harmful rather than beneficial. Pregnancy is an ideal time for parents to develop a critical attitude towards services that are likely to play a key part in their own and their children's futures. Antenatal education is therefore education for challenge and not for conformity.

By challenging the sickness model of pregnancy and childbirth, and the waste of resources associated with engaging inappropriate personnel and costly and unnecessary procedures (such as epidurals) in the process of pregnancy and birth, antenatal education is an essential part of the ecological agenda in midwifery. It aims to help women and men understand the natural process of pregnancy and birth, to recognize and trust the wisdom of the woman's body, to identify and utilize the woman's immense strengths to cope with childbirth, and to give them a critical framework within which to evaluate the numerous medical interventions they are offered during the childbearing year. It is one of the resources within a model of salutogenesis to which women can turn to achieve 'well-ness' in the childbearing year (Nolan 2002: 12).

Antenatal education and the ecology of labour and birth

I have found it is generally the case that women attending antenatal classes in the UK arrive at the first session with a great deal of 'medical knowledge' about drugs and interventions, but with very little 'real' understanding of what their bodies do during pregnancy and labour and how they might feel as a new mother. Yes, they may have read extensively and yes, they may have been exposed to a great deal of media coverage of birth, but only a fairly small number will have been close to another woman going through pregnancy; hardly any will have witnessed a birth, and only a few will have held a new-born baby. The educator has much work to do to transmit knowledge and develop understanding of how women's bodies are beautifully designed to grow a healthy baby and birth that baby without the need for any high-tech surveillance or procedures. She has to raise learners' awareness that every medical intervention in birth, even when necessary, has a down side as well as an upside and that *inappropriate* interventions have only down-sides. This is a whole new way of thinking for most clients attending antenatal classes.

Parents-to-be are amazed and thrilled, when, for example, they start to learn about the hormonal dance of labour. A debate about the appropriate place of birth is quickly generated as soon as they understand how oxytocin progresses labour, first gently and then more intensely, and how its action is subverted by adrenalin, which is too often stimulated by the frightening environment of the hospital, causing labour to go into stop/start mode. Drawing on the work of Tricia Anderson (2002), I invite parents to consider what conditions a cat needs to birth her kittens, and then explain how darkness, quiet and privacy stimulate the primitive centres of the brain to release hormones that encourage labour, while lights (especially neon ones!) noise, conversation and the presence of people unknown to the mother stimulate the neocortex of the brain, which suppresses the release of birthing hormones.

With this understanding in place, women may reconsider where they want to labour and make a decision to stay at home for as long as possible. They can easily identify the resources they will have available to them at home to help them cope. A survey (Nolan *et al.* 2009) that I undertook recently with colleagues in midwifery and psychology asked women in the UK to tell us what they did during the early part of labour. Responses from the nearly 2,000 women who completed the survey demonstrated that they had used a vast array of coping mechanisms to manage their labours while at home. These included taking a bath, showering, resting in a chair or on a sofa, distracting themselves by doing housework, meditation and yoga, playing with their children, listening to music and making love. These are everyday resources for coping with stress and discomfort, which are equally relevant in labour and have none of the drawbacks of pain-relieving medication. The role of antenatal education is to raise women's awareness that these are legitimate and effective ways of coping in labour and to reflect on how the place of birth will affect to what extent such strategies are available to them. Should they choose to birth in hospital, as many will, they can decide antenatally how best to overcome the limitations of the medical environment in order to continue to use their usual methods of managing pain.

In classes, I use relaxation sessions to help parents imagine themselves labouring at home. With the lights dimmed and some gentle background music, I ask them to visualize a room in their home where they feel particularly relaxed and safe. In the course of the visualization, they explore what they can see, hear and touch and whether there are any scents or tastes that they associate with the room. After achieving a mental picture of this familiar place, I invite parents to imagine labouring here. The women consider how they would make themselves comfortable if they were having a contraction, and the people who will be supporting them consider what they might be doing. Later in the course, we carry out the same relaxation exercise, but this time visualizing a hospital delivery room. The women imagine how they would manage a contraction there, and their supporters consider what their role might be.

In a hospital environment, oxytocin levels are compromised because women are repeatedly required to answer questions about their labours and to make decisions about interventions. When the *thinking* part of their brains is engaged, it is far harder for them to recognize what their bodies are telling them to do, and far harder to respond appropriately. When the instinctive response to labour is suppressed, women need to resort to *learned* behaviours and it is for this reason that it is necessary to *teach* physical skills for labour in antenatal classes.

When women come to classes, they are expecting information and may be shy of learning with their bodies as opposed to with their minds. Providing a rationale for practising physical skills for labour is therefore important. A very simple (but entirely accurate) rationale, which explains the role of gravity in helping a baby to be born, and how the space in the pelvis is enlarged when the woman is not sitting on her tailbone and is leaning forward, never fails to convince intelligent adults that lying on a bed is clearly not an effective way of achieving a straightforward labour and birth. The part played by a full bladder in impeding the progress of labour can be demonstrated by placing a blown up balloon in a model pelvis at the same time as a doll.

Once the rationale for learning physical skills is in place, women and the family members who are attending classes with them generally enjoy trying out different positions for labour, acquiring some easy massage skills and working with their breathing patterns to stay relaxed, conserve energy and provide optimum oxygenation for the baby during his journey into the world. Such skills require reinforcement at every session of the antenatal course if they are going to be used effectively in a hospital environment where there is an expectation that women will *not* be able to cope with labour using their own resources. As physical skills can only be acquired through practice, not to practise them reduces the resources that women can draw on during labour.

Antenatal educators promote the ecological agenda in midwifery through the language they use to build the woman's confidence in her ability to birth her baby. Language that portrays the woman as passive and acted upon ('you will be given'; 'when you have an internal examination'), rather than as being at the centre of her own labour, creates an expectation of dependence on people and procedures. This is contrary to the adult education mission, which is to enhance independence, and contrary to an ecology of birth that requires sustainability. Salutogenesis in antenatal education guides teachers to ensure that women understand how their emotions, relationships and worldview (their internal resources) play an influential part in labour. To separate the physical process of labour from its emotional, psychological and spiritual aspects is to perpetuate a Cartesian dualism that not only supports medical intervention (because what is done to the body is presumed not to harm the mind), but also diminishes the mother's understanding of the complexity of birth as a rite of passage.

Antenatal education therefore helps women reflect on the whole project of labour. In my classes, we discuss the women's philosophy of labour – whether they see it as a part of the continuum of their adult female lives: menarche, pregnancy, labour, birth, mothering, menopause – or whether they see it as an event outside that continuum, requiring intervention and supervision, and best experienced in a setting that is not part of their daily experience. Time is also given to considering who will be the best person to support them in labour and how many people they need. Birth stories, such as those in Ina May Gaskin's book *Spiritual Midwifery* (2002) can be powerful in demonstrating how 'unresolved issues' between women and the people with them in labour may impede the progress of the baby into the world. The effect of prolactin, along with oxytocin, adrenalin and endorphins, in the second stage of labour on creating the mindset that ensures that mother and baby respond immediately and positively to each other is explored at some length.

One of the key resources to which women will turn to meet the challenge of labour and birth is the person whom they have chosen to support them in labour. In the Western world, this person is often the woman's male partner. This can present difficulties in antenatal classes if the childbirth educator wants to share the research (and the ages-old experience of women) that women are more effective as birth companions than men. The study by Scott *et al.* (1999) drew together the results of 12 randomized controlled trials examining the benefits of women being supported by doulas in labour. The emotional and physical support provided by doulas decreased the length of labour and the need for interventions such as forceps, Caesarean, augmentation and epidural anaesthesia. However, support offered by fathers did not appear to produce the same obstetrical benefits. To help women maximize the effectiveness of the support they receive in labour, discussion needs to take place in antenatal classes both in plenary sessions and between the couples themselves. Each partner can reflect on their anticipated needs and on what the father feels he can offer to the mother and what he cannot. Women may decide, following classes, that they will choose a female birth companion to be with them, as well as their partner. In my experience, fathers are generally grateful to share the emotional load of labour with another person, and to be given permission to concentrate on their own rite of passage as well as supporting the woman through hers.

Cognitive dissonance and educational challenge

Antenatal education is about far more than simply transferring information, and should be hostile to the notion that 'informed choice' depends exclusively on having *facts*. If an ecology of birth is based on recognition of the complex interplay of individuals' internal and external resources, then informed choice for birth and parenting will take into account physical attributes, understanding of risk, life experiences and current relationships to determine which are the best choices for any individual mother. Teaching assertiveness skills for 'managing' health professionals is far less important than creating a learning environment in which women, in conversation with themselves, their partners and the other women in the class, discover how they feel about their bodies, their babies and their approach to the challenges of their lives.

Cognitive dissonance can often be very obvious while such discussions are taking place. Women can readily appreciate the rightness of treating pregnancy and labour as normal unless proved otherwise, and of the appropriateness of the home environment for a family event such as birth, while simultaneously arguing vigorously that in their particular cases, pregnancy and birth need hyper-vigilance and are best experienced in clinics and in hospital. Dissonance again becomes apparent when antenatal classes turn to the topic of pharmacological pain relief in labour. Women have often vigorously, and sometimes at great personal cost, eschewed the use of any kind of medication or recreational drugs during their pregnancies; however, discussion on drug use in labour highlights a different set of values. Women then argue not *whether* they will use pharmacological methods of pain relief, but only about the order in which they will use them.

To challenge this often comfortably maintained dissonance is one of the functions of antenatal education. In line with Paulo Freire's *Pedagogy of the Oppressed* (1973), adult education seeks to challenge the status quo by helping the oppressed – in this case, childbearing women – to understand how they are being oppressed, and then assisting them to combat oppression. Discussion on drugs in labour, which includes honest information on the problems with opiates and anaesthetics, is often perceived as threatening by learners. Part of the antenatal teacher's engagement with the adult education enterprise is to recognise that women may make choices that fly in the face of the facts, but which have an intuitive logic arising out of culturally induced fear of birth and the need to cope with a hostile birthing environment in hospital.

Challenging received views in antenatal education can be achieved in many ways: intellectually, emotionally and physically. The physical challenge, as has already been discussed, comes when classes move from *talking* about labour, to *practising* ways in which to help the mother work with her body. There are many approaches currently being used in antenatal education to challenge women's limited awareness of their bodies – from psychoprophylaxis to hypnobirthing; from yoga to natural childbirth preparation. The intellectual challenge may come through comparing statistics for interventions at different hospitals in the same area or the same country and asking why, in units serving very similar populations, some hospitals have a 14 per cent Caesarean birth rate and some a 34 per cent rate. Similarly, groups can discuss why women attending one hospital seem much less able to labour without the intervention of an epidural than in others, and why women labouring in midwife-led birth centres do not need the intervention of an epidural at all. Home birth rates provide the subject-matter for an important discussion on why it is far more prevalent in some areas of the country than in others.

The material for intellectual challenge may sometimes come from unlikely sources. In the UK, guidelines issued by government on best practice in maternity care are often far in advance of popular perceptions of what constitutes optimum care. The National Institute for Health and Clinical Excellence (NICE) advocates the use of intermittent auscultation with a Pinard's stethoscope or Doppler during labour for women who are in normal labour: '. . . your midwife . . . will use a small hand-held listening device to listen to your baby's heartbeat. There is no need for you to be connected to a monitoring machine even for a short period unless there is concern about your baby' (NICE 2007: 7). Yet the perception persists that both mother and baby are safest when the labour is being monitored continuously. Literature produced by the Royal Colleges may also surprise women, for example, the RCM casts serious doubts on the safety of both pethidine and epidurals in normal labour:

> Pethidine is the most commonly used opiate in labour . . . However, there are considerable doubts about its effectiveness and concerns about its potential maternal, fetal and neonatal side-effects . . . Epidural analgesia offers the most effective but most invasive and potentially hazardous method of pain relief in labour.
>
> (RCM 2008)

It is very challenging for pregnant parents to discover that information about labour care that they have received from a variety of sources (including midwives) may be considered incorrect and outdated by the most senior ranks of maternity care health professionals.

The *emotional* challenge in antenatal education revolves around eliciting women's intuitive understanding of the conditions under which women birth most easily. I sometimes ask women to draw a place in which they would like to labour. They draw a room with windows, lit by candles, furnished with cushions and with low tables bearing food and drink. If they draw anyone at all in the room, they draw themselves and a loved one. Sometimes, they place the midwife outside the door, although often, the room does not have a door at all; it is an enclosed space, which cannot be accessed by outsiders. Comparing this with photographs of delivery rooms at the local hospital is often challenging for women and their partners. They understand the disparity in the emotional charge of the two places, but are confused by what they have learned about the need for labour and birth to happen in a clinical environment.

Such emotional dissonance, when brought into consciousness, can be rich food for reflection and some women and their partners will be able to move forward in their thinking about where they want to give birth and about the meaning that they want labour and birth to have. Others will not be able to make such a conceptual leap, although they may shift their position when they come to be pregnant again, especially if their first experience of birth is emotionally traumatic.

Antenatal education and the ecology of parenting

The role of antenatal education in preparing women and men for the challenges of parenting is now increasingly being recognized in the UK. Again, this is to do with increasing awareness that pregnancy is a 'teachable moment' when it may be possible to promote positive parenting attitudes and behaviour before the stress of having a newborn baby in the house 24/7 makes reflection on one's approach to parenting far more difficult.

When applied to parenting education, salutogenesis suggest that educators need to help parents to recognize the pressures, both internal and external, which cause them to act in certain ways, and to identify renewable resources to maximize family cohesion, happiness and mental health. Many parents come to antenatal classes with a parenting agenda based on unrealistic and frankly brutal ideas of what a baby needs. The challenge provided by antenatal education centres on raising awareness of how contemporary approaches to parenting seem to demand that the baby should have a lifestyle that adults would never choose for themselves. For example, most adults like to share a bed with another person at night (because, whether they admit it or not, they are frightened of the dark just as they were as children); most adults in the affluent world expect to be able have snacks and meals at times of their own choosing; most expect that emotional distress on their part will be met with a loving response from family members.

A process of cognitive dissonance enables them to consider all of these as givens in their own lives while simultaneously feeling quite at ease with the idea of putting a baby down to sleep in a room on his own, restricting his feeding to certain times and ignoring his cries for attention. Ecological antenatal education helps participants identify to what extent parenting in the developed world is driven by needs other than the baby's (the 'busy-ness of adults' lives; the need to have sufficient sleep to cope with demanding jobs; wanting to control children so that they do not impose on adult time) and whether the prioritizing of these other needs may jeopardize the baby's physical, emotional and psychological development. When asked to consider what a baby 'learns' if he cries in the night and no-one responds to him, parents can easily identify that the baby learns only that no one comes to him when he is upset and frightened. He does not learn that it is naughty to waken his mother and father in the early hours of the morning. Building on the work of Darwin, evolutionists have described the 'separation cry' as the oldest form of vocalization, acting as a tracking device for mammals to locate each other in the dark, and used by young mammals to summon their mothers when threatened by predators (van der Kolk 1997). Babies separated from their mothers by the bedroom wall will use exactly the same cry; it is a mechanism for survival, not for manipulating parents!

Pregnancy provides a wonderful opportunity for parents to reflect on their own childhood and what events were most significant in bringing them happiness. Key parenting behaviours that stimulated contentment or self-esteem in themselves as children will be identified, such as having a bedtime story, being taken to the football match with Dad, or Mum keeping the bookmark made by the child at school in her diary. The ecology of such behaviours is that they are about having relationships rather than about having things (a bicycle, CD player, sports gear) and hence represent sustainable parenting, untouched by the vagaries of the global economic climate.

Challenging the oppression of both parents being out at work full time while they have young children is fraught and may be considered by antenatal teachers as too difficult in a time of economic stringency when many people are finding it hard to manage their lives within the finances they have available. Yet research is clear (Belksy and Rovine 1988; Leach 1997) that babies and small children who spend most of their time in nurseries are more likely to demonstrate antisocial behaviour when they get to school years. Antenatal classes may provide an opportunity for parents to consider whether they would be financially much worse off if one parent remained at home, and whether they would be mentally healthier – less guilt-ridden – if they were to make this choice.

Antenatal education and the ecology of community

It is often said that the Western world lacks communities, that people live in isolation and do not support each other. The results of this, it has been suggested, are loneliness, increased vulnerability of at-risk groups such as the elderly and disabled, and poor mental health (Putnam 2000). Poor mental health in women following childbirth has been demonstrated to compromise not only their own well-being but also the well-being of their babies if the mothers are not able to form and sustain a relationship with them (Kumar and Hipwell 1994). Boys seem to be especially affected by mothering that is distant and sporadic (Kraemer 2000).

The Cochrane Review by Gagnon and Sandall (2007) notes that the impact on women of support groups developed as a result of attending antenatal classes has never been researched. Yet antenatal teachers know well that the individual friendships and support groups formed at antenatal classes are particularly focussed and fruitful. The need to normalize what the woman is experiencing in pregnancy and early motherhood drives her to share her 'story' with other women more urgently than perhaps at any other time in her life. A learning environment in which women are gaining new and challenging information, and sharing some of their most profoundly held attitudes and cherished ideas, appears to facilitate the formation of lasting friendships. Ask any woman with a grown-up child whether she is still in contact with women from her antenatal classes, and the answer may very well be 'yes'.

Forming relationships and developing communities are essential parts of the ecology of sustainable, healthy human living. They are also related to salutogenesis in that they are the resources women can draw on to help them through the transition to parenthood and through the multiple challenges of the parenting years. Antenatal teachers need to ensure that friendships are formed during classes, that the conditions in which women can talk genuinely to each other about their fears and hopes, are created. These conditions stem from the teacher's own attitude towards the parents attending her classes – an attitude of complete respect, of valuing the individual life experiences of all present, and of partnership in the lifelong learning experience arising out of birthing our children. Antenatal education, delivered under these circumstances, and committed to challenging received views on the appropriateness of technology and materialism in childbirth and parenting, is an essential component of an ecological approach to midwifery.

References

Anderson, T. (2002) 'Out of the laboratory: back to the darkened room', *MIDIRS Midwifery Digest*, 21, 1: 65–69.

Antonovsky, A. (1987) *Unraveling the Mystery of Health: How People Manage Stress and Stay Well*. San Francisco: Jossey-Bass.

Belsky, J. and Rovine, M. J. (1988) 'Nonmaternal care in the first year of life and the security of infant-parent attachment', *Child Development*, 59: 157–67.

Enkin, M., Keirse, M. J. N. C., Neilson, J., Crowther, C., Duley, L. *et al.* (2000) *A Guide to Effective Care in Pregnancy and Childbirth*, 3rd Edition. Oxford: Oxford University Press.

Freire, P. (1973) *Pedagogy of the Oppressed*. London: Penguin Books.

Gagnon, A. and Sandall, J. (2007) 'Individual or group education for childbirth and parenthood, or both'. Cochrane database of systematic reviews. Online. Available at: http://mrw.interscience.wiley.com/cochrane/clsysrev/articles/CD002869/pdf_fs.html

Gaskin, I. M. (2002) *Spiritual Midwifery*, 4th Edition. Summertown: Book Publishing Company.

Knowles, M. S. (1990) *The Adult Learner: A Neglected Species*, 4th Edition. Houston: Gulf Publishing.

Kolk, B. A. van der (1997) *Psychological Trauma*. Arlington, VA: American Psychic Press.

Kraemer, S. (2000) 'The fragile male', *British Medical Journal*, 321: 1609–11.

Kumar, R. and Hipwell A. (1994) 'Implications for the infant of maternal puerperal psychiatric disorders', in M. Rutter, E. Taylor and L. Hersov (eds) *Child and Adolescent Psychiatry*, 3rd Edition. Oxford: Blackwell.

Leach, P. (1997) '"Infant care from infants" viewpoint: the views of some professionals', *Early Development and Parenting*, 6: 47–58.

McBride, C. M., Emmons K. M., Lipkus I. M. (2003) 'Understanding the potential of teachable moments: the case of smoking cessation', *Health Education Research*, 18, 2: 156–70.

National Institute for Health and Clinical Excellence (NICE) (2007) 'Care of Women and Their Babies During Labour', Clinical Guideline 55, London: NICE.

Nolan, M. (2002) '"Good enough" parenting', M. Nolan (ed.), *Education and Support for Parenting*. Edinburgh: Bailliere Tindall.

Nolan, M., Smith, J. and Catling, J. (2009) 'Experiences of early labour (2) Contact with health professionals', *The Practising Midwife*, 12, 9: 35–37.

Putnam, R. (2000) *Bowling Alone: The Collapse and Revival of American Community*. New York: Simon & Schuster.

Royal College of Midwives (RCM) (2008) *National Library of Guidelines: Care Guideline, 17 April*. London: Royal College of Midwives.

Scott, K., Klaus, P. H. and Klaus, M. H. (1999) 'The obstetrical and postpartum benefits of continuous support during childbirth', *Journal of Women's Health and Gender-Based Medicine*, 8, 10: 1257–64.

16 Co-sleeping

An ecological parenting practice

Sally Baddock

Midwives have a unique opportunity to share information with pregnant women and their family/whānau so that they can choose sustainable and ecologically-sound childcare practices. Practices that are established early in family life continue to have influence on later childcare decisions (Moon *et al.* 2004). The midwife is poised to have significant influence on these early decisions and to set the scene for practices in later life.

One of the most significant areas that midwives are positioned to influence is that of infant sleep practices. Co-sleeping may be part of a framework for a self-sufficient or sustainable parenting style. Infant–parent co-sleeping (or bedsharing) is an integral part of a traditional parenting style in many cultures and it is increasingly a parenting style of choice in Western societies (Arnestad *et al.* 2001; Ateah *et al.* 2008). It encourages a parenting style that is less dependent on consumer commodities such as cot mobiles, sleep aids, bottle feeding, etc., to care for the baby (Okami *et al.* 2002). Parents look to their own resources instead of to external solutions. The close contact of the mother is the tool for settling baby and breastfeeding provides nutrition.

There are some risks that have been associated with co-sleeping in relation to sudden unexpected death in infancy (SUDI), formerly known as sudden infant death syndrome (SIDS). Those risks are outlined below. Studies show that despite acknowledging the possible risk, many families still choose to co-sleep (Baddock *et al.* 2000; Ateah *et al.* 2008). For some this has a strong link to cultural practices and for others it is a parenting choice. Where risk factors are not present the net effect of co-sleeping can sustain not only the baby, but also the mother, and thus can have flow on effects for the well-being of the whole family/whānau. Mothers describe it as a strategy to facilitate breastfeeding, to settle a baby more quickly, to improve their own emotional well-being, and to reduce maternal tiredness. They report enjoying the close contact and a feeling of security (Baddock *et al.* 2000; Abel *et al.* 2001; Ball 2002).

Understanding co-sleeping

There are many reasons why parents choose to co-sleep and there are highly variable approaches to co-sleeping (or bedsharing). The wide variation in practices has implications for interpreting research, which treats the practice as a coherent entity and does not take into account the context of the co-sleeping or the value that families place on the practice. Differences in many aspects of co-sleeping, including the number of people in bed, the arrangement of the bedding, and the cultural background and motivation for co-sleeping, may influence the safety of the behaviour.

Studies have identified groups where co-sleeping is a common childcare practice yet the incidence of SIDS is low, for example Pacific families in New Zealand (Scragg *et al.* 1993) and the USA (Mathews *et al.* 2002), Bangladeshi in the United Kingdom (Gantley 1994) and families in Hong Kong (Lee *et al.* 1989), Japan (Nelson *et al.* 2001) and Thailand. However, among other groups, for example, New Zealand Māori and African Americans, co-sleeping is associated with a high risk of SIDS (Li and Daling 1991; Mitchell *et al.* 1993). This suggests that co-sleeping is not practised in the same way in all ethnic groups or perhaps that safety is compromised when families no longer adhere to traditional practice. For example, smoking is common among Māori (Mitchell *et al.* 1993) and African American women but is less common among Asian women.

Benefits of co-sleeping

Whether traditional or not, co-sleeping is often an integral part of a baby-centred parenting style and is perceived by parents to have substantial benefits. Data from 1,300 infants in the UK suggest at least 50 per cent of babies bedshared with their parents at some time in the first month, and that on any one night 25 per cent of babies slept with their parents. Bedsharing was more common in the first month of life among the more privileged families and was strongly associated with breastfeeding (Blair and Ball 2004). Studies of infants, who from birth commonly sleep all night with a parent, report fewer sleep difficulties (Latz *et al.* 1999; Okami *et al.* 2002).

Generally, the benefits that parents report are difficult to quantify, such as a sense of security and mother–infant bonding, but other outcomes can be measured. Observational studies have supported maternal reports that infants wake and feed more frequently compared to cot-sleeping infants (McKenna *et al.* 1997; Baddock *et al.* 2006). Total sleep time in either sleep arrangement is no different for infants, or their mothers (Mosko *et al.* 1997a). Bedsharing infants are seldom observed to sleep prone and when they do, it tends to be on the mothers chest (Richard *et al* 1996; Baddock *et al.* 2007). Infant and mother sleep cycles tend to coincide so that both are in the same sleep state at the same time (McKenna *et al.* 1994), and the number of maternal inspections per night is increased (McKenna *et al.* 1994; Baddock *et al.* 2006).

A longitudinal study following children from birth to 18 years of age has demonstrated that early childhood bedsharing is associated with improved cognitive competence at 6 years. This improvement is no longer evident at 18 years of age, but despite concerns by some, bedsharing in early childhood was not associated with sleep problems, sexual pathology, or any other problematic consequences at 6 or 18 years of age (Okami *et al.* 2002).

Cultural significance of co-sleeping

In cultures or families where bedsharing is the norm, interdependency between mother and baby tends to be valued over autonomy (Latz *et al.* 1999) and night waking is viewed as normal rather than problematic. A study utilizing focus groups of parents from different cultures in New Zealand (Abel *et al.* 2001) and another using semi-structured interviews of parents (Baddock *et al.* 2000), identified that Māori and Pacific families prefer to sleep in contact with their infants, and that these parents tend to value interconnectedness to foster an infant's physical, moral and spiritual development. This is illustrated by a quote from an interview with a Tongan mother:

> ... because of my whole Tongan upbringing and my Tongan background and culture ... I suppose you share everything and you do things together right from bedsharing to every other aspect of your life ... I think co-sleeping has a lot to do with that, cultivating that sense of unity and belonging and a part of one another.
>
> (Baddock *et al.* 2000)

Differences in values were identified between Pacific Island-raised and New Zealand-raised Pacific caregivers, and families were concerned with the negative impact of New Zealand's urban culture on traditional behaviours.

Pakeha (European) parents generally value development of independence and autonomy of their infants (Abel *et al.* 2001), however in a group who had chosen to bedshare, Baddock *et al.* (2000) reported that on the whole parents did not aspire to independent sleep regimes and they accepted frequent waking and feeding as part of the parenting style. Bedsharing was not part of their cultural heritage, but most were confident they had made an informed decision to adopt this practice.

A group of young single mothers who regularly bedshared were less confident and expressed guilt that they had chosen to bedshare for their own convenience – at what they feared was cost to the development of independent infant sleep practices. Despite commenting positively about bedsharing they appeared vulnerable to family and peer opinions and 'expert' advice. The following are quotes from these women:

> ... everyone I know had negative thoughts about having a baby in the bed.
>
> ... people thought ... she should learn to be in a bed by herself ... and I've got to put up with her crying
>
> ... she said the baby shouldn't even be in the same room as you because you were disturbing their sleeping pattern ...

Support did come from others:

> ... I didn't tell them at first ... quite a few of them said that they had done the same thing ... they found it quite neat sleeping with their child.

> ... mum said that she took us to bed occasionally ...

> ... I talked to a midwife about it and she said ... a whole list of things contribute to cot death for it to happen.

> (Baddock *et al.* 2000)

As circumstances change a traditional practice does not necessarily remain safe. In New Zealand, 50 per cent of Māori mothers and whānau (extended family) members from a group of 86 who were surveyed identified bedsharing as a strategy to increase breastfeeding. At the time of the study, 47 per cent of the mothers were smokers (Glover *et al.* 2009). They were aware of messages about risks associated with bedsharing but were not clear on the particular risks. This is a difficult issue to address in cultures such as Māori where maternal smoking rates are high and bedsharing is valued (Scragg *et al.* 1993).

Co-sleeping and sustainability

One of the most pertinent issues related to co-sleeping and sustainability is the encouragement of breastfeeding. Mother–infant bedsharing is a common strategy for night-time caregiving in the early months of an infant's life, particularly for breastfed babies (Ball *et al.* 1999; McCoy *et al.* 2004), and many studies have reported a positive association between bedsharing and breastfeeding (Ball 2003; Nelson *et al.* 2005; Tan 2009), although studies of low-income groups in Brazil (Galler *et al.* 2006) and the US (Brenner *et al.* 2003) did not find bedsharing was associated with breastfeeding.

Breastfeeding is a highly sustainable form of nutrition. It provides the infant with an optimal diet and has been shown in numerous studies to have many benefits to mother and baby. Benefits to babies include reduced risk of acute otitis media, non-specific gastroenteritis, severe lower respiratory tract infections, atopic dermatitis, asthma (young children), obesity, type 1 and 2 diabetes, childhood leukemia, SIDS, and necrotizing enterocolitis (Ip *et al.* 2007).

Maternal benefits include a reduced risk of type 2 diabetes, breast and ovarian cancer. Early cessation of breastfeeding or not breastfeeding is associated with an increased risk of maternal postpartum depression (Ip *et al.* 2007). Furthermore, as breastfeeding is reported to decrease overall post-neonatal mortality due to all causes, including infectious disease, SIDS, accidental death, and others (Chen *et al.* 2004), then actions that can encourage breastfeeding are advantageous. As such, the WHO recommends exclusive breastfeeding of all infants to six months of age. Breastfeeding also facilitates close maternal–infant contact and enhances maternal–infant bonding (Kennell *et al*. 2005).

Ball (2002) has investigated the behaviour of breastfeeding and non-breastfeeding infants and their mothers during bedsharing and reports that breastfeeding mothers adopt a protective position while bedsharing; that they sleep in a lateral position, with legs curled around the infant, and their arm in a position to prevent rolling onto the infant. By contrast, Ball suggests, when infants bedshare with a non-breastfeeding mother this may constitute a risk to their safety because mothers do not adopt this protective behaviour.

A number of small qualitative studies illustrate the perceptions mothers have of the impact of bedsharing on breastfeeding. Mayan mothers from Guatemala, where bedsharing is the norm, report they did not even need to wake when breastfeeding through the night and did not find breastfeeding disruptive. In contrast, a group of non-bedsharing middle-class mothers from the US reported having to stay awake for feeding, and the only mother from the group of 18 who said that nightly feedings did not bother her took her baby to bed to feed following the first awakening (Morelli *et al*. 1992). Of 40 UK mothers who began breastfeeding but stopped within five weeks, 20 per cent reported that frequent breastfeeding led to parental sleep disruption and was the reason for changing to bottle-feeding. Some mothers changed to bedsharing as a strategy to decrease the impact of feeding. This was evident from the fact that 21 per cent of bedsharing babies at three months had not bedshared at one month (Ball 2003).

Thus, bedsharing at night may be important to reduce barriers to continued breastfeeding. Waking and feeding poses less disruption in the bedsharing situation as mother and baby remain in bed, often with the mother feeding in a drowsy state (Baddock *et al*. 2007).

Bedsharing at night may also be an important time for increased infant–mother contact. Overnight monitoring of families co-sleeping in sleep laboratories and in their own homes has shown that the mother is almost exclusively the primary caregiver through the night whether the father or siblings are present or not. The mother–infant partnership involves sleeping in close proximity, facing each other, with the baby most often at the level of the mother's breast, in positions that facilitate breastfeeding. Mothers respond to infant cues throughout the night. Infant movements frequently initiate a maternal response, and the mother self initiates many checks through the night (Young 1999; Ball 2003; Baddock *et al*. 2007).

The physiology of co-sleeping

While most of our knowledge of infant sleep physiology has been established from studies of infants sleeping alone in a cot, there is a growing body of information about infant physiology during co-sleeping. McKenna has interpreted these findings to suggest bedshare infants are in a different physiological state, influenced by the continual sensory exchange between mother and baby (McKenna et al. 1994).

Studies have shown that infants are in a warmer environment within the bed but that healthy, low-risk infants are able to maintain normal core temperature nonetheless (Baddock et al. 2004; Young 1999). Bedshare infants are more often exposed to increased levels of carbon dioxide (and as a consequence, reduced levels of oxygen) during head-covering episodes, but healthy, low-risk infants are able to maintain normal blood oxygen levels (Baddock et al. 2004). Mosko et al. (1997b) demonstrated an increase in carbon dioxide at the infant's face due to the proximity of the mother, hypothesizing that maternal carbon dioxide may be beneficial as an added stimulus to infant breathing. Overnight axillary temperature (Richard 1999) and heart rate (Richard and Mosko 2004) have also been shown to be elevated in co-sleeping infants. These findings support the hypothesis that co-sleeping infants are in a different physiological state and a different sensory environment to solitary sleeping infants. In particular, McKenna and colleagues (McKenna et al. 1994; Mosko et al. 1997c) suggest that infants are more arousable in the co-sleeping situation, which may be protective. The implications of these findings are still not clear.

Risks associated with co-sleeping

In some situations co-sleeping has been identified as increasing the risk of SUDI, formerly known as SIDS. New Zealand has the highest rate of SIDS in the developed world and 40–50 babies succumb to this each year (1.1 deaths/1000 live births) (CYMRC 2009). Infants are found in an adult bed in approximately half of these deaths (CYMRC 2009). While many families enjoy the benefits of co-sleeping it is important they are aware of what risk factors might contribute to SUDI, so that they may make an informed choice of infant care practices.

Bedsharing with a mother who smoked during pregnancy has consistently been shown by large case-control studies from many countries, including New Zealand, as increasing the risk of SIDS (Mitchell et al. 1992; Carpenter et al. 2004; Horsley et al. 2007). Data has not been consistently collected in New Zealand on maternal smoking following the death of an infant (CYMRC 2009), however, international studies suggest that maternal smoking accounts for at least 85 per cent of SIDS deaths (Blair et al. 2006). It is possible that infants compromised by maternal smoking may not have adequate ventilatory (Campbell et al. 2001) or thermal responses (Tuffnell et al. 1995) to counter stresses arising in the bedsharing environment, such as head covering (Baddock et al. 2006). In New Zealand a disproportionate number of SIDS deaths are among Māori families (60 per cent of SIDS deaths in 2003–07) (CYMRC 2009) and maternal smoking is high among Māori (65 per cent) (Scragg et al. 1993).

Even though the mechanism is not clearly understood, the risk of bedsharing between adults and infants exposed to cigarette smoke *in utero*, or after birth, needs to be recognized and communicated to parents. At 2 weeks of age, infants of mothers who smoked in pregnancy and who bedshare have 27 times the risk of death compared to infants of non-smokers sleeping in a cot, while bedsharing infants of non-smoking mothers have twice the risk. By 6 months of age the risk associated with bedsharing and maternal smoking remains 10 times that of infants of non-smokers sleeping in a cot, while the risk to infants of non-smoking mothers who bedshare ceases to be statistically significant by 8 weeks of age (Carpenter *et al.* 2004). Other studies have suggested the risk for infants of non-smoking mothers continues to be small but significant until 11–16 weeks of age (Tappin *et al.* 2005; Ruys *et al.* 2007). These findings continue to be debated.

Maternal overtiredness, excessive bedding and household overcrowding also contribute to an increased risk of bedsharing (Blair *et al.* 1999; Carpenter *et al.* 2004; Ruys *et al.* 2007). Similarly, recent alcohol or drug use by parents, and sleeping on a couch are also associated with increased risk. In a study in the UK, the additional risk of bedsharing compared to cot sleeping was almost all explained by recent alcohol or drug use by parents prior to bedsharing, or by infants sleeping on a couch with an adult (Blair *et al.* 2009). Sleeping on a couch, chair or waterbed with a baby may increase the likelihood of the baby becoming trapped between adult and furniture (Blair *et al.* 2006).

Home studies of bedsharing show infants are more likely to have their head covered by bedding than during cot-sleep. Clearing the infant head has been observed as being due to intentional and unintentional movements by the mother and less frequently due to infant self-clearing (Baddock *et al.* 2007). Thus, it is important that the mother is unimpaired by alcohol or other mind-altering substances to enable her to respond to subtle infant cues during the night.

While the specific factors are still debated, because of the identified risk, safe sleeping advice in New Zealand (MoH 2009) and the UK, Foundation for the Study of Infant Death (FSID 2009) suggests the safest place for baby to sleep during the first 6 months is in a bassinette or cot beside the adult bed, while the American Academy of Pediatrics recommends that bedsharing is avoided for the first year of life (American Academy of Pediatrics Policy Statement 2005).

A study in the UK has provided evidence that clip-on bassinettes may provide a safer alternative to bedsharing in the hospital where there are risks associated with narrow, high hospital beds. Clip-on bassinettes may have similar benefits of maternal–infant proximity, increased breastfeeding and increased maternal satisfaction with mothers' post-natal experience in hospital (Ball *et al.* 2006). There is no research published to date investigating this type of sleeping arrangement in New Zealand or Australia.

Conclusions

Bedshare infants sleep in a warmer environment and experience more potentially dangerous events such as head covering and rebreathing air with a higher carbon dioxide content. However, it has been demonstrated that low-risk infants maintain normal rectal temperature and blood oxygen levels when they bedshare, suggesting they are protected by normal homeostatic responses. Infant safety is also facilitated by frequent maternal checking and maternal responses to infant movements. The proximity of mother and infant during co-sleeping allows prompt responses, reduces the time that infants are upset and minimizes disruption from frequent breastfeeding – aspects valued by many. It is not known if infants of smoking mothers or parents with impaired responses (for example, under the influence of alcohol) respond adequately to the potentially dangerous situations identified.

For healthy babies, who have not been exposed to cigarette smoke *in utero* or after birth, with mothers who are able to respond appropriately to the subtle cues of their baby, unimpaired by alcohol, drugs or overtiredness, co-sleeping may offer many advantages, particularly with respect to ease of breastfeeding and thus sustainability of baby and mother.

The role of midwives is to be able to acknowledge the context of each family, identify the potential risks and benefits and, before and after birth, share information on safe infant sleep. This needs to be shared in a way that has meaning within the family culture to enable informed decision making. This may also include sharing the information with family and whānau to gain appropriate support for the woman and her baby. It may also mean looking for alternative ways to maximize breastfeeding and contact while minimizing risks, for example, keeping the bassinette beside the bed.

References

Abel, S., Park, J., Tipene-Leach, D., Finau, S. and Lennan, M. (2001) 'Infant care practices in New Zealand: a cross-cultural qualitative study', *Social Science & Medicine*, 53, 9: 1135–48.

American Academy of Pediatrics Policy Statement (2005) 'The changing concept of Sudden Infant Death Syndrome: diagnostic coding shifts, controversies regarding the sleeping environment, and new variables to consider in reducing risk', *Pediatrics*, 116, 5: 1245–55.

Arnestad, M., Andersen, M., Vege, A. and Rognum, T. O. (2001) 'Changes in the epidemiological pattern of sudden infant death syndrome in southeast Norway, 1984–1998: implications for future prevention and research', *Archives of Disease in Childhood*, 85, 2: 108–15.

Ateah, C. A., Hamelin, K. J., Ateah, C. A. and Hamelin, K. J. (2008) 'Maternal bedsharing practices, experiences, and awareness of risks', *Journal of Obstetric, Gynecologic, & Neonatal Nursing*, 37, 3: 274–81.

Baddock, S. A., Day, H. F., Rimene, C. R., Moala, A. F., Taylor, B. J. *et al.* (2000) 'Bedsharing practices of different cultural groups'. 6th SIDS International Conference, Auckland, New Zealand.

Baddock, S. A., Galland, B. C., Beckers, M. G. S., Taylor, B. J. and Bolton, D. P. G. (2004) 'Bed-sharing and the infant's thermal environment in the home setting', *Archives of Disease in Childhood*, 89, 12: 1111–16.

Baddock, S. A., Galland, B. C., Bolton, D. P. G., Williams, S. and Taylor, B. J. (2006) 'Differences in infant and parent behaviors during routine bed sharing compared with cot sleeping in the home setting' *Pediatrics*, 117: 1599–607.

Baddock, S. A., Galland, B. C., Taylor, B. J. and Bolton, D. P. G. (2007) 'Sleep arrangements and behavior of bed-sharing families in the home setting', *Pediatrics*, 119, 1: e200–07.

Ball, H. L. (2002) 'Reasons to bedshare: why parents sleep with their infants', *Journal of Reproductive and Infant Psychology*, 20: 207–22.

Ball, H. L. (2003) 'Breastfeeding, bed-sharing, and infant sleep', *Birth*, 30, 3: 181–88.

Ball H. L., Hooker, E. and Kelly PJ. (1999) 'Where will the baby sleep? Attitudes and practices of new and experienced parents regarding cosleeping with their newborn infants', *American Anthropologist*, 101, 1: 143–51.

Ball, H. L., Ward-Platt, M. P., Heslop, E., Leech, S. J. and Brown, K. A. (2006) 'Randomised trial of infant sleep location on the postnatal ward', *Archives of Disease in Childhood*, 91, 12: 1005–10.

Blair, P. S. and Ball, H. L. (2004) 'The prevalence and characteristics associated with parent-infant bed-sharing in England', *Archives of Disease in Childhood*, 89, 12: 1106–10.

Blair, P. S., Fleming, P. J., Smith, I. J., Platt, M. W., Young, J. *et al.* (1999) 'Babies sleeping with parents: case-control study of factors influencing the risk of the sudden infant death syndrome', *British Medical Journal*, 319: 1457–62.

Blair, P. S., Sidebotham, P., Berry, P. J., Evans, M. and Fleming, P. J. (2006) 'Major epidemiological changes in sudden infant death syndrome: a 20-year population-based study in the UK', *Lancet*, 367, 9507: 314–19.

Blair, P. S., Sidebotham, P., Evason-Coombe, C., Edmonds, M., Heckstall-Smith, E. M. A. *et al.* (2009) 'Hazardous cosleeping environments and risk factors amenable to change: case-control study of SIDS in south-west England', *British Medical Journal*, 339: b3666.

Brenner, R. A., Simons-Morton, B. G., Bhaskar, B., Revenis, M., Das, A. *et al.* (2003) 'Infant-parent bed sharing in an inner-city population', *Archives of Pediatrics & Adolescent Medicine*, 157, 1: 33–39.

Campbell, A. J., Galland, B. C., Bolton, D. P. G., Taylor, B. J., Sayers, R. M. *et al.* (2001) 'Ventilatory responses to rebreathing in infants exposed to maternal smoking', *Acta Paediatrica*, 90, 7: 793–800.

Carpenter, R. G., Irgens, L. M., Blair, P. S., England, P. D., Fleming, P. *et al.* (2004) 'Sudden unexplained infant death in 20 regions in Europe: case control study', *Lancet*, 363, 9404: 185–91.

Chen, A., Rogan, W. J. and Chen, A. (2004) 'Breastfeeding and the risk of postneonatal death in the United States', *Pediatrics*, 113, 5: e435–39.

Child and Youth Mortality Revue Committee (CYMRC) (2009) *Fifth report to the Minister of Health: Reporting Mortality 2002–2008*. Wellington: Child and Youth Mortality Revue Committee.

Foundation for the Study of Infant Deaths (FSID) (2009) 'Reduce the risk of cot death leaflet'. Online. Available at: http://fsid.org.uk/Document.Doc?id=25 (accessed 12 March 2010).

Galler, J. R., Harrison, R. H. and Ramsey, F. (2006) 'Bed-sharing, breastfeeding and maternal moods in Barbados', *Infant Behavior & Development*, 29, 4: 526–34.

Gantley, M. (1994) 'Ethnicity and the sudden infant death syndrome – Anthropological perspectives', *Early Human Development*, 38, 3: 203–08.

Glover, M., Waldon, J., Manaena-Biddle, H., Holdaway, M. and Cunningham, C. (2009) 'Barriers to best outcomes in breastfeeding for Māori: mothers' perceptions, whanau perceptions, and services', *Journal of Human Lactation*, 25, 3: 307–16.

Horsley, T., Clifford, T., Barrowman, N., Bennett, S., Yazdi, F. *et al.* (2007) 'Benefits and harms associated with the practice of bed sharing: a systematic review', *Archives of Pediatrics & Adolescent Medicine*, 161, 3: 237–45.

Ip, S., Chung, M., Raman, G., Chew, P., Magula, N. *et al.* (2007) 'Breastfeeding and maternal and infant health outcomes in developed countries', *Evidence Report/Technology Assessment*, 153: 1–186.

Kennell, J., McGrath, S., Kennell, J. and McGrath, S. (2005) 'Starting the process of mother-infant bonding', *Acta Paediatrica*, 94, 6: 775–77.

Latz, S., Wolf, A. W. and Lozoff, B. (1999) 'Cosleeping in context: Sleep practices and problems in young children in Japan and the United States', *Archives of Pediatrics & Adolescent Medicine* 153, 4: 339–46.

Lee, N. N., Chan, Y. F., Davies, D. P., Lau, E. and Yip, D. C. (1989) 'Sudden infant death syndrome in Hong Kong: confirmation of low incidence', *British Medical Journal*, 298, 6675: 721.

Li, D. K. and Daling, J. R. (1991) 'Maternal smoking, low birth weight, and ethnicity in relation to sudden infant death syndrome', *American Journal of Epidemiology*, 134, 9: 958–64.

McCoy, R. C., Hunt, C. E., Lesko, S. M., Vezina, R., Corwin, M.J. *et al.* (2004) 'Frequency of bed sharing and its relationship to breastfeeding', *Journal of Developmental & Behavioral Pediatrics*, 25, 3: 141–49.

McKenna, J., Mosko, S., Richard, C., Drummond, S., Hunt, L. *et al.* (1994) 'Experimental studies of infant-parent co-sleeping – mutual physiological and behavioral influences and their relevance to SIDS', *Early Human Development*, 38, 3: 187–201.

McKenna, J. J., Mosko, S. S. and Richard, C. A. (1997) 'Bedsharing promotes breastfeeding', *Pediatrics*, 100 (2 Pt 1): 214–19.

Mathews, T. J., Mcdorman, M. F. and Menacker, F. (2002) 'Infant mortality statistics from the 1999 period linked birth/infant death data set', *National Vital Statistics Report*, 50, 4: 1–28.

Ministry of Health (MoH) (2009) 'Cosleeping and sudden unexpected death in infancy', Media release, 11 May 2009. Online. Available at: www.moh.govt.nz/moh.nsf/pagesmh/9023?Open (accessed 12 March 2010).

Mitchell, E. A., Stewart, A. W., Scragg, R., Ford, R. P., Taylor, B. J. *et al.* (1993) 'Ethnic differences in mortality from sudden infant death syndrome in New Zealand', *BMJ*, 306, 6869: 13–16.

Mitchell, E. A., Taylor, B. J., Ford, R. P., Stewart, A. W., Becroft, D. M. *et al.* (1992) 'Four modifiable and other major risk factors for cot death: the New Zealand Cot Death Study Group', *Journal of Paediatrics and Child Health*, 28 (suppl 1): S3–8.

Moon, R. Y., Oden, R. P. and Grady, K. C. (2004) 'Back to sleep: an educational intervention with women, infants, and children program clients', *Pediatrics*, 113, 3 Pt 1: 542–47.

Morelli, G.A., Rogoff, B., Oppenheim, D. and Goldsmith, D. (1992) 'Cultural variations in infants' sleeping arrangements: questions of independence', *Developmental Psychology*, 28: 604–13.

Mosko, S., Richard, C. and McKenna, J. (1997a) 'Maternal sleep and arousals during bedsharing with infants', *Sleep*, 20, 2: 142–50.

Mosko, S., Richard, C., McKenna, J., Drummond, S. and Mukai, D. (1997b) 'Maternal proximity and infant CO_2 environment during bedsharing and possible implications for SIDS research', *American Journal of Physical Anthropology*, 103, 3: 315–28.

Mosko, S. S., Richard, C. and McKenna, J. J. (1997c) 'Infant arousals during mother infant bedsharing – implications for infant sleep and SIDS research', *Pediatrics*, 100: 841–49.

Nelson, E. A., Taylor, B. J., Jenik, A., Vance, J., Walmsley, K. *et al.* (2001) 'International child care practices study: Infant sleeping environment', *Early Human Development*, 62, 1: 43–55.

Nelson, E. A., Yu, L. M., Williams, S. and International Child Care Practices Study Group Members (2005) International child care practices study: breastfeeding and pacifier use', *Journal of Human Lactation*, 21, 3: 289–95.

Okami, P., Weisner, T. and Olmstead, R. (2002) 'Outcome correlates of parent-child bedsharing: an eighteen-year longitudinal study', *Journal of Developmental & Behavioral Pediatrics*, 23, 4: 244–53.

Richard, C., Mosko, S., McKenna, J. and Drummond, S. (1996) 'Sleeping position, orientation, and proximity in bedsharing infants and mothers', *Sleep*, 19, 9: 685–90.

Richard, C. A. (1999) 'Increased infant axillary temperatures in non-REM sleep during mother-infant bed-sharing', *Early Human Development*, 55, 2: 103–11.

Richard, C. A. and Mosko, S. S. (2004) 'Mother-infant bedsharing is associated with an increase in infant heart rate', *Sleep*, 27, 3: 507–11.

Ruys, J. H., Jonge, G. A. de, Brand, R., Engelberts, A. C. and Semmekrot, B. A. (2007) 'Bed-sharing in the first four months of life: a risk factor for sudden infant death.' *Acta Paediatrica*, 96, 10: 1399–403.

Scragg, R., Mitchell, E. A., Taylor, B. J., Stewart, A. W., Ford, R. P. *et al.* (1993) 'Bedsharing, smoking and alcohol in the sudden infant death syndrome: New Zealand Cot Death Study Group.' *BMJ*, 307, 6915: 1312–18.

Tan, K. L. (2009) 'Bed sharing among mother-infant pairs in Klang district, Peninsular Malaysia and its relationship to breast-feeding', *Journal of Developmental & Behavioral Pediatrics*, 30, 5: 420–25.

Tappin, D., Ecob, R., Brooke, H. *et al.* (2005) 'Bedsharing, roomsharing, and sudden infant death syndrome in Scotland: a case-control study', *Journal of Pediatrics*, 147, 1: 32–37.

Tuffnell, C. S., Petersen, S. A. and Wailoo, M. P. (1995) 'Factors affecting rectal temperature in infancy', *Archives of Disease in Childhood*, 73, 5: 443–46.

Young, J. (1999) *Night-time Behaviour and Interactions Between Mothers and Their Infants at Low Risk for SIDS: A Longitudinal Study of Room-sharing and Bedsharing*. Bristol: University of Bristol.

17 How can birth activism contribute to sustaining change for better birthing for women, families and societies in the new millennium?

Rea Daellenbach and Nadine Pilley Edwards

Introduction

This chapter presents a critical evaluation of some aspects of maternity activism in New Zealand and in Britain, and examines how activism can be strengthened. It draws on our collective experiences and research interests as long-term birth activists and sociologists: Rea Daellenbach in New Zealand and Nadine Pilley Edwards in Scotland.

We begin the chapter by touching on the historical context of birth activism and maternity policies in order to acknowledge that any campaign is influenced by its social context. We suggest that birth activists are far from homogenous as a group. They may even campaign for opposing changes, based on their different and sometimes damaging birth experiences (for example, in Britain the Association for Improvements in the Maternity Services and the National Childbirth Trust have long supported campaigns for normal birth, whereas the Birth Trauma Association campaigns for all women to have access to epidurals for pain relief). We also look at how our current activities are set within competing global and local directions and agendas. We consider some of the impacts of some of these agendas (both their possibilities and limitations) and close with an exploration of the more recent concept of sustainability in respect of sustaining positive changes in maternity service that themselves are sustainable for women and midwives, for activists and for our decreasing resources.

The questions we consider are: how to develop and sustain movements that support women's and midwives' agency; how to develop and sustain a greater use of midwifery knowledge and skills; how to build on the knowledge and midwifery models that are already working well; how to encourage the above in ways that also support medical and surgical interventions when needed, quickly and expertly; and how to engage across a broad enough spectrum of groups to exert sustained political pressure. We hope that the discussion below will help place birth within global political debates about how we live our lives and future sustainability.

Historical context of birth activism

Early twentieth century

We have found that a consideration of historical contexts provides deeper insights into the contemporary issues facing maternity action groups. Women's activism over how to give birth, where and with whom has been a consistent feature of the wealthy, so-called democratic nations (De Vries *et al.* 2001; see Wolin 2008 for a critical analysis of current democracy). Over the previous century, with the rise of modernist ideas of maternal citizenship – the right to protection and services attendant on the responsibility to produce the nation's future citizens (Klaus 1993) – many women's organizations in both of our countries have taken an active interest in political lobbying to improve maternity services. But there has been significant historical variability in what women have considered to be 'improvements' in maternity services. For example, during the first half of the twentieth century, and even beyond, women's groups were rightly concerned about the high maternal and perinatal mortality rates associated with poverty such as poor health, the daily grind imposed by poverty and the crowded conditions in which women birthed at home. Their response to these concerns was significantly influenced by developments in medicine, thus they mainly campaigned for access to hospital beds and pain relief in labour for all women in childbirth (Garcia *et al.* 1990; De Vries *et al.* 2001; Donley 1998; Kedgley 1996). They believed that this would give women more control over previously uncontrollable aspects of childbirth – death, pain and suffering. However, as women entered into increasingly medicalized hospitals, they lost control over what was done to them by others during the birth process and post-natally. Thus, in the 1950s, 1960s and 1970s women formed new maternity groups and a new social movement emerged that challenged the medicalized and technocratic approaches to 'managing' labour and birth in maternity hospitals.

Maternity groups and their campaigns have been profoundly shaped by the welfare state provision of maternity care (Benoit *et al.* 2005) and, in Britain, the continued existence of (under resourced) community midwifery services for all. A nationalized health system in which women became entitled to free (at point of access) maternity services was introduced in New Zealand in 1938 and in the United Kingdom in 1948. This has meant that the political contestations about the shape of maternity services have been condensed around the state because it is the principal funder of maternity services. In comparison to the lay birth groups in the United States and Australia, where maternity services are primarily provided and funded by private organizations, and midwifery care is less available (Daviss 2001; Gosden and Noble 2000), the New Zealand and British movements have tended to work within local and national policy arenas in order to achieve their political goals (Bourgeault *et al.* 2001).

More recent campaigns in New Zealand and Britain

Childbirth activists in the 1980s and 1990s were influenced by the feminist and environmentalist social movements and were deeply critical of obstetric definitions and management of birth. Their campaigns focused on lobbying their respective governments for women's rights over their bodies, increased choices in childbirth, information for women and strengthening midwifery as an alternative to the over-medicalization of birth (Donley 1998; Garcia *et al*. 1990). Activists attested to women's capacity to make responsible, informed decisions. Thus, they challenged the paternalism of medical practice and saw midwives as allies in this struggle.

In New Zealand in the 1980s home birth women and midwives launched a concerted campaign to ensure the continuance of a state-funded home birth service and to improve conditions for midwives (Donley 1998; Kedgley 1996). This was greatly assisted when a Labour Government was elected and political opportunities opened up for childbirth activists to assume a larger role in policy-making for maternity services. As home birth activists became increasingly politically skilled they widened their agendas to include women-centred care in hospitals, support for midwives to establish a separate professional body from nursing (New Zealand College of Midwives (NZCOM)) and the reinstating of direct-entry midwifery education (Daellenbach 1999).

Drawing on the liberal feminist rhetoric of rights enabled home birth activists to form coalitions with other women's groups and midwives with a range of orientations to childbirth. They gained support from politicians who saw the welfare state as inflexible and suppressing individual preferences (Daellenbach 1999). In 1990, new legislation was introduced that enabled midwives to provide continuity of care to women through pregnancy, up to six weeks post-natally and included care for normal birth in hospital or at home, without medical supervision. Now almost 80 per cent of women access continuity of midwifery care for their childbirth experience funded from general taxation, and at no direct cost to the women (New Zealand Health Information Service 2007). When Helen Clark, who as the Minister of Health, brought in this legislation, she explained that she had wanted to address the inequitable position of midwives and the way medicalized childbirth had disempowered women. She also noted that she found 'surprising allies' among government officials and politicians who were pursuing a neoliberal agenda of introducing more competition within the health sector (1990: 3).

In Britain during a similar period, the *Winterton Report* (House of Commons 1992) was seen as a landmark report, signalling what many birth activists saw as a sea change towards socializing birth. The report recommended greater midwifery input and providing women with more information on which to base their decisions about maternity care. The policy document that stemmed from this, *Changing Childbirth* (Department of Health 1993), advocated a substantial restructuring of maternity services in order to provide women-centred care and access to continuity of midwifery-led care. It took up the theme of choice through the provision of information for women and strengthening midwifery options.

The shift in the New Zealand and British Governments' policies to support women's choices for childbirth was superimposed on obstetric ideology. This shift inevitably intensified debates about women's competence to make their own decisions about what is done to them during the childbearing process. These debates came to a head following a number of high-profile cases in Britain and in the United States in the mid 1990s when women were forced to undergo Caesarean sections against their wishes (Hewson 1994, 2004). Activists successfully secured formal legal recognition of women's capacities and the right to make decisions about how they wanted to give birth. This has also influenced practice in New Zealand (Pearce 1998), though choice in reality remains profoundly problematic (Kirkham 2004).

Childbirth activists believed that the focus on the right for women to make choices in childbirth was an important innovation and politically expedient. However, they were largely unaware of its concurrence with a rising neo-liberal project to dismantle the welfare state and the dangers of being recast as 'consumers' rather than citizens. This has had paradoxical consequences for maternity action groups, as can be clearly seen in the US, where choice is closely linked to wealth and class (Craven 2005).

The limited impact of birth activism

Neither the overwhelming research evidence showing the benefits of less interventionist birth, nor the campaigns focusing on rights, choice, control and (in New Zealand) continuity of midwifery care have led to the hoped for outcome – that is, a decrease in the over-use of technology for birth, more births in the community and an increase in births without interventions. On the contrary, in both our countries, almost a quarter of babies are now born by Caesarean sections, double the rates of 1990, and the rates of use of many obstetric interventions are continuing to increase rather than decrease (NHS Institute for Innovation and Improvement 2006; Ministry of Health 2009; BirthChoiceUK).

In Britain, the home birth rate remains very low and continuity of midwifery care is almost non-existent (Edwards 2005). The relatively few existing stand-alone birth centres are frequently threatened with closure (AIMS 2006) and most women have access only to large obstetric units (NCT 2009). In New Zealand the home birth rate has remained static at about 7 per cent, although, as only statistics on hospital births are collected, the real home birth rate is unknown (New Zealand Health Information Service 2007). Anecdotal evidence suggests that some midwives try to dissuade women from choosing a home birth on the grounds of potential risk factors and Maggie Banks suggests that there is a 'risk of [home birth] being accessible to only the elite few who escape medicine's vast list of 'abnormal'" (2000: 123; see also Hungerford 2003).

Barriers to normal birth

Current ideology

We are finding that the more we understand about the broader influences in our societies, the more we understand about why campaigns to increase straightforward births with midwives and to support women's decision-making capacities have been limited (Murphy-Lawless 2006; Edwards 2008). From this work, it is apparent that the campaigns of childbirth organizations in New Zealand and in Britain, as in other wealthier nations, are struggling not to be completely overtaken by the unfolding (and largely irresistible) forces of globalized neoliberal ideology.

This ideology has had diverse local impacts (Harvey 2005), but has generally led to the commodification of all areas of life (Ehrenreich and Hochschild 2002; Hochschild 2003) in which capitalism and thus privatization are inevitable (Pollock 2004; Edwards and Murphy-Lawless 2006; Murphy-Lawless 2006; Edwards 2008). Our governments have attempted to package these complex global shifts and make them palatable through the notion of choice. Thus, both the New Zealand and British governments promise women 'choice' within maternity services. But, as the state sheds its responsibilities in relation to equality, as privatization increases, and as choice becomes an individualized responsibility, the promised choice becomes a privilege for increasingly few (See Murphy-Lawless (Chapter 1) and Meleo-Erwin and Katz-Rothman (Chapter 4) in this volume). These developments tend to fragment resistance to maternity policies that fail to address the central issues of supporting women's and midwives' agency.

Another aspect of how neoliberal thinking impacts on governments is the relentless search for standardized, streamlined 'efficient' health services through the increasing reliance on guidelines that decrease the very choices promised by our governments' rhetoric. The choices available to women are increasingly determined by the National Institute of Clinical Excellence (NICE) for example, which informs practice in both New Zealand and Britain. NICE Guidelines are convenient for governments attempting to extricate themselves from the politics attendant on health service provision and serve to maintain the overriding role of mainstream science and technology, rather than increase normal birth supported by midwifery knowledge and skills. Importantly, they are based on risk-management strategies that reflect the current risk-aversion imperative that permeates our societies.

Risk

Ulrich Beck's (1992) analysis of the 'risk society' enables us to identify how risk as a powerful discourse is increasingly deployed to limit women's decision making through obstetric risk. The focus on risks and the attendant moral responsibility to avoid risky outcomes, which affects society broadly, has a particular salience in maternity care. Risk calculations apparently offer an objective and scientific basis for decision making. However, the risks commonly identified in relation to childbearing tend to be obstetrically rather than socially defined, and experts tell us both what they are and what should be done (Edwards and Murphy-Lawless 2006). When a risk indicator is found there is a general expectation that 'responsible' women and midwives will take all preventative measures to avert these risks and they may be blamed or censured if they choose not to (Anderson 2004). As Nikolas Rose suggests, 'once known to fall within a risk group, the individual may be treated – by others and by themselves – as if they were, now or in the future, certain to be affected in the severest fashion' (2001: 10).

Obstetric definitions of risk are thus coercing some women to make the 'right' choices against their better judgement, though mostly these choices are internalized and rationalized, obscuring the fact that choice is an illusion. In Britain sanctions on women who stray outside obstetric ideology and advice are increasing: some are reported to Social Services, which is attempting to define this as negligent and is then placing their babies on the 'at risk register' for monitoring, or even removing them from their mothers at birth (AIMS 2009). Thus, through the focus on risk and risk-management guidelines, obstetric power 'can . . . be achieved through individual freedom (in the form of consumer freedom to be precise) and not through its suppression' (Bauman[1] 1992: 51).

Critical analyses by birth activists and midwives discuss the limitations and oppressive nature of the obstetric risk discourse (Kirkham 2004; Symon 2006). For example, if we consider the potential short-term and long-term negative physical and psychological impacts of dehumanized, technocratic birth on mother, baby and family and the consequences on the women's ability to mother, risk may look very different (Davis-Floyd *et al.* 2009: Edwards 2005, see Chapter 8 by Carolyn Hastie in this volume).

Potential spaces

Coalitions

While we might deplore neoliberal ideology and its impact on health services, birth activists have attempted to open up spaces within these troubling regimes through working in coalitions with other interest groups. In Britain, one of the coalitions put in place as part of the Changing Childbirth policies was the multidisciplinary Maternity Services Liaison Committees (MSLCs). Each geographical locality in Britain was encouraged to set these up in order to influence local maternity services policies. Over the last two decades these have become more formalized and MSLC Guidelines (Department of Health 2006) suggest that a third of the membership should be lay people, though these are often women who have very recently had babies and may be unaware of the politics of childbirth. Research on the experiences of women on these

Committees suggested that while women often felt welcomed and were able to voice some of their views, they were usually unable to influence the broader agenda and policy decisions that might have increased normal birth such as introducing or increasing caseloading midwifery, birth centres, water births and home births (Edwards 2008).

In New Zealand, there are no policymaking forums equivalent to the MSLCs. Overall, there has been a move away from utilizing consumer reference and advisory groups in national and local health policymaking arenas with the shift to a more market-oriented approach to health service delivery (New Zealand Guidelines Group 2004). The main arena in which childbirth activists have opportunities for participation in maternity policy debates is through the NZCOM, the professional organization for midwives (Daellenbach 1999). At regional and national levels, NZCOM is inclusive of representatives from childbirth groups. However, within NZCOM they participate in the collective lobbying efforts of midwives and not as legitimate representatives of community interests within government forums.

For childbirth activists who promote undisturbed, normal birth, working in coalitions may have costs as well as benefits. For example, in the US birth activists have had to form coalitions in order to secure legislation to enable midwives to practice, but in some states this has entailed midwifery having to relinquish care of women having breech births, twin births and vaginal births following Caesarean section (Davis-Floyd and Johnson 2006).

On the MSLCs, obstetric ideology and its views on safety and risk remain powerful. Thus, when women or lay members appeal to the overwhelming evidence that caseloading midwifery and community-based birth improve outcomes and satisfaction, and suggest that existing resources could be used more creatively, they are mostly ignored. Childbirth activists working with NZCOM are also often drawn into compromises in their support of midwifery in a context in which midwives are often subject to public criticism (Daellenbach 1999; Cole 2006; Guilliland 2008).

Sustaining moves towards better birthing

The questions we asked in our introduction included questions about: supporting women's and midwives' agency; building on existing midwifery knowledge; skills and models that are working well (while also supporting the availability of expert medical and surgical interventions when needed); and forging collective activities that exert political pressure for sustaining positive changes in maternity service that themselves are sustainable for women and midwives, for activists and for our decreasing resources.

The justification for normal, or undisturbed, birth supported primarily by skilled midwives providing continuity of carer as a public aspiration is manifold and includes benefits across a range of outcomes. Pregnancy and the act of giving birth and being born without unnecessary pharmacological and technical interventions have tangible physiological, emotional and spiritual benefits, while the use of these interventions carry tangible risks (see Tracy, Chapter 3 in this volume; Huber and Sandall 2006; Davis-Floyd *et al.* 2009).

Increasing normal birth impacts positively on families and communities and as long as women are listened to, and provided with care that is sensitive to them, it is perhaps the only change that would improve birth for women. For many midwives it would provide a sustainable way of working that might encourage some of the most committed and skilled to remain in midwifery and return to midwifery (Ball *et al.* 2002). One of the ingredients for exerting influence is finding ways of making our voices heard.

Agency: finding and defining our own voices

Citizens' voices are frequently fragmented between the conflicting agendas of our complex societies in ways that undermine their voices and thus question which, if any of these, should be given legitimacy. For example, in their efforts to reject the term 'patient' (Lane 2000), with its connotations of passivity and lack of knowledge, New Zealand and Australian activists adopted the terms 'consumer' and 'consumer groups' to signify those who access maternity services and those who mobilize to represent a collective voice. This further implied that 'the rightness of a service or its credibility can be judged on its consequences for consumers' (Lane 2000: 44). In Britain, activists have been referred to as 'users' as well as 'consumers'. While the adoption of terms such as 'consumer' may have seemed useful in the 1980s, it is clearly disempowering in the contemporary context of birthing. Women are redefined as consumers who make choices in a marketplace of birthing services rather than citizens who are vested with rights to 'justice, representation, participation and (more recently) equal opportunities' (Pollitt 1990: 129) in relation to the welfare state (see also Bauman 1998). Thus, the term 'consumer' confines pregnant women and mothers to recipients of maternity services rather than agents and policy shapers and makers.

Additionally, there are increasingly complex debates about who can legitimately represent women's views about maternity services and take part in policymaking. Charlotte Williamson (1992, 2010) has put forward the idea that there are different lay voices with varying degrees of awareness, depending on experience. For example, the views of women who have recently had babies will usually be more unique and therefore limited than those of the birth activist who has listened to women's experiences over many years, read the literature and has had opportunities to reflect on these. The latter will probably have a more politically critical stance. Thus all voices have their own agency and legitimacy, but we need to know about the person's experiences and find ways of including different voices, and resist attempts to fragment our voices and pit them against each other so that they can be ignored.

The power and sustenance of cohesive political action

Our work to improve maternity services for women has made us acutely aware of the need for and the importance of alliances and collective action to define, promote and achieve sustainable midwifery practices that safely support women and babies. This is captured by the catchphrase 'women need midwives need women'. Collective action (by women and midwives) is imperative if we want to impact on policy, as shown by the writings about other community initiatives in health and welfare (Jones 1994; Wainwright 2003). In order to do this, activists need 'political scripts' that define the issues and articulate the possibilities for better alternatives (Swidler 1995).

From our experiences of activism, we believe that the midwifery models that support and sustain physiological birth are the very models that sustain political action. Caseloading, small birth centres and home birth midwifery models not only promote and increase undisturbed birth (Kirkham 2003; Walsh 2007; Davis-Floyd *et al.* 2009; Walsh and Byrom 2009), greater individual agency for women and midwives (Hunter and Deery 2009) and are valued by women, families, communities and midwives, but the ongoing relationships that usually develop from these models provide the collective awareness and confidence for cohesive political action. Thus they are sustaining at both local and political levels.

For example, the Birth Project Group is a collaboration between the Pregnancy and Parents Centre in Scotland, the University of Edinburgh, Edinburgh Napier University and Trinity College Dublin in Ireland set up in 2008. It came together to look at how women, doulas, student midwives and newly qualified midwives and experienced midwives could work sustainably together to improve birth for women, babies, families and birth workers. Its work to date suggests that women and birth workers need similarly supportive environments: those that foster positive relationships, which enable midwives to provide skilled midwifery care, and that encourage continuity of care and promote engagement between all concerned with birth (Mander *et al.* 2009, 2010).

Another very recent and poignant example involves a conflict between women, families, and a Hospital Trust over the internationally renowned Albany Midwifery Practice in south London. Since 1997, the Practice has served around 200 women each year in one of the most deprived areas in Britain and achieved outstanding outcomes in terms of lower than average perinatal mortality rates, greatly increased numbers of normal births and breastfed babies, a lower than average Caesarean section rate and a 43 per cent home birth rate (Reed and Walton 2009). The local Trust abruptly terminated the contract with the Albany Midwifery Practice amid outcries and with no consultation with the community in November 2009. A 700-strong group of mothers formed 'Albany Mums' and an online petition collected over 4000 signatures (www.savethealbany.org.uk). The Trust has so far refused to reinstate the Practice, but the campaign remains vigorous and

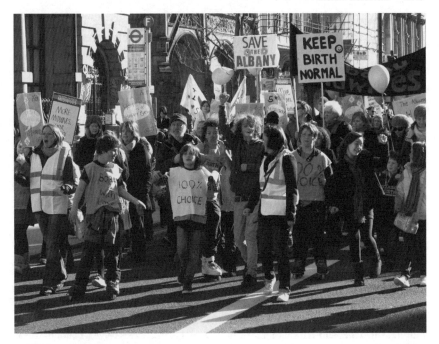

Figure 17.1 Reclaiming Birth March, London 2009, courtesy of Wayne Mitchell.

has now engaged national and international support for the wider issues of change: particularly one-to-one care from known and trusted midwives, more midwives, and more birth centres and home births. A rally in March 2010 to highlight these calls was supported by the Royal College of Midwives, the National Childbirth Trust, the Association for Improvements in the Maternity Services, the Association of Radical Midwives, Independent Midwives UK, Albany mums and the Albany Action Group. It is this sort of collective, cohesive action that might impact on maternity services.

Resources

In terms of ecological sustainability, technologically intensive approaches to birth are no longer sustainable for entire populations. Protecting and enhancing knowledge and practices to support natural physiological birth processes has become a pressing necessity. There are, in addition, issues of equitable deployment of resources: though complex, in the main, there is a need to reduce the level of technological interventions in the wealthier nations and to make necessary interventions more available when needed in poorer nations, though there is still a crucial need to support existing low-tech midwifery practices in poorer nations, as well as improve access to appropriate medical help when needed.

The sustainability and global justice movements have cast a spotlight on issues of allocation and misuse of resources, vested financial interests and how these are used to shape research and policy agendas. These movements have also highlighted that markets cannot be left unchecked and that we (the public) urgently need to engage with these debates. These movements create new political scripts for childbirth activism that validate the aspirations for undisturbed natural birth and midwifery care as an ethical position that pays attention to the social dimensions of childbirth, and insists on the need to take into account the future consequences of present actions, not just for the individuals concerned but for the wider community as well.

Note

1   Baumann states this in relation to the reproduction of consumer capitalism.

References

AIMS (2006) 'Free standing and proud', *AIMS Journal*, 18: 3.
AIMS (2009) 'Social services', *AIMS Journal*, 21: 2.
Anderson, T. (2004) 'The misleading myth of choice', in M. Kirkham (ed.), *Informed Choice in Maternity Care*. Houndsmills: Palgrave Macmillan.
Ball, L., Curtis, P. and Kirkham, M. (2002) 'Why Do Midwives leave?' London: Royal College of Midwives. Online. Available at: www.rcm.org.uk/info/docs/Why%20midwives%20leave%20full%20report.pdf (accessed 27 March 2010).
Banks, M. (2000) *Home Birth Bound: Mending the Broken Weave*. Hamilton: Birthspirit.
Bauman, Z. (1992) *Intimations of Postmodernity*. London and New York: Routledge.
Baumann, Z. (1998) *Work, Consumerism and the New Poor*. Milton Keynes: Open University.
Beck, U. (1992) *Risk Society: Towards a New Modernity*. London: Sage.
Benoit, C., Wrede, S., Bourgeault, I., Sandall, J. De Vries, R. *et al.* (2005) 'Understanding the social organization of maternity care systems: midwifery as a touchstone', *Sociology of Health & Illness*, 27, 6: 722–37.
BirthChoice UK (n.d.) 'Where to have your baby?' Online. Available at: www.birthchoiceuk.com/Frame.htm (accessed 18 March 2010).
Bourgeault, I., Declercq, E. and Sandall, J. (2001) 'Changing birth, interest groups and maternity care policy', in R. De Vries, C. Benoit, E. van Teijlingen and S. Wrede (eds), *Birth by Design, Pregnancy, Maternity Care, and Midwifery in North America and Europe*. New York and London: Routledge.
Clark, H. (1990) 'Opening Address', *New Zealand College of Midwives Conference Proceedings*, Dunedin: NZCOM.
Cole, S. (2006) 'Anyone who is not against us is for us', *Midwifery News*, 43: 7–12.
Craven, C. (2005) 'Is reproductive healthcare access a "consumer right"', *Anthropology News*, 46, 1: 16–19.
Daellenbach, R. (1999) 'The paradox of success and the challenge of change: home birth associations of Aotearoa/ New Zealand', unpublished thesis submitted for the degree of Doctor of Philosophy in Sociology at the University of Canterbury, Christchurch.
Davis-Floyd, R. and Johnson, C. B. (2006) *Mainstreaming Midwives: The Politics of Change*. New York and London: Routledge.

Davis-Floyd, R., Barclay, L., Daviss, B. and Tritten, J. (2009) 'Introduction', in R. Davis-Floyd, L. Barclay, B. Daviss and J. Tritten (eds), *Birth Models That Work.* Berkeley, CA: University of California Press.

Daviss, B. (2001) 'Reforming birth and (re)making midwifery in North America', in R. De Vries, C. Benoit, E. van Teijlingen and S. Wrede (eds), *Birth by Design, Pregnancy, Maternity Care, and Midwifery in North America and Europe.* New York and London: Routledge.

Department of Health (1993) *Changing Childbirth, Part 1: Report of the Expert Maternity Group.* London: HMSO.

Department of Health (2006) *National Guidelines for Maternity Services Liaison Committees MSLCs.* London. Online. Available at: www.dh.gov.uk/prod_consum_dh/groups/ dh_digitalassets/@dh/@en/documents/digitalasset/dh_4128340.pdf (accessed 18 February 2010).

De Vries, R. Salveson, H. B., Wiegers, T. A. and Williams, A. S. (2001) 'What (and why) do women want?' in R. De Vries, C. Benoit, E. van Teijlingen and S. Wrede, (eds), *Birth by Design, Pregnancy, Maternity Care, and Midwifery in North America and Europe.* New York and London: Routledge.

Donley, J. (1998) *Birthrites, Natural vs Unnatural Childbirth in New Zealand.* Auckland: Full Court Press.

Edwards, N. (2008) 'Safety in birth: the contextual conundrums faced by women in a "risk society" driven by neoliberal policies', *MIDIRS Midwifery Digest*, 18, 4: 463–70.

Edwards, N. and Murphy-Lawless J. (2006) 'The instability of risk: women's perspectives on risk and safety in birth', in A. Symon (ed.), *Risk and Choice in Maternity Care: An International Perspective.* Edinburgh: Churchill Livingston.

Edwards, N. P. (2005) *Birthing Autonomy: Women's Experiences of Planning Home Births.* New York and London: Routledge.

Ehrenreich, B. and Hochschild A. R. (2002) *Global Woman: Nannies, Maids and Sex Workers in the New Economy.* London: Granta Books.

Garcia, J., Kirkpatrick, R. and Richards, M. (eds) (1990) *The Politics of Maternity Care Services for Childbearing Women in Twentieth-Century Britain.* Oxford: University Press.

Gosden, D. and Noble, C. (2000) 'Social mobilization around the act of childbirth: subjectivity and politics', *Annual Review of Health Social Sciences*, 10, 1: 69–79.

Guilliland, K. (2008) 'Midwifery into the future', *Midwifery News*, 51: 6–8.

Harvey, D. (2005) *A Brief History of Neoliberalism.* Oxford: Oxford University Press.

Hewson, B. (1994) 'Court-ordered caesarean: ethical triumph or surgical rape?' *AIMS Journal*, 6, 2: 1–5.

Hewson, B. (2004) 'Is it murder to refuse a caesarean section?' *AIMS Journal*, 16: 1. Online. Available at: www.aims.org.uk/Journal/Vol16No1/murderToRefuse.htm (accessed 18 February 2010).

Hochschild, A. R. (2003) *The Commercialization of Intimate Life: Notes from Home and Work.* Berkeley, CA: University of California Press.

House of Commons Health Committee (1992) *Maternity Services Second Report Volume 1.* London: HMSO.

Huber, U. and Sandall, J. (2006) 'Continuity of carer, trust and breastfeeding', *MIDIRS Midwifery Digest*, 16, 4: 445–49.

Hungerford, R. (2003) 'Are all home births created equal?' *Waikato Home Birth Association Newsmagazine*, October. Online. Availalble at: www.homebirth.org.nz/articles/Are%20all%20home%20births%20created%20equal.pdf (accessed 2 March 2010).

Hunter, B. and Deery, R. (eds) (2009) *Emotions in Midwifery and Reproduction*. London: Palgrave Macmillan.

Jones, J. (1994) *Private Troubles and Public Issues: A Community Development Approach to Health*. Edinburgh: Community Learning Scotland.

Kedgley, S. (1996) *Mum's the Word, The Untold Story of Motherhood in New Zealand*. Auckland: Random House.

Kirkham, M. (ed.) (2003) *Birth Centres: A Social Model for Maternity Care*. Oxford: Books for Midwives, Elsevier.

Kirkham, M. (ed.) (2004) *Informed Choice in Maternity Care*. Houndsmills: Palgrave Macmillan.

Klaus, A. (1993) *Every Child a Lion, The Origins of Maternal and Infant Health Policy in the United States and France*. Ithaca, NY: Cornell University Press.

Lane, K. (2000) 'Multiple visions or multiple aversions? Consumer representation, consultation and participation in maternity issues', *Annual Review of Health Social Sciences*, 10, 1: 43–52.

Mander R., Murphy-Lawless J. and Edwards N. (2009) 'Reflecting on good birthing: an innovative approach to culture change Part 1', *MIDIRS Midwifery Digest*, 19, 4: 481–86.

Mander R., Murphy-Lawless J. and Edwards, N. (2010) 'Reflecting on good birthing: an innovative approach to culture change Part 2', *MIDIRS Midwifery Digest*, 20, 1: 25–29.

Ministry of Health (2009) *Maternity Snapshot 2007*. Wellington: Ministry of Health.

Murphy-Lawless, J. (2006) 'Birth and mothering in today's social order: the challenge of new knowledges', *MIDIRS Midwifery Digest*, 16, 5: 439–44.

NCT (2009) 'Location, location, location: making choice of place of birth a reality', London: NCT. Online. Available at: www.nctpregnancyandbabycare.com/choice (accessed 18 February 2010).

New Zealand Guidelines Group (2004) *Effective Consumer Voice and Participation for New Zealand, A Systematic Review of the Evidence*. Wellington: New Zealand Guidelines Group.

New Zealand Health Information Service (2007) *Report on Maternity 2003*. Wellington: Ministry of Health.

NHS Institute for Innovation and Improvement (2006) *Focus On: Caesarean Section*. Coventry: NHS Institute for Innovation and Improvement.

Pearce, J. (1998) 'Informed consent: issues for midwives', *NZCOM Journal*, 19: 10–12.

Pollitt, C. (1990) *Managerialism and the Public Services*. Cambridge: Basil Blackwell.

Pollock, A. M. (2004) *NHS plc: The Privatization of Our Health Care*. London: Verso.

Reed, B. and Walton, C. (2009) 'The Albany Midwifery Practice', in R. Davis-Floyd, L. Barclay, B. Daviss and J. Tritten (eds), *Birth Models That Work*. Berkeley, CA: University of California Press.

Rose, N. (2001) 'The politics of life itself', *Theory Culture and Society*, 18, 6: 1–30.

Swidler, A. (1995) 'Cultural power and social movements', in H. Johnston and B. Klandermans, *Social Movements and Culture*. Minneapolis: University of Minnesota Press.

Symon, A. (ed.) (2006) *Risk and Choice in Maternity Care, An International Perspective.* Edinburgh: Churchill Livingstone.

Wainwright, H. (2003) *Reclaim the State: Experiments in Popular Democracy.* London and New York: Verso.

Walsh, D. (2007) *Improving Maternity Serivces: Small is Beautiful – Lessons from a Birth Centre.* Abingdon: Radcliffe Publishing.

Walsh, D. and Byrom, S. (2009) *Birth Stories for the Soul: Tales From Women, Families and Childbirth Professionals.* London: Quay Books.

Williamson, C. (1992) *Whose Standards? Consumer and Professional Standards in Health Care.* Buckingham, PA: Open University Press.

Williamson, C. (2010) *Towards the Emancipation of Patients: Patients' Experiences and the Patient Movement.* Cambridge: Policy Press.

Wolin, S. (2008) *Democracy Incorporated: Managed Democracy and the Spectre of Inverted Totalitarianism.* Princeton, NJ: Princeton University Press.

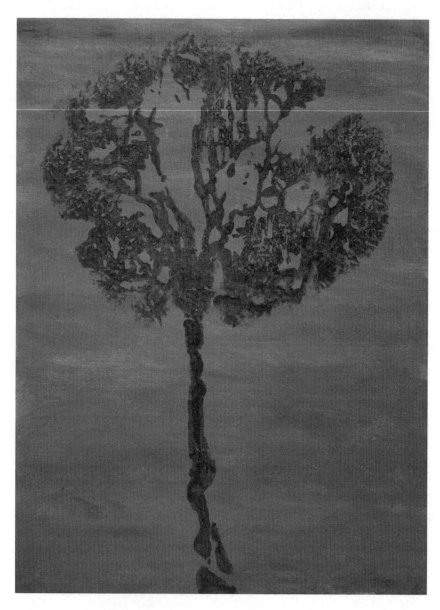

Placenta print image, courtesy of Richard Grevers.

Epilogue
Planet and placenta

A cycle of seasonal correspondence between two old friends

Jenny L. Meyer

Inspired by the phenomenon of climate change and reflections of the personal and political consequences for future generations, this story is presented as a platform to promote debate about caring for women who struggle with body image through pregnancy, and the possible impact on their babies.

Originally presented as an audio play, the story is informed by the work of Dr Jane Harding and Dr Peter Gluckman at the Liggins Institute and their work into placental functioning; and Dr David Barker's body of research into maternal nutrition and adult disease.

The privilege and intimacy of working with families at the Auckland Regional Eating Disorders Service, and currently at the Wellington Neonatal Unit, has focussed my interest in growth-restricted newborns.

My personal background, raised as a daughter of blind parents and growing up in South Auckland, has given me an appreciation of listening to stories and an admiration for Māori culture. This tale is deliberately non-visual in an effort to evoke imagination and offer an alternative 'view' on an image-based problem; thus providing food for thought.

Autumn

Dear Planet,

I would like to book a womb please.

I have been feeling the urge to pull myself together lately and get a life. I know I've got the makings of a good placenta; humble, humane, hungry and a little bit horny.

I understand it's not all about me, and that my job is caring and sharing. But I am feeling the need to be. I am getting more and more desperate by the day to get on, get in and get out.

Hope you can find me a nice young couple with a good heritage, as I don't want to be wasting my time, and would like to make this cycle a fruitful one.

Yours sincerely,
Potential Placenta

Dear Potential Placenta,

Thank you for your letter requesting a womb.

As you may be aware my resources are becoming more and more limited, and this decade has been particularly difficult. Quality wombs are a bit harder to come by these days. People are just not breeding like they used to. Its just work, work, work, money, money, money.

I can tell you I am becoming exhausted. I am sick and tired of being taken for granted. Sometimes I feel like I can hardly breathe. Everybody has to drive and fly everywhere. Nobody is getting outside into the garden. Here we are in the middle of autumn, the planting season, and I'm feeling breathless already! All that jolly carbon, it's just suffocating.

Anyway, sorry to rant, I will keep your request in mind, and let you know as soon as a suitable womb becomes available.

Yours truly,
Planet

Winter

Dear Placenta,

Sorry it has been a while, good things come to those who wait. I know it hardly even feels like winter, it has been so unseasonably warm, but don't worry, there is a polar blast on the way soon to a spot near you.

Great news! I think I have found you a womb. A bit of background bio, so you know who you're getting into: Theresa is twenty-seven years old, lives in Wellington New Zealand, is a high powered career woman in banking, and a recovering bulimic. Not ideal, but salvageable. At least she knows she has a problem, and is working on it, sort of. Anyway there is not as much choice as there used to be, what with all that contraception. So controlling . . .

Theresa's mate is a bloke called Wiremu, unusual name, but a fabulous soul. He is part Māori on his mother's side, plays touch rugby, likes a beer, and works as a recycling contractor. He is twenty-six and has just gone through a tough time splitting up with his ex, so he is a bit sad, which is how I came to know him.

There is just one hitch. This couple have not actually met yet. But their stars are about to line up, it is just a question of timing. So be ready.

Kind regards,
Planet

Dear Planet,

Wow! Thank you very much for the womb. It is early days, but I think I am in, in fact I know I am. The whole thing was so romantic. When I first saw them both, I thought I had the wrong planet, and you were off on a tangent completely. And then it happened. Love at first sight! Who would have thought?

There was Theresa, corporate chic trying to reverse her SUV out of the driveway, when she nearly backs into the recycling truck (it being a Monday and her running late over a fight with the hair straighteners). And then there is Wiremu, fit as a fiddle, dashing and darting between the bins and the truck, sorting and clearing as he goes, pure poetry in motion . . . She revs into reverse, he is dodging and distracted, then . . .

BANG! She hits him!

Suddenly there is blood everywhere. He has gashed himself on the lid of her lemon and pepper tuna can, and he has a haemorrhage on his hands. She leaps out in her high heels and starts out with a load of expletives . . . then, then, then . . . Oh Planet, it was the moment, the synchronized shared heart beat, the gasping breath of deep involuntary connection as those two souls looked, locked and lived! Fantastic, I knew I was in.

Like you promised the polar blast turned up, so what with her first aid, his longing, their loving and, credit where it is due, your power cut, complete with candles and extra blankets, it was all on!

A couple of lost souls found each other and I'm on my journey. I have to hand it to you Planet, you know your stuff. What an awesome force you are.

My only hesitation is the womb's stores. Theresa's bulimia has been a greedy little blighter by all accounts, raiding her body of nutrients, and her personal pantry is certainly not full. Still she is truly in love with Wiremu, and I reckon with him and the baby on my side, we will beat the bulimia hands down.

We are just going to hibernate here. It is so exciting, I love surprises! Thanks again for all your help with the womb. I feel like a new person.

Be in touch,
Love Placenta

Spring

Dear Placenta,

So pleased you made the connection with Theresa and Wiremu. I guess it must be a hive of activity there in Wellington now that it is spring. Although to be honest, sometimes I feel like there are only two seasons these days; wet and dry. Not like the old times when you knew what you were in for.

Hope you and your people are coping with the rain. I have just felt so tense with all these emissions lately, that in the end I'd had enough! All this me, me, me, more, more, more! I tell you my friend, I am fed up with this spoilt, senseless, selfishness. It is sending me into such a spin. So I have pulled the plug. Made some mayhem and whipped up a storm. Well, I would call it a storm, those humans might call it a hurricane. Let's just say I am hoping some havoc might bring them to their senses. Get them to actually notice their neighbours, and take stock of their naughtiness. Let's hope enough of them get the hint that they can't just keep trashing the place, otherwise I will have to up the anti even more.

I really would love this climate of excess to change. I am just getting exhausted. I wish a few more folk would get up in the morning and look out of the window to admire my beauty, rather than stare in the mirror at themselves all the time. At the end of the day, I do love these people, and I don't want to be a lonely old planet.

Anyway enough of me, I expect you will be nice and cosy tucked up in your warm womb. So the storm should not bother you too much.

Do let me know how you are getting on.

Lots of love,
Planet

Dear Planet,

Sorry to hear you have been having such a hard time. I have heard about the rain.

Funnily enough it has been pretty damp around here too. As you can imagine, my secret is out now. Theresa and Wiremu were, well ... 'shocked', I guess sums it up, by the arrival of me and my companion. Tears, tantrums, tirades ... What a messy trimester! Thankfully Theresa, bless her heart, is totally smitten with the wonderful Wiremu, and we successfully averted termination. Thank goodness, especially after the effort we have all put in.

So now it is growing time. It is actually a lot trickier than you would think. My companion, the baby, is beautiful. Loads of fun, and a joy to live with. But, I have to say, needy. It is 'want this' and 'want that', sustenance here, space there. Honestly, I hardly get a moment's peace.

What with processing the food Theresa gives me, sorting my little friend's waste out, not to mention trying to keep my own self in good running order; life is pretty demanding.

Like I mentioned to you before, that bossy bulimia has not exactly left a full tank of gas here. However, I do think I might have sent it packing. Once my little cute partner started to dance around the womb, good old Theresa spilt the beans about her eating disorder to her man!?

What a hero, he was gorgeous about the whole thing. He gave us all a huge hug, and she just let the tears flow. What a relief I can tell you. The atmosphere around here has been a lot less stressful. The best part is the menu has improved immensely. Wiremu is an amazing cook. So hopefully the baby and I can build some strength and max up on our potential.

Anyway, I had better get some rest now.

See you in the summer.

Love,
Placenta

Summer

Dear Placenta,

Great to hear things are growing well for you.

I can hardly believe we are nearly at the end of summer already. I love summer. Birds singing, bees pollinating, people playing, solar panels basking in the sun . . . Long, lovely days, and warm, dreamy nights, happy holidays, and humans getting back in touch and nurturing my nature. It all makes me feel so free, full and fertile.

Which reminds me, you must be getting pretty ripe yourself? I hope you have enjoyed your cycle and new lease of life Placenta.

I would imagine that Wiremu will be keen to return you back to the land with your burial when your job is done. You know, from one whenua to another.

I will keep an eye out for a good location for you. Somewhere with a coastal view perhaps, good soil, pedestrian only access; where you can put down some roots and have the grandchildren come and visit.

Good luck with your delivery.

Love as always,
Planet

Dear Planet,

Stress, stress, stress!!! Crikey, things are hotting up now. Here we are, at the full term of this pregnancy, and I can tell you, I have had enough!

That baby, who it turns out is going to be a girl, has been so stroppy lately. She is keeping me up 24/7 with her demands, always wanting more fuel. Then when I give it to her, what do I get but more rubbish to sort out, and even more cramped accommodation.

In her spare time she wants to practise her gymnastics, suck on her thumbs to look cute, and try out different styles of wearing her umbilical cord.

'Careful you don't strangle yourself' I said to her. That sent her into a sulk for about five seconds. Just as well one of us has got a grip around here!

I have had a gutsful. 'Time is up' I said to myself. I did not want to turn nasty on such a sweet baby, but the honeymoon is over, and we just have to go our separate ways now. So Planet, do you know what I did? I do feel a little bit guilty, but I was at the end of my tether . . . cord . . . whatever. Anyway, I went on strike! Well more like a grow slow . . . And I made her feed me! I know, I know, call me a traitor. But everyone has their limits.

Well it seems to have worked, because Theresa and Wiremu have just followed the 'hot curry, hot shower, hot sex' recipe, so I should be out before tomorrow's sunset.

See you soon!

Love,
Placenta

Autumn

Dear Planet,

What a trip! Once the baby headed on out, I knew it was my turn. A pretty exciting ride I can tell you. Thank goodness you chose a strong womb, I felt the momentum, and in the end I just let go and went with the flow.

The baby, they have called her 'Grace', was true to her name and thanked me for my services and support. Of course I could not have done it without you, Planet. Growing all that good food for us, organizing our couple, and being there at the end.

Grace also thanked me on behalf of her children and her grandchildren. You know, the eggs within the eggs. That is the special thing about providing for a girl, you get that lovely echo effect of all your hard work.

Anyway, once I was out Wiremu did the Dad thing and cut the cord between Grace and me. The last thing I said to her; 'You might feel like you are on your own without me, but you have got two wonderful breasts to rely on now'. And she looked pretty happy as she tucked in and sucked. Those two are so much more attractive than me. I guess it is just a fact of nature.

Did I mention Grace's hair? The most awesome orange colour shining away like a beautiful sun, a throw back to his Scottish side Wiremu said. It gives me goose bumps seeing Grace in the light of day.

So Planet, thanks for everything. It has been a fantastic cycle this time around. But, I am so depleted. I think my burial is tomorrow, so I look forward to connecting up with you then.

Yours truly,
Placenta

Dearest Placenta,

Here you are at last. Returned to your home and in your element, with all of your ancestors, and most of your descendants. I have to say, you did look a bit bedraggled, even for you.

The burial service was a wonderful crisp autumn day. A light breeze, early morning sky, and just a few clouds to the south. Such a spiritual location out on the point, over looking the sea. Wiremu, Theresa and Grace were there, and most of their families as well, all to pay their respects to you. They have given you a pohutukawa tree to bond with, which is nice, as Grace is a summer baby and those red flowers are kind of like more pretty versions of yourself. They also placed a large piece of local stone next to your tree, to mark the spot, with a message from each parent carved into it. Theresa's message is an old one from her family; 'Luceo non uro' I shine not burn. Wiremu's words 'E whenua au whenua' From the placenta to the land.

There was a prayer from Theresa's father, and a song from Wiremu's mother. I had to have a little cry, it was so emotional. So the ceremony ended rather abruptly, as everyone was getting soaked. The pohutukawa was pleased though, as it was getting really thirsty.

Enjoy your rest and recovery my friend.

See you next time around.

All my love,
Planet

Index